NURSING TODAY

Transition and Trends

JoAnn Zerwekh, Ed.D., R.N., C.A.R.N., C.A.D.A.C.

University of Phoenix, Tucson
Tucson, Arizona

El Centro College
Dallas, Texas

Jo Carol Claborn, M.S., R.N.

El Centro College
Dallas, Texas

Executive Directors
Nursing Education Consultants
Dallas, Texas

W. B. SAUNDERS COMPANY
A Division of Harcourt Brace & Company
Philadelphia London Toronto Montreal Sydney Tokyo

W. B. SAUNDERS COMPANY
A Division of Harcourt Brace & Company
The Curtis Center
Independence Square West
Philadelphia, PA 19106

Library of Congress Cataloging-in-Publication Data

Nursing today : transition and trends / edited by JoAnn Zerwekh, Jo
  Carol Claborn. — 1st ed.
      p.   cm.
  Includes index.
  ISBN 0-7216-3645-4
  1. Nursing — Vocational guidance.   2. Nursing — Social aspects.
I. Zerwekh, JoAnn Graham.   II. Claborn, Jo Carol.
  [DNLM: 1. Nursing.   WY 16 N97874 1994]
RT82.N874   1994
610.73'06'9 — dc20
DNLM/DLC   93-22603

NURSING TODAY Transition and Trends   ISBN 0-7216-3645-4

Printed in the United States of America

Last digit is the print number: 9 8 7 6 5 4 3 2 1

In memory of
Margie N. Slaughter
A dear friend and colleague
who shall be greatly missed.

PREFACE

Nursing Today: Transition and Trends evolved out of the authors' experiences with nursing students in their final semester and the students' transition into the realities of nursing practice. There is a need for the graduating nurse to become aware of the transition process *before* graduation. It is our belief that the beginning nurse can benefit from practical, down-to-earth guidelines about how to make the transition from student to effective practice at the entry level.

The experience of other nursing faculty, Marlene Kramer's research on Reality Shock, and Patricia Benner's work with performance characteristics of beginning and expert nurses have initiated the development of transition courses. These courses focus on trends and issues, along with information to assist the new graduate to be better prepared to practice nursing in today's world. We have written this book to be used in these transition type courses, as well as by the individual student.

Each chapter begins with *student objectives* and a *cartoon*—by John Wise, R.N.,—as a visual introduction to the content. As you read through a chapter, you will find practical application to the concepts discussed. Information is highlighted by boxes within the text to draw emphasis to the point being discussed. Using a *Question approach,* material is presented in a logical, easy to read manner. There are also opportunities to respond to *thought-provoking questions* and *student exercises* to facilitate self-evaluation.

The reader is given an overall view of the nursing profession from past historical events that influenced nursing to its present day image and the legal, ethical, political, and on-the-job issues today's nurse must be aware of. Communication in the workplace, time management, how to write an effective resume, interviewing tips, employee benefits, and self-care strategies are among the sound career advancement tools provided.

For Nursing Faculty:

Our key goal in developing this book has been timely information, applicable to current practice and fun to read. To this end, we will provide, to nursing faculty teaching a transition course, a semi-annual *update newsletter* regarding current events and their implications to nursing.

An instructor's manual is available from the publisher to assist faculty in planning and promoting a positive transition experience for their students.

Contact your W.B. Saunders representative to obtain copies of the Instructor's Manual and the Newsletter. For the name of the sales representative in your area, call (215) 238-8405 or 238-8406 between 9 a.m. and 5 p.m. Eastern Time.

ACKNOWLEDGMENTS

We are grateful for the contributions and efforts of our chapter contributors who provided their expertise and knowledge.

We thank the wonderful faculty members who reviewed chapters and shared their insights and experiences:

Teresa M. Bianco, MSN, RN
Coordinator, School of Nursing
Essex Community College
Baltimore, Maryland

Sharon S. Fulling, MSN, RN
Assistant Dean and Director of Nursing
Mississippi County Community College
Blytheville, Arkansas

Frazine Jasper, JD, MEd, RN
Chairperson, School of Nursing
Community College of Southern Nevada
Las Vegas, Nevada

Adele D.S. Mitchell, PhD, MSN, RN
Director, School of Nursing
Hawaii Loa College
Kaneohe, Hawaii

Carla Randall, MSN, RN
School of Nursing
Salish Kootenai College
Pablo, Montana

Patricia Finder-Stone, MS, RN
School of Nursing
Northeast Wisconsin Technical College
Green Bay, Wisconsin

Mary E. Hazzard, PhD, FAAN, RN
Head, Department of Nursing
Western Kentucky University
Bowling Green, Kentucky

Carol J. McFadyen, PhD, RNC
Director, Nursing Programs
Sheridan College
Sheridan, Wyoming

Carol Ann Morris, EdD, MS, RN
Director, School of Nursing
Northeastern Oklahoma A&M College
Miami, Oklahoma

Adelia M. Shelton, MSN, RN
Director, ADN School of Nursing
Wharton County Junior College
Wharton, Texas

And we thank

Debby Hanry, word processor and desktop publisher, extraordinaire, for her support, editing, and preparation of the manuscript.

Ilze Rader, Senior Editor, W.B. Saunders, for her patience, encouragement, and persistence in completing this project.

Kay Eggleston, PhD, RN, and Carol Speyerer, EdD, RN, El Centro College AD Nursing, for their willingness to continue to provide us with a creative and flexible teaching schedule.

Our children, Tyler, Ashley, Jaelyn, Michael, and Kim, for tolerating another publishing project their mothers started.

Our parents, Charles and Marie Graham, and Frank and Hazel Cooper, for providing us support during our life transitions.

Tom and Robert, for feeding us, meeting plane schedules, late night manuscript deliveries and continued support and encouragement.

CONTRIBUTORS

Linda T. Anglin, D.A., R.N.C.
Associate Professor, Nursing,
College of Education and Health
Sciences, Bradley University, Peoria,
Illinois

Historical Perspectives: Influences of the Past

Linda Camin, M.S.N., R.N.
Lecturer, Professionalism in
Nursing, Director, Continuing
Nursing Education, The University
of Texas at Arlington, School of
Nursing, Arlington, Texas

Time Management

Jo Carol Claborn, M.S., R.N.
El Centro College, Dallas, Texas.
Executive Director, Nursing
Education Consultants, Dallas,
Texas

*NCLEX-RN and the New Graduate;
Reality Shock*

Mary E. Foley, R.N., B.S.N.
Immediate Past President, California
Nurses Association, San Francisco,
California. American Nurses
Association, Chair, Constituent
Assembly, Washington, District of
Columbia. Staff Nurse, Saint Francis
Memorial Hospital, San Francisco,
California

A Collective Voice in the Workplace

Susan Houston, Ph.D., R.N.
Clinical Associate Professor, Texas
Woman's University, St. Luke's
Episcopal Hospital, Nurse
Researcher, Houston, Texas

*Contemporary Healthcare Delivery:
Trends and Economics*

**Lynette Jack, Ph.D., R.N.,
C.A.R.N.**
Assistant Professor, Health and
Community Systems Department,
School of Nursing, University of
Pittsburgh, Pittsburgh,
Pennsylvania

Effective Communication

Joan Jones, M.S., R.N.
Adjunct Faculty, The University of
Texas at Arlington, School of
Nursing, Arlington, Texas. Director
of Obstetrics, Gynecology, Urology,
St. Luke's Episcopal Hospital,
Houston, Texas

Contemporary Healthcare Delivery:
Trends and Economics

Karlene Kerfoot, Ph.D., R.N.,
C.N.A.A., F.A.A.N.
Executive Vice President, Patient
Care and Chief Nursing Officer, St.
Luke's Episcopal Hospital, Houston,
Texas

Nursing Service and Healthcare
Delivery

Barbara Michaels, Ed.D., R.N.
Instructor, El Centro College,
Dallas, Texas. Therapist, Private
Practice, Neighborhood Youth
Services, Richardson, Texas

Self-Care Strategies

Nellie Nelson, M.S.N., R.N.,
C.A.R.N.
Nursing Faculty, Scottsdale
Community College (ADN),
University of Phoenix (BSN),
Phoenix, Arizona. Chairperson,
Addictions Nursing, Certification
Board of the National Nurses
Society on Addictions, Chicago,
Illinois

Image of Nursing: Influences of the
Present

Alice B. Pappas, Ph.D., R.N.
Assistant Professor, Baylor
University School of Nursing,
Baylor, Texas. Staff Nurse (part
time), Children's Medical Center,
Dallas, Texas

Ethical Issues; Interviewing for
Employment

Carol Singer, Ed.D., R.N.
Director, Division of Nursing and
Health Sciences, Manatee
Community College, Bradenton,
Florida

Challenges of Nursing Management

Betty Skaggs, Ph.D., R.N.
Assistant Professor of Clinical
Nursing, Director, Learning Center,
The University of Texas, Austin
School of Nursing, Austin, Texas

Political Action in Nursing

Kathleen M. Speer, P.N.P., Ph.D., R.N.
Adjunct Assistant Professor, The University of Texas at Arlington, Arlington, Texas. Clinical Affiliation Liaison, Children's Medical Center of Dallas, Dallas, Texas

Employment Considerations: Opportunities and Resumes

Sarah L. Stark, J.D., R.N.
Division Head, Health and Public Services, Doña Ana Branch Community College, Las Cruces, New Mexico

Legal Issues

Gayle P. Varnell, Ph.D., R.N., C.P.N.P.
Coordinator/Instructor, El Centro College, Dallas, Texas

Nursing Education

JoAnn Zerwekh, Ed.D., R.N., C.A.R.N., C.A.D.A.C.
University of Phoenix, Tucson, Tucson, Arizona. El Centro College, Dallas, Texas, Executive Director, Nursing Education Consultants, Dallas, Texas.

Conflict Management; Reality Shock

CONTENTS

UNIT I

ROLE

TRANSITIONS

1

Reality Shock

JoAnn Zerwekh, Ed.D., R.N., C.A.R.N., C.A.D.A.C.
Jo Carol Claborn, M.S., R.N.

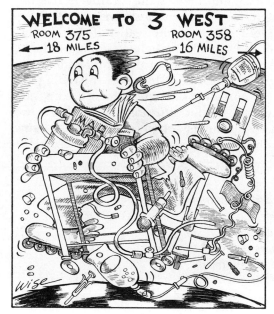

Role transition can be a complex experience.

If only dreams and reality were not so far apart.
—Cervantes

After completing this chapter, you should be able to:

◆ Identify the characteristics of reality shock.

◆ Compare and contrast the phases of reality shock.

◆ Identify your perception of reality shock.

◆ Describe four possible resolutions for reality shock.

This book is for YOU! That's right, you—student-almost-graduate nurse. It will help make your life easier during the transition period when you adjust both personally and professionally to completing nursing school and starting your first job as a professional nurse. We have designed this book to help you keep your feet on the ground and your head out of the clouds, as well as to boost your spirits when the going gets rough. There are many down-to-earth tips offered that will save you time and energy.

As you thumb through this book, you will notice that there are cartoon illustrations and places for you to respond to some questions. Don't be alarmed! These questions are not meant to be graded; instead, their purpose is to guide you through some of the content in a practical, participative manner. Our intention is to add a little humor here and there while giving information on topics such as reality shock, the image of nursing, finding that first job, politics in nursing, nursing education programs, nursing management skills, communicating effectively, ethical and legal issues, career planning, and avoiding burnout, just to name a few. We want you to be informed on the controversial issues affecting nursing today. After all, the future of nursing rests with YOU!

Are you ready to begin? Then, let's start with the real stuff. You are beginning to see the light at the end of the tunnel. It has been a long struggle. You are *almost* there. Nursing is one of the most rewarding professions you could possibly pursue. However, it can also be one of the most frustrating. As with marriage, raising children, and the pursuit of happiness, there are ups and downs. We seldom find the world or our specific situation the exact way we thought it would or should be. Often your fantasy of what you think nursing should be is not what you will find nursing to be.

You will cry, but you will also laugh.
You will share with people their darkest hours of pain and suffering, but you will also share with them their hope, healing, and recovery.
You will be there as life begins and ends.
You will experience great challenges that lead to success.
You will experience failure and disappointment.
You will never cease to be amazed at the resiliency of the human body and spirit.

The paradox of nursing becomes obvious to you *early* in your career. This realization usually occurs during the first six months of your first job. Your control over the basic conditions of your work life is usually limited, but your ability and skill in creating your *experience* of your work life can be unlimited. Therein is the key to your successful **role transition.**

The role transition process does not take place automatically. Having the optimum experience during role transition requires lots of attention and determination on your part. How you perceive and handle the transition will determine how well you progress through the process. So, let's get started. We will first define an important term—**reality shock.**

REALITY SHOCK

What Is Reality Shock?

Reality shock is a term used to describe the reaction experienced when one moves into the work force after several years of educational preparation. The new graduate is caught in the situation of moving from a familiar, comfortable educational environment into a new role in the work force where the expectations are not clearly defined or may not even be realistic. For example, as a student you were taught to consider the patient in a holistic framework, yet in practice you often do not have the time to consider the psychosocial or teaching needs of the patient even though they must be attended to and documented.

The new graduate in the work place is expected to be a capable, competent nurse. That sounds fine. However, sometimes there is a hidden expectation that the graduate nurse function as though she or he had five years of nursing experience. This situation may leave the graduate with feelings of powerlessness, depression, and insecurity over an apparent lack of effectiveness in the work environment. Needless to say, the process of reality shock and transition is not unique to nursing. It is described in many professions as the graduate moves from the world of academia and begins to adjust to the expectations and values of the workforce.

What Are the Phases of Reality Shock?

Kramer (1974) described the process of reality shock as it applies to nursing (Table 1–1). Adjustments begin to take place as the graduate nurse adapts to the reality of the practice of nursing. The first phase of adjustment is the **honeymoon phase** (Fig. 1–1). The new graduate is thrilled with completing school and accepting the first job. Life is a bed of roses, because everyone knows nursing school is much harder than nursing practice. No more writing nursing care plans deep into the night. No one watching over your shoulder while you insert a catheter or give an intravenous medication. You're no longer a "student," but now a NURSE! During this exciting phase, the perception of the situation may feel unreal and distorted, and the graduate may not be able to understand the overall picture.

I just can't believe how wonderful everything is! Imagine getting a paycheck—money, at last! It's all great, really, it is.

TABLE 1-1 *Phases of Reality Shock*

HONEYMOON	SHOCK AND REJECTION	RECOVERY
Sees the world of nursing looking quite rosy	Has excessive fear and mistrust	Beginning sense of humor is the first sign
Often fascinated with the thrill of "arriving" in the profession	Experiences increased concern over minor pains and illness	Decrease in tension
	Experiences decrease in energy and feels excessive fatigue	Increase in ability to objectively assess and evaluate work setting
	Feels like a failure and blames self for every mistake	Increase in competence
	Bands together and depends on people who hold the same values	Crucial period for conflict resolution
	Has a hypercritical attitude	
	Feels moral outrage	

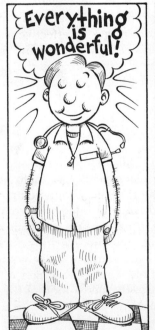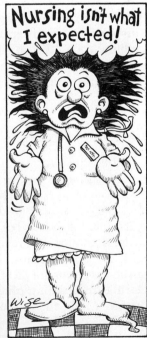

FIGURE 1-1 *Reality shock. The honeymoon's over.*

The honeymoon phase is frequently short lived as the graduate begins to identify the conflicts between the way she or he was taught and the reality of what is done. The graduate may cope with this conflict by withdrawing and/or rejecting the values from nursing school. This may mark the end of the honeymoon phase of transition. The term "going native" was used by Kramer and Schmalenberg (1977) to describe new graduates as they begin to cope and identify with the reality of the situation by rejecting the values from nursing school and beginning to function like everyone else does.

Mary was assigned ten patients for the morning. There were numerous medications to be administered. It was difficult to carry all of the medication administration records to each room for patient identification. Because she "knew the patients" and the other experienced nurses did not check identification, she decided she no longer needed to check patient identification prior to administering medication. Later in the day, she gave insulin to Mrs. James, a patient she "knew"; unfortunately, the insulin was for Mrs. Phillips, another patient she "knew."

With experiences such as this in transition, the graduate begins to feel like a failure, taking the blame for every mistake. The graduate may become morally outraged at having been put in such a position. When the bad days begin to outnumber the good days, the graduate nurse may experience frustration, fatigue, anger, and develop a hypercritical attitude toward nursing. Some graduates become very disillusioned and drop out of nursing altogether. This is the period of *shock and rejection*.

I had just completed orientation in the hospital where I had wanted to work since I started nursing school. Immediately, I discovered the care there was so bad that I did not want to be a part of it. I went home at night very frustrated that the care I had given was not how I was taught to do it. I cried every night. I hated to go to work in the morning. I did not like anyone I was working with. My stomach hurt; my head throbbed; I had difficulty sleeping at night. It was hard not to work a double shift because I was worried about who would take care of those patients if I was not there.

The transition period is successfully managed when the graduate is able to objectively evaluate the work situation and effectively predict the actions and reactions of other staff. Nurturing the ability to see humor in a situation may be a first step. As the graduate begins to laugh at some of the situations encountered, tension decreases, and *perception* increases. It is during the critical period of **recovery** that conflict resolution occurs. If this resolution occurs in a positive manner, it enables the graduate to grow more fully as a person. Also, it enables the graduate to meet the work expectations to a greater degree, and to see that she or he has the capacity to change a situation. If the conflict is resolved in a less positive manner, however, the graduate's potential to learn and grow is limited.

Kramer (1974) described four groups of graduate nurses and the options they took toward resolution of their experienced reality shock. The graduates who were considered to be most successful at adapting were those who "made a lot of waves," within both their job setting and their professional organizations. Accordingly, they were not content with the present state of nursing, but worked to effect a better system. This group of graduates was able to keep worthwhile values from school and integrate them into the work setting. Often they returned to school, but not too quickly.

I am really glad I became a nurse. Sure, there are plenty of hassles, but the opportunities are there. Now that I am more confident of my skills, I am willing to take risks to improve patient care. Why, last week my head nurse, who often says jokingly, "I'm a thorn in her side," appointed me to the Nursing Standards Committee. I feel really good about the recognition.

Another group limited their involvement with nursing by just putting in the usual eight hour day. This group seldom belonged to professional organizations and cited as their reasons for working "to provide for my family," "to buy extra things for the house," and "to support myself." Typically, this type of conflict resolution would lead to burn-out, where conflict would be turned inward, leading to constant griping and complaining about the work setting.

I was so happy, at first. Gee, I was able to buy my son all those toys he wanted. Things here always seem to be the same. I get so upset with the staff and the care that is given to patients. I wonder if I will ever get the opportunity to practice nursing as I was taught. Well, I'll hang on till my husband finishes graduate school, then I'll quit this awful place!

Another group of graduates seemed to have found their niche and were content within the hospital setting. However, their positive attitude toward the job did not extend to nursing as a profession; in fact, it was the opposite. Rather than leave the organization during conflict, these "organization women" would change units or shifts—anything to avoid increased demands for professional performance.

During those first few months as I was just getting started, I sure had a tough time. It was difficult learning how to delegate tasks to the aides and

LVNs. But, now that I have started working for Dr. Travis, everything is under my control. I just might go back to school someday.

The last group of graduates job hopped. After a short-lived career in hospital nursing, this group would pirouette off to graduate school where they could "do something else in nursing" (i.e., "I can't nurse the way I've been taught; I might as well teach others how to do things right"). Achieving a high profile in professional nursing organizations was common for these graduates along with seeking a safer, more idealistically structured environment in which the values learned in school still prevailed.

Finally, I got so frustrated with my head nurse, I just resigned. What did she expect from a new graduate! I couldn't do everything! Cost containment, early discharge, no time for teaching, rush, rush, rush, all the time. Well, I've made up my mind to look into going back to school to further my career.

The job expectations of the hospital and the educational preparation of the graduate nurse are not always the same. This discrepancy, according to Schempp and Rompre (1986), is the basis for reality shock. Relationships among staff, nurse professionalism, job satisfaction, and employee alienation were studied by Ahmadi, Speedling, and Kuhn-Weissman (1987). What is of interest in this study—as well as those of Myrick (1988), Wolfgang (1988), Lund (1988), and Horsburgh (1989)—is that the issues of reality shock and role transition described by Kramer in the early 1970s are still around twenty years later. We need to search for a way out.

BOX 1–1

Think About . . .

What is your greatest concern about your transition from school to practice?

BOX 1–2

Reality Shock Inventory

All students, as well as new graduates, experience reality shock to some extent or another. The purpose of this exercise is to make you aware of how you feel about yourself and your particular life situation.

Directions: To evaluate your views and determine your self-evaluation of your particular life situation, respond to the statements with the appropriate number.

1 Strongly Agree
2 Agree
3 Slightly Agree
4 Slightly Disagree
5 Disagree
6 Strongly Disagree

1. ☐ I am still finding new challenges and interests in my work.
2. ☐ I think often about what I really want from life.
3. ☐ My own personal future seems promising.
4. ☐ Nursing school and/or my work has brought stresses for which I was unprepared.
5. ☐ I would like the opportunity to start anew knowing what I know now.
6. ☐ I drink more than I should.
7. ☐ I often feel that I still belong in the place where I grew up.
8. ☐ Much of the time my mind is not as clear as it used to be.

It might seem to you right now, after reading all of this information, that reality shock is a life-threatening situation. Be assured it is not. You may, however, experience a number of physical as well as psychological symptoms in varying degrees of intensity. For example, you may feel stressed out, have headaches, insomnia, gastrointestinal upset, or a bout of *poststudent blues*. Just remember, it takes time to adjust to a new routine, and sometimes even after you've gotten used to it, you still may feel overwhelmed, confused, or anxious. The good news is, there are various ways to get through this critical phase of your career while establishing a firm foundation for future professional growth and career mobility. Try the assessment exercise in Box 1–2: Reality Shock Inventory.

BOX 1–2

Reality Shock Inventory Continued

---

9. ☐ There's no sense of regret concerning my major life decision of becoming a nurse.
10. ☐ My views on nursing are as positive as they ever were
11. ☐ I have a strong sense of my own worth.
12. ☐ I am experiencing what would be called a crisis in my personal or work setting.
13. ☐ I can't see myself as a nurse.
14. ☐ I must remain loyal to commitments even if they have not proven as rewarding as I had expected.
15. ☐ I wish I were different in many ways.
16. ☐ The way I present myself to the world is not the way I really am.
17. ☐ I often feel agitated or restless.
18. ☐ I have become more aware of my inadequacies and faults.
19. ☐ My sex life is as satisfactory as it has ever been.
20. ☐ I often think about students and/or friends who have dropped out of school or work.

To compute your score, reverse the number you assigned to statements 1, 3, 9, 10, 11 and 19. For example, 1 would become a 6, 2 would become a 5, 3 would become a 4, 4 would become a 3, 5 would become a 2, and 6 would become a 1. Total the numbers. The higher the score, the better your attitude. The range is 20–120.

Adapted from White, E. Doctoral dissertation, April 23, 1986. Chronicle of Higher Education, p. 28.

ROLE TRANSFORMATION

Remember when . . . you first started nursing school. The war stories everybody told you. The changes that occurred in your family as a result of your starting nursing school. Seems a long time ago, doesn't it? Believe it or not, you have already experienced a role transition—to student nurse. Now as you draw nearer to the successful completion of that experience, you are ready to embark on a new one. Take a minute to read the thoughts of one of your peers about her transition into nursing. (I'm sure you will smile at her satire.)

BOX 1–3

Survival Techniques

You finally did it, you have decided nursing is what you want to do for the rest of your life. After all, who would go through all this anguish if you only wanted to do this as a pastime? If you are taking this like everyone else, you are probably going to do this by trial and error, "war" stories, or by helpful hints from the nursing staff.

You need to prioritize your time. This is a familiar and much used term which you will hear often. It is also easier said than done!

If you are single, you have an advantage—maybe. You can decide right now that single is "where it's at" and stay that way for the duration. Of course this means literally living the "single" life. There are no "dinners-for-two," no telephone conversations, no movies at the cinema (rarely any TV), in other words no physical contact with the opposite sex. I know you weren't thinking about it anyway but in case you are studying anatomy and physiology and hormonal thoughts pervade your consciousness, dismiss them.

If you are married, I am not suggesting divorce, just abstinence. Hopefully, you kissed your spouse goodbye when you came to school for your first day of class because your next chance will be on your breaks or when you graduate.

If you happen to be a parent, do as I did. I put pictures of myself in all rooms of my house when I started to school so my kids wouldn't forget me. My children, in return, helped me by plastering their faces on my fridge (they know I'll look there) or on my mirror (another sure spot).

I have acquired a son-in-law, a daughter-in-law, and five grandchildren in the past two and a half years and I usually don't recognize them if I run into them on the rare occasions when I go to the store for essentials (like food) or out to pay our utility bills. Christmas is fun though, because each year I get to spend a few days getting to know the family again. But we all must wear name tags for the first day!

If your children are small, buy them the Fisher Price Kitchen and teach them how to "cook" nourishing "hot" cereal on the stove that doesn't heat up. For the infant, hang a TPN (hint: Total *Parental* Nutrition) of Similac with iron at 40 cc/hr that the baby can control by sound! Crying should do it! Instead of a needle, use a nipple . . . .

Diapers—what would we do without those disposable diapers that stay dry for two weeks at a time? You can even buy the kind that you touch the waist band and Mickey Mouse and his friends jump off to entertain your baby.

BOX 1–3

Survival Techniques Continued

Some of you may feel guilty about not fixing those delicious meals your family once enjoyed. Don't! We get two "breaks" a year and during that time fix barrels of nourishing liquid (you can add a few veggies) and when your family gets hungry, just take out enough to keep fluids and lytes balanced. Remind them that this is only going to last another year or two. Have I covered everything? Oh, I forgot dust . . . Dust used to bother me, but not anymore. I use it to write notes to my 17 year old, to let him know what time I am going to be in the house so he won't mistake me for a burglar, and to say *I Love You*.

On a serious note, each semester you will get regrouped with new classmates. They will become your family, your support group. You will form a chain and everyone is a strong link. This is a group effort. These are people who will laugh with you and cry with you. You will form friendships that will last a lifetime. Take advantage of these opportunities.

On a closing note—do not listen to all the "war stories" that go around— just to the credible ones . . . like mine!

Reprinted with permission from Beagle, B. (1990): Survival techniques. *AD Clin Care* May/June, p. 17.

Give yourself a well-deserved pat on the back for what you have accomplished thus far. It is important to learn early in your practice of nursing to take time to reflect on your accomplishments. Now back to the present. Let's look at the current role transition process at hand, from student to graduate nurse RN (Real Nurse!!).

When Does the Role Transition to Graduate Nurse Begin?

At graduation? No. It started when you began to move into the *novice* role while in your first nursing course (Table 1–2). According to Benner (1984, p.20), "Beginners have no experience of the situation in which they are expected to perform. To get them into these situations and allow them to gain experience also necessary for skill development, they are taught about the situation in terms of objective attributes, such as weight, intake/output, temperature, blood pressure, pulse, and other objectifiable, measurable parameters of a patient's conditions— features of the task world that can be recognized without situational experience." For example, the instructor will give the novice or student nurse specific directions on how to listen for bowel sounds. There will be specific rules on how to guide their actions—rules that are very limited and fairly inflexible. Remember

TABLE 1–2   *From Novice to Expert*

STAGE	CHARACTERISTICS
Novice Nursing student Experienced nurse in a new setting	◆ No clinical experience in situation expected to perform ◆ Need rules to guide performance ◆ Experience difficulty in applying theoretical concepts to patient care
Advanced Beginner Last semester nursing student Graduate nurse	◆ Demonstrates ability to deliver marginally acceptable care ◆ Requires prior experience in actual situation to recognize it ◆ Begins to understand the principles that dictate nursing interventions ◆ Continues to concentrate on the rules and takes in minimum information regarding the situation
Competent 2-3 years clinical experience	◆ Conscientious, deliberate planning ◆ Begins to see nursing actions in light of clients long term plans ◆ Demonstrates ability to cope and manage different and unexpected situations that occur
Proficient Nurse clinicians Nursing faculty	◆ Ability to recognize and understand the situation as a whole ◆ Demonstrates ability to anticipate events in a given situation ◆ Holistic understanding enhances decision making
Expert Advanced practice nurse clinicians and faculty	◆ Demonstrates an understanding of the situation and is able to focus on the specific area of the problem ◆ Operates from an indepth understanding of the total situation ◆ Demonstrates highly skilled analytical ability in problem solving, performance becomes masterful

Adapted from Benner, P. (1984): *From Novice to Expert*. Menlo Park, CA, Addison-Wesley, pp. 20-36.

your first clinical nursing experiences? Your nursing instructor was your shadow for patient care. As nursing students enter a clinical area as novices, they have little understanding of the meaning and application of recently learned textbook terms and concepts. Students are not the only novices; *any* nurse may assume the novice role upon entering a clinical setting in which they are not comfortable functioning or have no practical experience.

By graduation, most nursing students are at the level of *advanced beginner*. According to Benner (1984, p. 22), "Advanced beginners are ones who can demonstrate marginally accepted performance, ones who have coped with enough real situations to note (or to have pointed out to them by a mentor) the recurring meaningful situation components. . . ." To be able to recognize characteristics that can only be identified through prior experience is the signifying trait of the advanced beginner. Thus, when directed to perform the procedure of checking bowel sounds, the students at this level are learning how to discriminate bowel sounds and understand their meaning. They do not need to be told specifically how to perform the procedure.

Let's look at what you and your nursing instructors can do to promote your well-being and success during the role transition experience. These activities reinforce the progress and movement along the continuum from advanced beginner to competent nurse.

No more "mama management." It's time to have your nursing instructor cut the umbilical cord and allow you to function more independently the last semester of clinical training.

More realistic patient care assignments. Start taking care of increased numbers of patients to help you with time management and work organization. Evaluate the nursing staff's assignments to determine what is a realistic workload for a new graduate.

Clinical hours that represent realistic shift hours. Obtain experience receiving shift reports, and with closing charts, completing patient care, and communicating with the oncoming staff. It will be a rude awakening as a new graduate if you have never had the opportunity to work a full shift.

Perform nursing procedures instead of observing. Take an inventory of your nursing skills. If there are nursing skills or procedures you lack or are uncomfortable with, take this opportunity while you are still in school to gain the experience. Identify your clinical objectives to meet your personal needs. Request from your instructor and staff nurses opportunities to practice.

More truth about the real work setting experience. Identify resource people to objectively discuss with you the dilemmas of the work place. Talk to graduates from previous semesters. Ask them what do they know now that they wish they had known the last semester of school.

Look for opportunities to problem solve and to practice critical thinking. No more "spoon feeding" from your instructor—telling you what to do and how to do it. Now is the time to stand on your own two feet while there is still a backup—your instructor—available.

Request constructive feedback by staff as well as by instructors. Stop avoiding evaluation and constructive criticism. Find out now how you can improve your nursing care. Evaluate your progress on a periodic basis. The consequences may be less severe now than later with your new employer.

How Can I Prepare Myself for This Transition Process?

▼

Attitude is the latitude between success and failure.

▲

Think Positive!!   Be prepared for the reality of the work place environment, including both its *positives* and *negatives*. You have certainly encountered by now the "ole battle axe" nurse who has a grudge against new graduates.

> *I don't know why you ever decided to be a nurse. Nobody respects you. It's all work, low pay. I guess as long as you've a good back and strong legs, you'll make it. Boy, do you have a lot to learn. I wouldn't do it over again for anything!*

When you find these nurses, tune them out, and steer out of their way! They have their own agenda to deal with, and it doesn't include providing supportive assistance to you. Eventually, you will learn how to work with this type of individual (more on conflict management in Chapter 8), but for now, concentrate on identifying nurses who share with you a common philosophy. Surround yourself with nurses who have a positive attitude.

Another way to keep a positive perspective is to focus on the good things that have happened during the shift, rather than on the frustrating events. When you feel yourself climbing onto the proverbial, "pitty pot," ask yourself "who's driving this bus?" and turn it around! Review the job duties of the nurse from the year 1887 (Fig. 1–2)—and be grateful!

Anticipate small irritations and disappointments, keep them in perspective; don't let them mushroom into major problems. Turn disappointments and unpleasant situations into learning experiences. Once you have encountered an unpleasant situation, the next time it occurs you will recognize it sooner, anticipate the chain of events, and be better able to handle it.

▼

Don't major in a minor activity.

▲

Be Flexible!!   Procedures, policies, and nursing supervisors are not going to be the same as experienced in school. Be prepared to do things differently than you learned as a student. You do not have to give up *all* the values you learned in school, but you will need to reexamine them in light of the reality of the work place setting.

Duties of the Floor Nurse
Circa 1887

In addition to caring for your 60 patients, each nurse will follow these regulations:

1. Daily sweep and mop the floors of your ward, dust the patient's furniture and window sills.

2. Maintain an even temperature in your ward by bringing in a scuttle of coal for the day's business.

3. Light is important to observe the patient's condition, therefore, each day fill kerosene lamps, clean chimneys, and trim wicks. Wash the windows once a week.

4. The nurse's notes are important in aiding the physician's work. Make your pens carefully, you may whittle nibs to your individual taste.

5. Each nurse on day duty will report every day at 7am and will leave at 8pm, except on the Sabbath on which day you will be off from 12 noon to 2pm.

6. Graduate nurses in good standing with the Director of Nurses will be given an evening off each week if you go regularly to church.

7. Each nurse should lay aside from each pay day a good sum of her earnings for her benefits during her declining years, so that she will not become a burden. For example, if you earn $20 a month you should set aside $10.

8. Any nurse who smokes, uses liquor in any form, gets her hair done at a beauty shop, or frequents dance halls will have given the Director of Nurses good reason to suspect her worth, intentions, and integrity.

9. The nurse performs her labors, serves her patients and doctors faithfully and without fault for a period of 5 years will be given an increase by the hospital administration of 5 cents a day providing there are no hospital debts that are outstanding.

FIGURE 1–2 *The duties of a floor nurse, 1887.*

....

School learned ideal: *Never prepare a medication ahead of time; always prepare it immediately prior to administration.*

Work place reality: *Staff nurses set up medications for the entire 3 PM.–11 PM shift at 4 PM.*

Compromise: *Your value system does not allow you to feel comfortable about setting up medications this early in the shift. However, your time organization tells you the necessity of planning ahead in order to complete medications on time. Therefore, in light of the reality of the workplace, you compromise by preparing medications at 3:30 PM for the 4 PM and 6 PM medications and at 7:30 PM for the 8 PM and 10 PM medications. Your primary objective is to administer medications according to the Five Rights. You have appropriately and effectively adapted your value system to meet the challenges of the workplace without losing sight of your values.*

....

Get Organized!!   Does your personal life seem organized or chaotic, calm or frantic? Sit back and take a quick inventory of your personal life. How do you expect to get your professional life in order, when your personal life is in turmoil? For some helpful tips in organizing your personal life, review the ten suggestions for getting organized in Figure 1–3. How many do you currently use?

Stay Healthy!!   Have you become a "couch potato" since you finished school? Too tired or not enough time to exercise when you get home from work? Candy bars during break . . . pepperoni pizza at midnight . . . Twinkies PRN. . . . How have your eating habits changed while you were in school? Your routine should include exercise, relaxation, and good nutrition. Becoming aware of the negative habits that can have detrimental effects on your state of mind and overall physical health is important in developing a healthy lifestyle.

Find a Mentor!!   Negotiating this critical transition as you begin your nursing career should not be done in isolation.

Today, the evidence suggests that close support relationships are a key, if not *essential*, ingredient in the career development of a successful, happy, new graduate (Campbell-Heider, 1986). In addition to your family and close nursing school friends, it will be important to develop professional support relationships. An important step that will help in your transition process is finding a mentor.

A mentor is an established professional (one that you select) who takes a long-term personal interest in your nursing career. The mentor not only serves as a role model or counselor for you, but actively advises, guides, and promotes you in your career. A mentor can be any successful experienced nurse who is

10 Ways to Get Organized

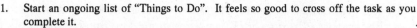

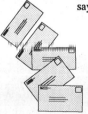

1. Start an ongoing list of "Things to Do". It feels so good to cross off the task as you complete it.

2. If you don't already have a file-folder system, then start one immediately. If you can't keep up with magazine and journal articles, or if you don't have time to put your notes together — file them. Get to them when you can.

3. Post a large calendar on the refrigerator door. It is a great way to keep track of a busy family's schedule. Assign each person to write down his or her meetings, practices, etc. in a different colored ink.

4. Keep a shopping list posted on your refrigerator. When you run out of something, write it down right away. This will eliminate extra trips to the grocery store for forgotten items, and it will keep your cabinets fully stocked.

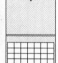

5. Don't spend a lot of time in card shops searching for birthday and annivesay cards. Keep a supply of attractive blank cards on hand for those last minute greetings to be made. Or, buy a bunch of greeting cards and keep them in a letter holder with dividers indicating month and day that cards should be mailed.

6. Set a food timer or alarm clock — and make time for yourself. Tell the children that this is your time to read, watch TV, relax.

7. Neighborhood teenagers are often willing to run errands, mow lawns, wash cars or clean house. Call on them.

8. Check to see if your cleaner, drug store, or grocer has free delivery — and use it.

9. Do your shopping by mail, TV, or phone. Make use of the numerous catalogs around; get on a mailing list and do your buying from your armchair, or by watching Home Shopping on TV.

10. Learn to say "NO". Remember, "No" is a complete sentence! It's so easy to get involved in too many activities. Set priorities and do just one to two activities that please you — say "No" to the rest.

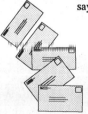

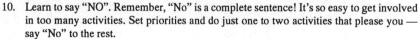

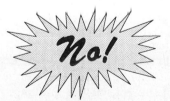

No!

FIGURE 1–3   *Ten suggestions for organizing yourself.*

committed to a professional nursing career and to being a key figure in your life for a number of years. Mentors should have your best interest at heart and bolster your self-confidence. Mentors should be able to give criticism in a highly constructive, supportive atmosphere. As a result, trust and caring are hallmarks of the bonding that occurs between mentor and graduate. In short, a mentor is "a wise and trusted advisor."

A mentoring relationship is an evolving, personal experience for both mentor and graduate. It involves a personal investment of the mentor in the direction of the graduate's professional development. The mentor also benefits from the association by gaining an awareness and perspective of the new graduate's role in nursing. Take note of the following characteristics of successful mentors:

- Have experienced role transition and maintained a positive attitude.
- Are trustworthy.
- Are sincere.
- Share mutual respect.
- Are not in a position of authority over the graduate.
- Promote an easy, give-and-take relationship.
- Are experienced.
- Have compatible values and goals with the graduate.
- Are nurturing.
- Have good sense of humor and enjoy nursing!

Many relationships that have value to the graduate may not be classified as mentor-type relationships because of their short duration. One example of this type relationship is that with the preceptor. The preceptor is most often assigned by the institution to orient the graduate and to be available as a resource on the nursing unit.

Have Some Fun!!   Do something that makes you feel good. This is life, not a funeral service! Nursing has opportunities for laughter and for sharing life's humorous events with patients as well as coworkers. Surround yourself with people and friends who are lighthearted and merry, and who bring that feeling out in you. Remember, the return of humor is one of the first signs of a healthy role transition. Loosen up a little bit. Go ahead, have some fun!

Know What Is Expected!!   How can you expect to do a job correctly if you don't know what the expectations are? Learn the rules of the road early. While still in school, it may be helpful to interview nurse managers to determine their perspectives of the role of the graduate nurse during the first six months of employment. This will give you a base of reference when you interview for your first job. How do you measure up to some of the common expectations nurse managers may be looking for in a graduate nurse? Are you

◆ Excited and sincere about nursing?

◆ Open-minded and willing to learn new ideas and skills?

◆ Comfortable with basic nursing skills?

◆ Able to keep a good sense of humor?

◆ Receptive to constructive criticism?

◆ Able to express your thoughts and feelings?

◆ Able to evaluate your performance and request assistance?

◆ Comfortable talking with your patients regarding their individual needs?

What Are the "Rules of the Road" for Transition?

To summarize, the role transition process can be likened to a stoplight. There is the green light for **GO**—move ahead, you are going in the right direction. The yellow light denotes **CAUTION**—proceed slowly, be sure to look around (CYA—cover your actions—nursing and otherwise, Milazzo, 1990). The red light means **STOP**—do not proceed ahead, your career direction may need to come to a screeching halt.

The following are some helpful tips (i.e., "rules of the road") from graduates who have made the transition successfully:

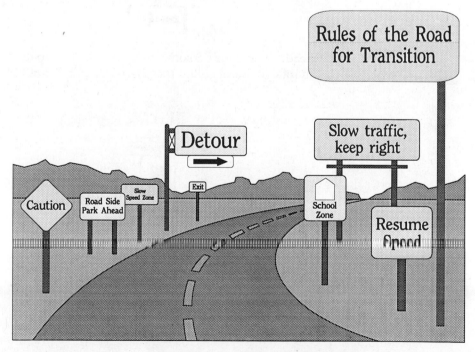

FIGURE 1–4 *Rules of the road.*

Stop.   Take care of yourself. Take time to plan your transition. Get involved with other new graduates; they can help you. Don't be afraid to ask questions.

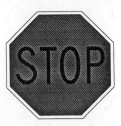

Detour.   You will make mistakes; recognize them, learn from them, and put them in the past as you move forward. Regardless of how well you plan for change there are always detours ahead. Detours take you on an alternate route; they can be scenic, swampy, or desolate, or bog you down in heavy traffic. Don't forget to look for the positive aspects—the detour may open your eyes to new horizons and new career directions.

Curve Ahead.   Get your personal life in order. Anticipate changes in your schedule. Be adaptable, because the transition process is not predictable.

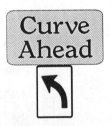

Yield.   You don't always have to be right. Consider alternatives and make compromises within your value system.

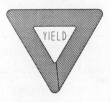

Resume Speed.   Maintain a positive attitude. As you gain experience you will become better organized, and begin to really enjoy nursing. Be aware; sometimes as you resume speed, you may be experiencing another role transition as your career moves in a different direction.

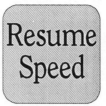

Exit.   Pay attention to your road signs; don't take an exit you really don't want. Before you exit your job, critically evaluate the job situation. "Look before you leap"; make sure the change will improve your work situation.

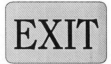

Slow Traffic, Keep Right.   Your career direction may be more comfortable in the slower traffic lane. Take all the time you need—it's okay for everyone to travel at different speeds. Don't get run over in the fast lane.

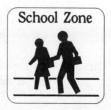

School Zone.   Plan for continuing education, whether it be an advanced degree program or one to maintain your clinical skills or license. Allow yourself sufficient time in your new job before you jump back into a full-time student role.

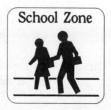

Slow Speed Zone.   Take time to get organized before you resume full speed! Have a daily organization sheet that fits your needs and works for you both on the job and in your personal life.

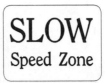

Caution.   Don't commit to anything you are not professionally or personally comfortable with. Think before you act. Don't react. Don't panic. If in doubt, check with another nurse.

Roadside Park Ahead.   Take a break—whether it's fifteen minutes while working or thirty minutes a day to indulge yourself, or a week to do something you really want to do.

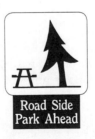

▼

Look for the humor in each day, take time to laugh. You will be surprised at how good it makes you feel!

▲

REFERENCES

Ahmadi, K.S., Speedling, E.J., Kuhn-Weissman, G. (1987): The newly hired hospital staff nurse's professionalism, satisfaction and alienation. *Int J Nurs Stud* 24 (2), 107–21.

Benner, P. (1984): *From Novice to Expert*. Menlo Park, Addison-Wesley.

Blanchard, S. L. (1983): The discontinuity between school and practice. *Nurs Manag* 14 (4), 41–3.

Bygrave, D. (1985): The shock of transition. *Nurs Time* 81 (2), 32–3.

Campbell-Heider, N. (1986): Do nurses need mentors? *Image* 18 (3), 110–13.

Carroll, T.L. (1989): Role deprivation in baccalaureate nursing students pre and post curriculum revision. *J Nurs Educ* 28 (3), 134–9.

Charron, D.C. (1982): Save the new graduate. *Nurs Manag* 13 (11), 45–6.

Gambacorta, S. (1983): Head nurses face reality shock, too! *Nurs Manag* 14 (7), 46–8.

Glennon, T.K. (1983): An additive model to promote biculturism . . . resolves the conflicts between the worlds of academy and clinic. *Nurs Manag* 14 (8), 28–31.

Goldfarb, S. (1986): Reality shock for new OR nurses. *Today's OR Nurse* 8 (6), 21–3.

Horsburgh, M. (1989): Graduate nurses adjustment to initial employment: natural field work. *J Adv Nurs* 14 (8), 610–17.

Johnson, S. (1986): Bridging the gap: a new graduate nurse program that works. *J Nurs Staff Devel* 2 (4), 166.

Kramer, M. (1974): *Reality Shock*. St. Louis, C.V. Mosby.

Kramer, M., Schmalenberg, C. (1977): *Path to Biculturalism*. Rockville, MD, Aspen Publications.

Locasto, L. W., Kockanek D. (1989): Reality shock in the nurse educator. *J Nurs Educ* 28 (2), 79–81.

Lund, P.Z. (1988): *Role Concepts and Role Discrepancies of Senior Baccalaureate Nursing Students Following Selected Summer Work Experiences*. New York, NY, Columbia University Teachers College.

Medendorp, S.J. (1990): A new grad wonders: can I handle nursing? *J Christian Nurs* 7 (3), 32–4.

Milazzo, V. (1990): *How to Easily Avoid Lawyers' Traps*. Houston: Medical-Legal Consulting Institute, p. 12.

Myrick, F. (1988): Preceptorship: a viable alternative clinical teaching strategy. *J Adv Nurs* 13 (5) 588–91.

Naughton, T.J. (1987): Effect of experience on adjustment to a new job situation, part 2. *Psychol Rep* 60 (3), 1267–72.

Sayeed, N.A. (1983): You may feel wonderfully free . . . problems facing newly qualified staff nurses. *Nurs Times* 79 (4), 56–8.

Schempp, C.M., Rompre, R.M. (1986): Transition programs for new graduates: how effective are they? *J Nurs Staff Develop* 2 (4), 150–6.

Swayne, M. (1986): Why we work side by side with student nurses. *RN* 8 (6), 44–5.

Vance, C. (1989): Is there a mentor in your career future? *Imprint* 36 (5), 41–42.

Wolfgang, A.P. (1988): Job stress in the health professions: a student of physicians, nurses, and pharmacists. *J Human Stress* 14 (1), 43–7.

UNIT II

NURSING:
A
DEVELOPING
PROFESSION

2

HISTORICAL PERSPECTIVES: INFLUENCES OF THE PAST

Linda T. Anglin, D.A., R.N.C.

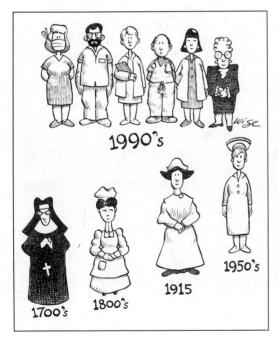

Nursing has come a long way—It is not what it used to be.

. . . I am sufficiently up-to-date to recognize that anything written in the 1890s must be nonsense. But I am not yet advanced enough to view anything that is written in the 1950s as necessarily making sense.
—Edward Hallet Carr, 1961

History repeats itself because each generation refuses to read the minutes of the last meeting.
—Anonymous

After completing this chapter, you should be able to:

◆ Explain the early European contributions to nursing.
◆ Explain the forces that affected the roles of American nurses.
◆ Discuss what nurses do.

So you have to study the History of Nursing. Generally, the topic is known for being boring. Well, be prepared for a different approach to the topic. Knowing the history of our profession guides our understanding of why we do what we do today. This understanding can be useful in directing our planning for our professional goals. Many times understanding the history can help in deciding what changes are needed, what changes are helpful, and what changes may be unnecessary. Let's begin with a look at where nursing began.

NURSING HISTORY: PEOPLE AND PLACES

Where Did It All Begin?

Most nurse historians agree that nursing, or the care of the ill and injured, has been done since the beginning of human life and has generally been a women's role. A mother caring for a child in a cave on a plain and someone caring for another ill adult by boiling willow bark to relieve fever both are examples of nursing. In early times, women generally worked as gatherers while men hunted, thereby providing food for the family. The word nurse actually is derived from the Latin word *nutricius,* meaning nourishing. Roman mythological figures included the goddess Fortuna, who was usually recognized as being responsible for one's fate, and also served as Jupiter's nurse (Dolan, 1969).

Even before Greek and Roman times, ancient Egyptian physicians and nurses assembled voluminous pharmacopoeia with more than 700 remedies for numerous health problems. Great emphasis was placed on the use of animal parts in concoctions that were generally drunk or applied to the body. The physician prescribed and provided the treatments, and usually had an assistant who provided the nursing care (Kalisch and Kalisch, 1986). Much of ancient medicine was based on driving out the evil spirit rather than curing or treating the malady. The treatments were often very foul and many times included fecal material. By now you may be thinking of the saying, "the treatment was successful, but the patient died."

There is little to report on advances in nursing specifically during the Greek and Roman eras. Even the advancement of medical knowledge halted abruptly during the fall of the Roman Empire. Any medical and healthcare knowledge that survived these dark times survived only through the efforts of Jewish physicians who were able to translate the Greek and Roman works (Kalisch and Kalisch, 1986). One bright spot was the establishment in Salerno of a school of medicine and health that not only trained physicians, but also trained women to assist in childbirth. In fact, a midwife named Trotula wrote what may be considered the first nursing textbook on the cure of diseases of women (Dalton, 1900; Jamieson and Sewall, 1949).

Generally nursing was performed by designated priestesses and was associated with some type of temple worship. The temples were centers for men's activities and seldom included women. Little information has survived about this early period. Historians have assumed that Hippocrates was assisted by women, but there is little to support that assumption. Generally women had little value in society and few educational opportunities. Some Roman women, however, were able to wrest themselves from their lowly status, become educated, and own property. Out of these roots nursing began to develop as a recognized and valued service to society (Jamieson and Sewall, 1949).

Why Deacons, Widows, and Virgins?

Paralleling the fall of the Roman empire was the rise of Christianity. The early organization of the young Christian church, which was directly affected by the vision of Paul, included a governing bishop and seven appointed deacons. These individuals assisted the apostles in the work of the church (the word deacon means *servant*). The deacon was directly responsible for distributing all the goods and property that apostles relinquished to the church before they "took up the cross and followed." The apostles were required to give up all material resources in order to achieve full status in the church. Women sympathetic to the Christian cause of aiding the poor were encouraged in this work by the bishops and deacons. Eventually the deacons relinquished aiding the poor to women and established the position of deaconess for that purpose. In order to maintain a pure heart these women were required by the church to be either virgins or widows. The stipulation for widows, however, was that they had only been married once (Jamieson and Sewall, 1949). The deaconesses carried nursing forward as they ministered to the sick and injured in their homes. Phoebe, a friend of Paul and the very first deaconess in the young Christian church is considered to be the first visiting nurse (Dana, 1936). Their treatments continued to be a mixture of scientific fact, home remedies, and magic. Eventually an Order of Widows evolved, composed of women who were free from home responsibilities and thus able to give a total commitment to work among the poor. The Widows, although not ordained, continued to do the same work as the deaconesses. This was soon followed by the creation of the Order of Virgins as the church began placing greater value on purity of body. Although in the Mediterranean the deaconess orders were abolished, in Europe they thrived. The traditional commitment to care for the poor and sick become invaluable in a society that generally had neither time nor inclination to aid them. Eventually these women became known as nuns (*non nuptae*, not married).

What is important to keep in mind is that during this time tremendous upheavals were constantly occurring in the world. Wars, invasions, and battles were constant, and as a result of all these encounters the number of widows was significant. Society during this time did not have the sophistication nor the

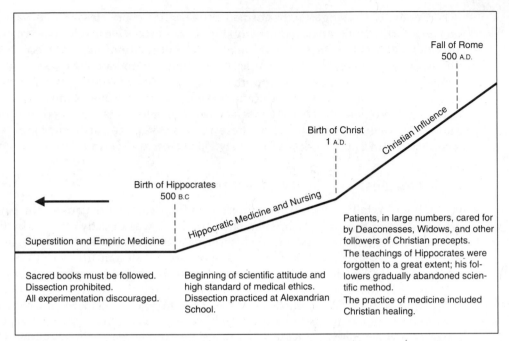

FIGURE 2–1 *Medicine and nursing of ancient civilizations, 5000 BC-500 AD.*

(Reprinted with permission from Jamieson, E.M., Sewall, M.F. (1949): *Trends in Nursing History*. Philadelphia, W.B. Saunders, p. 121.)

means to deal with the dependents of the soldiers killed in battle. As a means of survival, women joined the nuns as a form of protection from starvation and poverty. The world crashed into a dark and dreary time in which superstition, witchcraft, and folklore were predominant influences. Out of the need for physical protection, convents were built to shelter these women (Jameison and Sewall, 1949). The convents became a haven to which women could withdraw from the ignorance and evil and be nurtured in the traditional Christian beliefs (Donahue, 1985). The deaconesses, Widows, and Virgins continued to minister to and nurse the ill within the safety of the convent.

Why Was Knighthood Important?

The Holy Wars furthered the development of nursing in a rather interesting way. Because many Christian crusaders became ill while in Jerusalem, a hospital known as the Hospital of St. John was built to accommodate them. Those who fought in these Holy Wars were known as knights, men who had taken oaths of chivalry, justice, and piety. They often had men trained in the healing arts accompany them into battle to care for them should they be stricken. These male nurses usually wore a red cross emblazoned on their tunics so that in the heat of battle they could be easily identified and hopefully avoid injury or death (Bullough and Bullough, 1978). It became apparent that the Hospital of St. John gave excellent nursing care. Many of the nurses who survived stayed to work with the hospital organizers. As the battles in the Holy Land continued the nurses and knights organized a fighting force with a code of rules and a uniform consisting of a black robe with a white maltese cross, the symbol of poverty, humility, and chastity. They ventured out to rescue the sick and wounded and transported them to the hospital for care and thus they became known as the Hospitalers (Kalisch and Kalisch, 1986). Male nurses dominated these orders. Other orders that emulated the Hospitalers developed in Europe, and more hospitals were opened using the Hospital of St. John as a model (Donahue, 1985).

The altruistic spirit of nursing was seen also in the craftsmen's guilds. Although their primary purpose was to provide training and jobs through the practice of apprenticeship, the guilds provided care and aid for their members when they became old and could no longer work at their trade. The guilds also assisted members and their families in times of illness and injury. The apprenticeship system—in which experience is gained on the job but no formal education is given—once served as a model for training of nurses (Donahue, 1985); it is no longer used, however, and is now considered to have been detrimental to the evolution of nursing.

What nursing gained from this period of history was *status*. The altruistic ideal of providing care as a service performed out of humility and love became the foundation for nursing. The recognition of the value of hospitals grew, and all across Europe cities were building their own hospitals. A general resurgence in the demand for trained doctors and nurses contributed to the building of medical schools and the development of university programs in the art and science of healing.

What About Revolts and Nursing?

Revolts—not the kind that incurred battles, but revolts of a social nature—were common. There were battles too, however the social revolts had a more direct impact on nursing. The revolution of the spirit, more commonly known as the *Renaissance*, ushered in new concepts of the world—the discovery of laws of nature by Newton, exploration of unknown lands, and the growth of secular interests *(humanism)* over spiritual ones. In this era emerged several outstanding humanists who were to become saints (Donahue, 1985). Interestingly, in depictions of these saints, they are shown as needing nursing care or as giving care to a wounded or injured person.

The religious revolution, the *Protestant Reformation*, began primarily as a reform movement but ended with revolt within the Church. Many hospitals in Protestant countries were forced to close, and those loyal to the Church who operated them were driven out of the country, which resulted in a significant shortage of nurses (mostly nuns) to care for the ill and injured. The poor and ill were considered a burden to society, and those hospitals that remained operational in the Protestant countries became known as "pest houses." To fill the need for nurses, women, many of whom were alcoholics and former prostitutes, were recruited. Generally, a nurse was a woman serving time in a hospital rather than a prison (Donahue, 1985; Jamieson and Sewall, 1945).

The industrial and intellectual revolutions that followed the Reformation all had a significant impact on nursing. During the Industrial Revolution, as production of much-needed goods was streamlined through industrial innovation, craftsmen left the rural life to work in factories. The intellectual contributions of scientists—many of whom were physicians—combined with the inventions of the microscope, thermometer, and pendulum clock, advanced knowledge and understanding of the world. The invention of the printing press allowed for easier sharing of information, which further contributed to experimentation. Finally, a disease that was feared worldwide was conquered when Edward Jenner (1749–1823) proved the effectiveness of the smallpox vaccination.

Throughout these revolutions, however, the maternal and infant death rates continued to be high. In fact, prior to his pioneering work in antisepsis in obstetrics, Ignaz Phillipp Semmelweis (1818–1865) observed that patients of educated physicians giving birth in hospitals had significantly higher death rates than those women giving birth at home or at clinics with the assistance of midwives. Despite all of the knowledge gained during this time of revolution, society was generally callous to the plight of children. Children were abandoned without apparent remorse, and infanticide was practiced by poor families desperate to reduce the number of mouths to feed. Remember, they had no reliable form of birth control except abstinence. Additionally, because it was common practice for the woman hired as a wet nurse to sleep with the infant, many infants were inadvertently suffocated. Donahue (1985) reported that during this period 75% of all children baptized were dead before they reached the age of five years. With the persistence of these sad conditions, children's and foundling hospitals were established; eventually, laws were enacted to aid these unfortunate victims (Donahue, 1985).

Existing healthcare conditions for the ill and injured continued to yield high mortality rates. Some sources report hospital mortality rates as high as 90%. Conditions in the armies were no better. In any military action, mortality rates were high. Reports from the battle front during the Crimean War suggested that battles were postponed because there were too few able-bodied soliders to fight. Dysentery and typhoid were the military nemeses. If a soldier was wounded, infection invariably resulted, and hospitals generally offered no guarantee of survival. In any event, these occurrences had a serious effect on military strategies. If men are ill or injured, battles cannot be won.

Upon this gruesome scene entered Florence Nightingale.

Florence Nightingale—the Legend and the Lady

First let's discuss the legend. Published works about Florence Nightingale prior to the 1960s generally presented the legend. Most authors agree that she was beautiful, intelligent, wealthy, socially successful, and educated. She certainly had an ability to influence people and used every Victorian secret to accomplish her desires. Although Nightingale believed it improper for her to accept payment for her services, she did demand financial support for materials, goods, and staff to accomplish her programs and goals. Some historians believe that it was through Nightingale's influence that Henri Dunant, a Swiss gentleman, provided the aid to the wounded that laid the foundation for the organization of the International Red Cross (Bullough et al., 1978; Dodge, 1965). Regardless of what actually happened between her and Dunant, Nightingale's interest and ambition lay in becoming a nurse. Her family was in an uproar over this decision. After all, hospitals were terrible places to go and nurses were, in most cases, the dregs of society. Hospitals were certainly not places for women of proper social upbringing. Though she was forbidden to go, Florence studied nursing in secret. Finally, after a fortuitous meeting, a relationship developed between Nightingale and Sidney and Elizabeth Herbert, an influential couple who were interested in hospital reform. Impressed with Nightingale's analytical mind and her ability to apply nursing knowledge to the critical situation in the hospitals (Bullough et al 1978; Bullough & Bullough, 1990), they encouraged her to study nursing at the Kaiserwerth School, run by Lutheran deaconesses (Dolan, 1969). Her family, of course, was very unhappy; in fact, Dodge (1965) reported that the event precipitated a family crisis as they threatened to withdraw her financial support.

Nightingale accepted a position as administrator of a nursing home for women, the Institution for the Care of Sick Gentlewomen in Distressed Circumstances. She hired her own chaperon and went to work at reforming the way things were done. Florence's interest in hospital reform was unsatiable. She visited hospitals and took copious notes on nursing care, treatments, and procedures. She sent reports on the hospital conditions to Sidney Herbert a very important cabinet minister, who assigned her other hospitals to review. The reviews always included recommendations for improving nursing care. From this early background of experiences, Florence was now ready for her greatest mission, the Crimean War. The legend was on the way.

In 1854, soldiers were dying, more from common diseases than from bullets. Bullough, Bullough, and Stanton (1990) reported that the Crimean War was a series of mistakes. No plan was made for supplying the troops. There was no planning to maintain the environment in camps and there were no provisions to care for the injured after the battle. When Herbert appointed Nightingale as head of a group of nurses to go to the Crimean, she had already developed a plan of action. In fact, some historians believe that she was already planning to go in an unofficial capacity. The announcement caused a sensation, and when Nightingale began a rigorous selection process for accepting nurses, many volunteered but few were chosen. She cleaned up the kitchens, the wards, the patients and the mess. From there the legend grew.

She was clever: after demonstrating the effectiveness of her methods, she withdrew her services. Naturally all that she had accomplished was done under scrutiny, skepticism, suspicion, and anger of the physicians. Without the services of the nurses, the abominable conditions quickly returned, and finally the physicians begged her to do whatever she wished—just help! Naturally, Nightingale responded to the pleading. The actual number of soliders who benefitted from the care of her nurses is innumerable.

▼

The nurses made rounds day and night, and the legend of the lady with the lamp was born.

▲

Nightingale's great success prompted her to begin developing schools of nursing based on her knowledge of what was effective nursing. Eventually, many schools in Europe and America used the Nightingale model for nursing education. The program was generally one year in length and classes were small. Many women wanted to become nurses, however, only fifteen to twenty applicants were accepted. The goals of her programs included training hospital nurses, training nurses to train others, and training nurses to work in the district with the sick poor (Dolan, 1969). In any event, Nightingale had changed society's view of the nurse to one of dignity and value, and worthy of respect.

In any legend, the truth is often mixed with myth. The stories surrounding Florence Nightingale are many. What is interesting is that prior to the 1970s, authors tended to deify Nightingale, or establish her as a saintly person. These myths make for interesting reading. Early nurse historians also contributed to these myths by their interpretations of Nightingale's work. But myths have a purpose. They can be used to explain world views of groups of people or professions at a given time and they provide explanations for practice beliefs or natural phenomena. Myths tend to maintain a degree of accuracy when the truth is lost. The trick is to separate myth from fact, and story from legend, and draw conclusions regarding the occurrences. This is no easy task when one studies Florence Nightingale. Therefore, it is important to read a variety of studies across several time periods before drawing conclusions about the legend and the lady, Florence Nightingale.

In summary, Florence Nightingale had certain characteristics that assisted her in becoming successful during the strict Victorian times in which she lived. She was extremely well-educated for her time. She had traveled throughout the world and had the advantage of personal wealth as well as a gift for establishing relationships with persons of influence and philanthropic spirit. Most portraits depict her as an attractive woman with pleasant features. Contemporary historians agree she had tremendous compassion for all who suffered. She was very strong-willed and determined, characteristics that carried her through the period of the Crimean War. She had the ability to analyze data and draw relevant conclusions on which she based her recommendations. Her students of nursing received better preparation than most physicians. She was thirty-six at the end of the war, and when she returned home she became a virtual recluse until she died at age ninety. She did have some physical ailments: Crimean fever, sciatica, rheumatism, and dilatation of the heart, each of which could have crippling side effects and contribute to her becoming bedfast (Bullough et al., 1990). In any event, the legend and the lady had a significant effect on American nursing as we know it today (Dodge, 1965; Dolan, 1969; Bullough et al., 1978, 1990).

AMERICAN NURSING: CRITICAL FACTORS

What Was It Like in Colonial Times?

In colonial times nursing responsibilities were shared by all able-bodied persons, however, if there was a choice, women were preferred to do the nursing. Early colonial historians described care for the ill, as well as house chores, as the responsibilities of nurses. While most women of this era were considered dainty (Bradford, 1898), nurses were usually depicted as willing to do hard work. Some colonies had organized nursing services which sought out the sick and provided comfort to those who were ill with smallpox and other diseases (Bullough and Bullough, 1978). Generally, however, there were few trained nurses, and most of the individuals who delivered nursing care in the five largest hospitals were men (Dolan, 1969). Eventually women were hired at the command of George Washington to serve meals and care for the wounded and ill. The era ended with the enactment of the first legislation to improve health and medical treatment as well as provide for formal education for society as a whole (Dolan, 1969).

What Happened to Nursing During
the Period of the Civil War?

The period of the Civil War witnessed an improvement in patient care through control of the environment in which the patient recovered. The greatest problems for the army stemmed from the poor sanitary conditions in the camps, which bred diseases such as smallpox and resulted in deaths from inadequate nutrition, impure water, and general lack of cleanliness.

Nurses who had some formal training were recognized as being major contributors to the relative success of hospital treatment. It was in this era that the value of *primary prevention*, or the prevention of the occurrence of disease by measures such as immunization and the provision of a pure water supply, became understood. Volunteer nurses, mostly women, who served in hospitals caring for those wounded soldiers fortunate to have survived the trip from the battlefield, knew that when their patients were nursed in a clean environment and were provided adequate nutrition, the likelihood of their recovering was significantly improved. Astute physicians observed that patients cared for by nurses generally recovered well enough to return to the battlefield. Families, too, saw that when nurses had control over the environment, their ill or injured loved one was more likely to recover—and return home.

As the United States moved into the industrial age of the early 1900s, Victorian values began to permeate the middle and upper middle classes. Social concerns focused on protecting families from the diseases of the crowded urban areas and the demand for improved healthcare increased.

How Did the Roles of Nurses and Wives Compare During the Victorian Era?

The Victorian era had a significant effect on nurses primarily because they were women. The parallelism between the traditional Victorian woman and the nurse is stunning (Table 2–1). The effect of many of the values and beliefs of this era, some historians report, is still felt by women today.

The typical Victorian household consisted of a husband, who earned a living outside of the home and maintained total control of the family finances, and his wife, who maintained harmony within the home and raised their children. Women's work was generally restricted to philanthropic and voluntary work; they attended teas and other social functions to raise money for organizations and people in need. Most women were considered fragile and dainty. They were often ill. It has been suggested that their illnesses and frailty were used as a form of birth control to prevent the numerous pregnancies that most women experienced. Some historians concluded that it was through their weakness that women gained control and attention. If the wife was ill or frail, maids or servants were hired, but if the wife was healthy, the husband would expect more from her. In summary, the Victorian wife was expected to "be good." She was esteemed by her husband and had limited positional power within the confines of the home and society. She was expected to be hard-working and able to maintain harmony, while at the same time be submissive to the demands of her husband. Generally, this fostered dependence on the dominant male figure—the Victorian husband.

TABLE 2–1   *Comparison of Health Care System and Victorian Family*

HEALTH CARE SYSTEM	VICTORIAN FAMILY	COMMENTS
Doctor or hospital administrator	Father has power and position as head of the family	Generate income, see to the welfare of the system
The good nurse	The good wife	Maintains harmony within the system or family, hard working, compliant, submissive, few choices
Client rewarded for being ill	Rewarded for being frail, female, or ill; save my child	Attention, caring, curing, escape from drudgery or work
Paid for treating and curing ills	Frail wife needed servants and maids to assist with the household	Society expectations
Health promotion does not generate income	I want to live forever and I'm willing to pay	Societal expectation to save lives, no focus on self-care
Development of an illness care system	Belief that all is curable	Can buy a cure for every illness

Let's examine nursing during this same time, especially within the hospital organization. Nurses generally were women who wanted to avoid the drudgery of a Victorian marriage. They were required to be single in order to make a complete commitment to their vocation. Women, who had been schooled in submission, were expected to be equally accommodating within the hospital organization. A good nurse worked for harmony within the hospital. She was expected to be hard working, compliant, and submissive. The doctor and the hospital administrator were frequently the same person, usually a man—who expected position and power to go hand in hand. Patients were only admitted if they had income and could afford to pay for the services. It was the physician who generated income, and good nurses were expected to help them continue to maintain their power. Since the system rewarded people for being ill, there was little incentive to be healthy. Again, the social values contributed to dependence on the healthcare system. Out of the milieu came the reformers (Bullough and Bullough, 1978; Davis, 1961; Kalisch and Kalisch, 1986; Stewart, 1950).

Who Were the Reformers?

The Victorian era, while a time of repression for women, was also an era of reform. A list of important names in nursing reform would have to include M. Adelaide Nutting, Minnie Goodnow, Lavinia L. Dock, Annie W. Goodrich, Isabel

Hampton Robb, Lilian D. Wald, Isabel M. Stewart, and Sophia Palmer, among others (Jamieson and Sewall, 1949; Kalisch and Kalisch, 1986). These women, who had in common a comfortable upper middle class background, intelligence, and education, also had in common a desire to reach beyond the constraints that society imposed upon them. As society began to realize the important role that nurses played in treating the ill and injured, it also began to understand the need for training programs that would turn out better nurses. These reformers focused on establishing standards for nursing education as well as practice. Among their accomplishments were the organization of the American Nurses Association and creation of its journal, the *American Journal of Nursing*, as well as the enactment of legislation to require the licensure of prepared nurses in order to protect the public from inadequate care from people who were not trained to nurse (Christy, 1979; Dock, 1900).

THE NURSE'S ROLE: THE STRUGGLE FOR DEFINITIONS

What Do Nurses Do?

As a student, you study nursing texts that explain theories, skills, principles, and care of clients. Every text has at least one introductory chapter that describes nursing and its significance. By examining many of these introductory chapters of nursing texts a rather extensive list of roles can be generated (Anglin, 1990). From this list of roles, six major categories can be determined (Table 2–2). The most traditional role for nurses is that of **caregiver.** The nurse as **teacher** is often referred to when discussing client care or nursing education. The role of **advocate** has been very controversial since 1900. Nurses, on the other hand, were expected to be **managers** ever since the first formal education or training program was instituted. Another interesting role for nurses is that of **colleague.** The final role is that of **expert.**

TABLE 2–2   *What Nurses Do*

CAREGIVER	TEACHER	ADVOCATE	MANAGER	COLLEAGUE	EXPERT
Care provider	Patient educator	Interpreter	Administrator	Change agent	Academician
Comforter	Counselor	Learner	Coordinator	Collaborator	Historian
Handmaiden	Patient teacher	Protector	Decision maker	Communicator	Nursing instructor
Healer		Risk-taker	Evaluator	Facilitator	Professional educator
Helper			Initiator	Peer reviewer	Researcher
Nurturer			Leader	Professional	Research consumer
Practitioner			Planner	Specialist	Teacher
Rehabilitator					Theorist
Support agent					Practitioner

What Is the Traditional Role of a Nurse?

The role of the nurse as caregiver has engendered the least amount of controversy. This role has been thoroughly documented, not only in writing but through art, since early times (Donahue, 1985). Nurses and nursing leaders agree that this is their primary role, and as students your caregiving skills will be measured constantly through skill laboratories, clinical evaluation proficiency, and eventually, through licensure testing and staff evaluations. All of these mechanisms attempt to evaluate your ability to be a caregiver. When we think of the role of caregiver, we think of someone who is moved to take action so that suffering can be relieved. What is difficult to measure is the level of feeling related to caring. There is a great debate in nursing as to whether nurses can be taught to care. However, despite this controversy, the majority of nurses agree that they are caregivers. Since our current education is based on Nightingale's principles of caring, it is no surprise that all of you believe that you will provide care to those in need. You may choose to provide this care in various settings, but basically, all of you desire to be caregivers and are expected to be so.

▼

Caregiving is probably the only role on which there is agreement as to what it means and how we do it.

▲

Imagine a nurse giving care. Generally, the picture that most often comes to mind is someone, usually female, in a white uniform caring for a patient who is ill. This picture is the romanticized version of caregiving continually portrayed in movies, television, and novels. We know that caregiving takes place in many settings: clinics, homes, hospitals, offices, businesses, schools, among others. We can probably agree that caregiving is an important role for nurses and is probably why most of us chose nursing. Research into the role of caregiver continues and our understanding of the role is expanding (Leininger, 1984; Watson, 1985; Gaut, 1984; Benner, 1984). Without a doubt, this is an important role, one that is essential to nursing.

Who Says Nurses Can Teach?

When you take care of clients, it soon becomes apparent that certain information must be shared with them so that they can participate in their care. Teaching a client about their therapy, condition, or choices is critical to the successful outcome of some prescribed treatments. For example nurses have learned through research that knowledge can reduce anxiety before and after surgery. We teach patients about everything. Knowledge can enhance compliance with medications and can encourage healthy lifestyles and behaviors. Teaching becomes especially important when clients have to make treatment choices and decisions about their care. With the volumes of information available regarding healthcare, it is even more important that nurses help the client understand what they need to know to make wise decisions. Without exception, standardized care plans include as a nursing action patient or client education. Most discharge plans also provide for patient education. Agency charting procedures all include required documentation for patient education. All nursing textbooks include sections on what the nurse needs to emphasize regarding patient education. With all this evidence, there is little doubt that teacher is an important role for the nurse.

The role of the nurse as teacher of other nurses is rooted in the evolution of nursing education, however, as schools of nursing developed, nurses were taught by physicians. Gradually, nurses began supervising students of nursing and taught them on the job. Eventually, the influence of Nightingale resulted in qualified nurses teaching students about nursing. This model has prevailed for some time in schools that have the greatest degree of credibility.

In America, the greatest impetus to nurses as teachers occurred in 1948 when recommendations from the Brown report included the separation of the nursing schools from hospital administrative budget. This was a major step in nurses' gaining control over the budget and the educational processes of students. Numerous nursing curricula, since 1900, have included sections on what the nurse needs to teach the patient about the illness. This continues to be a very important role for the nurse at a time when treatment choices and lifestyle choices are numerous. In many ways the nurse as teacher is also an interpreter of information, and this leads us to the next role for discussion.

Who Will Advocate?

A useful definition of the term advocate is one who pleads the cause before another. The first advocacy issue, arising early in the 1900s, concerned nursing practice. Public health and visiting nurses were the majority (approximately 70%) and the minority (approximately 30%) were hospital nurses. Working as a private duty nurse or visiting nurse was a source of income for women who had no other means of support. Since there was no way to determine the credentials of the visiting nurse, many impostors worked in that capacity. Lavinia L. Dock, Sophia Palmer, and Annie Warburton Goodrich, three nursing leaders, deplored this situation and endeavored to protect the public from unscrupulous "nurses" (Dolan, 1983; Goodnow, 1936). Dock was an excellent nurse who believed in fairness to qualified nurses and to the public. She advocated that all practicing nurses be measured by a "fair-general-average standard," as determined by written examination, and rewarded with licensure upon attainment of the standard (Christy, 1979).

Palmer's proposed solutions were similar. Many hospitals were sending out inexperienced undergraduates to do private duty while keeping the income. She advocated a training school in which students of nursing would learn to give care under a qualified nurse and supported the implementation of a registration process for all qualified nurses in order to protect the public from these incompetent, unqualified nurses.

Goodrich advocated compulsory legislation that would ensure that graduates or trained nurses would be the only ones who could work as nurses. She pleaded for the registration of qualified nurses, not only for the protection of the nurse, but for the protection of the community. Goodrich also fought against correspondence or home study programs for nurses, which were a greater menace to the public safety than people realized. Such legislation, she believed, would encourage talented young women who were intellectually prepared for scientific education to select nursing as a career. The role of the advocate as understood by these three early nursing leaders was to protect the public from unqualified nurses (Dock, 1900; Christy, 1969; Palmer, 1900).

From this beginning the role of advocate grew. Public health nurses served as advocates in factories as well as communities during the industrial revolution. Many municipal boards of health hired trained visiting nurses to work as inspectors in the factories in order to protect the workers from health hazards and to help prevent accidents. Communities were finding that the nurse as advocate for the factory worker had inestimable value. Visiting nurses were also proving very effective in preventing the spread of communicable diseases.

In hospitals nurses also worked as advocates for the patients while giving care. Nurses were critical in protecting the patient from harm when they were too ill to protect themselves (Riddle, 1900). Nurses were responsible for providing measures to relieve pain, and strove to make their patients happy and comfortable, even if it meant breaking the rules (Hill, 1900).

During the 1970s and 1980s the responsibility of the nurse as advocate was expanded to include speaking for their clients when they could not speak for themselves (Sovie, 1978). Nurses are now responsible for explaining the treatments and choices in such a way that the patient could understand the options. Nurses are also expected to help the patient understand the benefits and risks involved so that the patient can make an informed choice (Ozimek, 1974).

However, consumers, administrators, and the courts do not share the perception of the nurse as advocate. Findings of a study done in 1983 indicated that consumers do not recognize the nurse as an initiator of health care (Miller et al., 1983). It also found that consumers believe that the *physicians* will protect the rights of the patient. Miller et al. (1983) found that while nurses were serving as mediators between the patients and the institutions, rarely did changes occur within the institution's structure as a result of this role. Patient advocacy was directly related to the power and authority allowed the nurse by the particular system; generally nurses became advocates whenever the issue was care, however, they had little power to truly be effective as an advocate when the concerns involved the medical regime or healthcare services (Miller et al., 1983). Examples of advocacy include questioning doctors orders, promoting client comfort, and supporting patient decisions regarding health care choices.

▼

Advocacy is a critical role for nurses today. Nurses are in a vital position to be effective in this role.

▲

With the need for informed consent, advanced directives, and treatment choices, more than ever patients need an advocate to interpret information, identify the risks and benefits of the various treatment options, and support the decision they make. Being an advocate does involve taking personal and professional risks. When the issue is care, nurses are willing advocates, but when the issue is professional, nurses seem reluctant (Anglin, 1991).

Why Should Nurses Manage?

Even Florence Nightingale recognized the need for nurses to be managers. She insisted that nurses needed to organize the care of the patient so that other nurses could carry on when they were not present. There were four major eras in the development of the nurse as manager. During the first period lasting until about 1920, the nurse was known as the *charge nurse*. Charge nurses were responsible for teaching the nursing students what they needed to know as well as directing the care that the students gave. The charge nurse was autocratic and had absolute authority over the student.

The second era, lasting until 1949, the term *supervisor* was used to describe the role. The supervisor continued to be responsible for the students, however, the role had expanded to include enforcing agency policies, developing improvements in the care of the ill, and being responsible for the effective use of the ward's resources. The supervisor served on hospital committees, but had no vote. Supervisors continued their autocratic management styles and established high standards of nursing practice. At the end of this period, management techniques were beginning to focus on a more humanistic approach, which was a more effective use of human resources. Nurses were more involved in the patient care process. Hospital administrators were relying on nursing expertise to establish policies for patient care and hospital administration. This era ended with the publishing of Esther Lucille Brown's report recommending that nursing education be separated from hospital administration.

During the third period, lasting until 1970, the nurse was referred to as a *coordinator*. The nurse coordinator no longer had responsibility for nursing education of the students, but was expected to motivate staff, be innovative, and solve problems. Coordinators were active in improving patient care and expected to maintain the harmony within the institution. Many nurse coordinators had few skills and little knowledge for this middle manager position and basically learned by trial and error how to be effective.

The last period brings us up to the present. The term *manager* is now most often used in the nursing literature but can be used to describe all four periods.

▼

**No matter what time frame you might study the expectation is that the
nurse manager will coordinate patient care and supervise nurses in the
delivery of quality care.**

▲

The knowledge and skills required for the nurse as manager have become increasingly complex. Nurse managers are expected to solve problems, evaluate
care and personnel, be able to develop budgets, delegate responsibility, negotiate, and be critical thinkers, in an effort to maintain harmony within the institution. Without a doubt, the role of the nurse as manager has evolved into a
complex one that includes organizing patient care, directing personnel to achieve
agency goals, and the allocation of resources.

Can Nurses be Colleagues?

The role of colleague is a vital role for any profession. The status of colleague
within health care generates pictures of nurses, doctors, pharmacists discussing
on an equal basis problems and concerns related to health care. In nursing,
however, a review of our history reveals that we have not quite achieved the
status of colleague. Interdisciplinary collegial relationships currently are ten-
uous. Even more surprising is that even among nurses intradisciplinary collegial
relationships are strained. Three periods in the evolution of this role can be
identified.

The first period, that of the *assistant* role, ended in 1940. This early category
of colleague was clearly defined by nursing leaders as one who was cooperative,
loyal, and obedient to the physician and the hospital (Anglin, 1990). These
characteristics were considered critical to being a competent nurse. In 1905 Jan
Hodson actually set the standard by insisting that loyalty to the doctors was the
most important factor for a faithful nurse to be successful. Hodson supported
blind faith in carrying out doctors' orders, no matter how different or unusual.
She also recommended a strong sense of responsibility when working with
subordinates and superiors (Hodson, 1905; Anglin, 1990). However, she encouraged collegial exchange of information and emphasized asking for advice
in serious or delicate matters (Hodson, 1905). Obviously, physicians encouraged
and rewarded this type of subordinate role (Lawman, 1907; Aikens, 1935; Hamilton, 1940).

From 1941 to 1959, the role of colleague fell under the title of *coordinator*.
A major effort to evaluate nursing service delivered during World War II revealed
this more authoritarian principle of management (Brown, 1948). Nurses were
caught between their hospital's administration and the physicians, and, unfortunately, the highly authoritarian managers within their own profession. Few
contributions from nurses were incorporated into the planning of the organizations. In public health nursing, however, the role of colleague was fully re-

alized (Brown, 1948). Public health nurses served on boards of health and were major contributors in public health planning and programs within local health departments. One important recommendation that came from the Brown report (1948) was that nurses should work to improve their actions and words based on their understanding of human behavior and learn to deal effectively with people. Brown continued by recommending an even more important goal for nurses. Once nurses learned to deal effectively with people, they could make major contributions to the total effort of healthcare delivery and other disciplines (Brown, 1948). Great emphasis was placed on developing collegial relationships for the good of the healthcare system. From these significant recommendations came team nursing approaches to care and coordinate activities for improved patient care. However, the theme of cooperation remained (Anglin, 1990).

Between 1960 and the present, the term *collaborator* has been adopted for this role. The root of this word means "to exchange information with the enemy." This may be the most fitting description of the role. Nursing was interested in developing collaborative relationships with doctors, pharmacists, and other health professionals. The literature is abundant with discussions of these relationships and consistently describes these relationships as collaborative (Hahm and Miller, 1961; Quint, 1967; Seward, 1969; Kelly, 1975; Wisener, 1978; Tourtillott, 1982; Moloney, 1986).

Where Does This Leave the Role of Colleague?

Nursing education has promoted the term collaborator over colleague. The dilemma is that employers do not recognize nor reward the role. Students in their educational experiences are seldom offered opportunity to practice the role of colleague and therefore have only a vague understanding of the role. However, public health nurses throughout American history have not only understood the role, but probably have attained a greater degree of collegiality than any other practice area of nursing. Public health nurses are not the majority within the profession. Nevertheless, they continue to enjoy and maintain the essence of the role (Anglin, 1990). As a colleague one recognizes nurses with expertise and relies on those nurses for their expertise in the interest of improving patient care and advancing the profession. The essence of the role is mutual respect and equality among professionals both intradisciplinary and interdisciplinary (Anglin, 1990). Until nurses can respond to each other with respect, it will be difficult to move from the collaborator to true colleague.

What About Experts?

There is one other role in which nurses are often found. For lack of a better name, this role is called expert. It is a conglomerate of advanced formal or informal education and acquired or recognized expertise, and includes academicians, historians, nursing educators, clinicians, professional educators, researchers, research consumers, theorists, and leaders within the profession. The

American Academy of Nurses recognizes some of these individuals and votes to bestow upon them the honor of Fellow. There are many nurses who are experts in their areas of practice, whether it be in clinics, at the bedside, in nursing homes, or in other settings. As nurses with special expertise, they are called upon to provide testimony in courts and at government hearings, or to share information and knowledge with other nurses, which is their obligation to the profession. This sharing can be done through mentoring, guest speaking, performing in-services, continuing education programs, contributing to publications, and writing technical papers. These experts are usually the nurses who create the momentum that moves the profession forward. This is a role that should be recognized, encouraged, and rewarded.

THE BEGINNING

What do nurses do? There is no simple answer. We agree that nurses care for patients or clients, and so are caregivers. We agree that nurses teach clients what they need to know to make informed choices, and so are teachers. We also agree that the role of manager exists in some form, and so we manage our practice and clients' care. We even can define the role of advocate, although based on the history of the role nurses are reluctant to take risks to fully carry the role forward into the future. The role of colleague is less clear. We are consistent in using the term collaborator, however the term colleague is deemed more fitting for *professionals*, that is, the role to which we should aspire. Finally, we have experts, who we may or may not recognize, and who the profession expects to provide the leadership for the whole. These roles merely provide a beginning for you to understand the profession you have chosen, nursing. May you become proficient in these roles and develop into an expert, and then provide the leadership for nursing in the future.

> The future is not the result of choices among
> alternative paths offered;
> It is a place that is created,
> Created first in the mind and will,
> Created next in activity.
> The future is not some place we are going to,
> But one we are creating.
> The paths to it are not found, but made.
> And the activity of making them
> Changes both the maker and the destiny.
>
> *—Anonymous (1987)*

REFERENCES

Aikens, C.A. (1935): *Studies in Nursing Ethics*. Philadelphia, WB Saunders.

Anglin, L.T. (1991): *The Roles of Nurses: A History, 1900 to 1988*. Ann Arbor, MI, University of Michigan.

Benner, P. (1984): *From Novice to Expert*. Menlo Park, CA, Addison-Wesley. 1984.

Bradford, W. (1898): *History of Plymouth Plantation. Book II* (1620). Wright & Potter.

Bullough, V., Bullough, B. (1978): *The Care of the Sick: The Emergence of Modern Nursing*. New York, Prodist.

Bullough, V., Bullough B., Stanton, M.P. (1990): *Florence Nightingale and Her Era: A Collection of New Scholarship*. New York, Garland.

Carr, E. H. (1961): *What is History?* New York, Vintage Books.

Christy, T. (1969): Portraits in nursing: Isabel Hampton Robb. *Nurs Outlook* 17:28.

Christy, T. (1975): Nurses in American history: The fateful decade, 1890–1900. *Am J Nurs* 75:1163.

Christy, T. (1979): The first fifty years. *Am J Nurs* 71:1778.

Dalton R. (1900): Hospitals: Their origins and history. *Dublin J Med Sci* 109:17.

Dana, C.L. (1936): *The Peaks of Medical History*. New York, Paul B. Hoeber.

Davis, M.D. (1961): I was a student over 50 years ago. *Nurs Outlook* 61:62.

Degler, C.N. (1980): *At Odds*. New York, Oxford University Press.

Dock, L. (1900): What may we expect from the law? *Am J Nurs* 1:9.

Dodge, B.S. (1989): *The Story of Nursing*. 2nd ed. Boston, MA, Little, Brown.

Dolan, J.A. (1969): *History of Nursing*. Philadelphia, WB Saunders.

Donahue, M.P. (1985): *Nursing: The Finest Art*. St. Louis, CV Mosby.

Goodnow, M. (1936): *Outlines in History of Nursing*. Philadelphia, WB Saunders.

Hahm, H., Miller D. (1961): Relationships between medical and nursing education. *Journal of Medical and Nursing Education* 39:849.

Hamilton, J.A. (1949): Success or failure in nursing administration. *American Journal of Nursing* 49:496.

Hill, J. (1900): Private duty nursing from a nurses point of view. *American Journal of Nursing* 2:129

Jamieson, E.M., Sewall, M.F. (1949): *Trends in Nursing History*. Philadelphia, WB Saunders.

Kalisch, P.A., Kalisch, B.J. (1986): *The Advance of American Nursing*. Boston, Little, Brown.

Kelly, L.Y. (1975): *Dimensions of Professional Nursing*. 3rd ed. New York, Macmillan.

Lawman, J.H. (1907): The evolution and development of the nurse. *American Journal of Nursing* 8:8.

Leininger, M. (1972): The leadership crisis in nursing: A cultural problem and challenge. *J Nurs Admin* p. 62.

Leininger, M. (1984): *Care: The Essence of Nursing and Health*. Thorofare, NJ: Charles B. Slack.

Miller, B.K., Mansen, T.J., Lee, H. (1983): Patient advocacy: Do nurses have the power and authority to act as patient advocate? *Nurs Leadership* 6:56.

Ozimek, D. (1974): *The Baccalaureate Graduate in Nursing: What Does Society Expect?* New York, National League for Nursing.

Palmer, S. (1900): The editor, *Am J Nurs* 1:166.

Ryan, M.P. (1979): *Womanhood in America: From Colonial Times to the Present*. New York, New Viewpoints.

Quint, G.C. (1967): Role models and the professional nurse identity. *Journal of Nursing Education* 6:11.

Riddle, M.M., (1900): Prophylactics. *American Journal of Nursing* 1:29

Shattuck, L. (1948): *Report of the Sanitary Commission of Massachusetts, 1850.* Cambridge, MA, Harvard University Press.

Seward, Sister J.M. (1969): Role of the nurse: Perceptions of nursing students and auxiliary nursing personnel. *Nursing Research* 18:164.

Stewart, I.M. (1950): A half-century of nursing education. *Am J Nurs* 50:617.

Stille, C.J. (1863): *History of the United States Sanitary Commission: Being the General Report of Its Work During the War of Rebellion.* Philadelphia, JB Lippincott.

Tourtillott E.A. (1986): *Commitment—A Lost Characteristic.* New York, J.B. Lippencott

Watson, J. (1985): *Nursing: Human Science and Human Care—A Theory of Nursing.* East Norwalk, CT, Appleton-Century-Crofts.

Wisener, S. (1978): The reality of primary nursing care: risks, roles and research. *Role Changes in Primary Nursing.* New York, National League of Nursing.

Wormeley, K.P. (1863): *The United States Sanitary Commission: A Sketch of Its Purposes and Its Work.* Boston, Little, Brown.

3

Image of Nursing: Influences of the Present

Nellie Nelson, M.S.N., R.N., C.A.R.N.

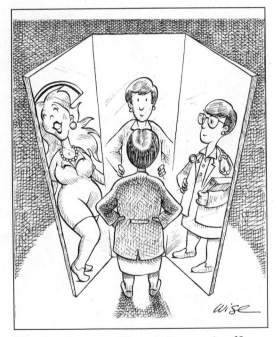

Nursing image—How is it perceived?

Oh the power the gift He give us, to see ourselves as others see us.

—Robert Burns, 1786

We write our own destiny . . . We become what we do.

—Madame Chiang Kai-Shek

After completing this chapter, you should be able to:

◆ Identify selected historical educational studies and literature that have influenced the image of professional nursing.

◆ Describe different sociological models that characterize "professionalism."

◆ Apply Pavalko's characteristics as a framework to describe modern-day nursing practice.

◆ Identify the role that nursing organizations have in professional practice.

◆ Review the scope of nursing literature in today's healthcare marketplace.

◆ Describe the role of credentialing and certification in professional practice.

◆ Examine two controversial issues affecting nursing practice: entry into practice and the nursing shortage.

W hat does it mean to be a professional nurse? How does the public view nursing? How does nursing define and view itself?

Within the profession of nursing there is no single definition of nursing on which all nurses agree. To describe the current image of the professional nurse would be analogous to the old Indian folk tale in which three people attempt to define an elephant by blindly touching three separate parts of the animal. Modern-day nursing has many exciting professional dimensions, one of which includes the debate surrounding its identification as a profession. A current movement in nursing is to change the public image of the nurse. This chapter discusses the development of nursing into a profession and explores present and future dimensions of the "image." Let's continue with nursing's historical journey by beginning with the question "What constitutes a profession?" Historical knowledge about our "rites of passage" gives us an appreciation of where nursing is today as a profession and what the future of nursing may hold for you, the new graduate, in our complex and evolving healthcare world.

IMAGE OF NURSING

What Do We Mean By the "Image" of Nursing?

Nursing has been identified as an "emerging profession" for at least 150 years. The image of professional nursing continues to evolve and is significantly impacted by the media, women's issues/roles, and a high-technology healthcare environment. How nursing views itself in the evolution of the profession and how actively nurses are involved in the definition process will determine the "image" of nursing in the future.

Some authors say the image of nursing is directly related to what the profession offers society and the value placed on that service (Shaffer, 1989). Nursing leaders have recognized that role behavior in professional nursing is related to the image of the nurse held by the consumer (i.e., the public). The most significant changes in the public's image of nursing have occurred within the past 50 years. Typically, the public image of nursing does not accurately reflect the nurse's expertise and does not recognize the contributions nursing makes to healthcare. Until the image of nursing as portrayed by the media is modified nursing will not be recognized as a profession. Lynn Licardo (1991), a journalist for *Soap Opera Weekly*, wrote that no profession gets depicted very accurately in the soaps:

> Look at how physicians are portrayed . . . it's just as ridiculous as the way nurses are portrayed. The problem for nurses is that the public doesn't have a frame of reference to filter through the reality. If they see nurses doing something totally uncharacteristic, they figure that must be what nurses do.

Ideally, 1990s nurses will be thought of as autonomous and competent decision makers within their nursing practice areas (Kaler, 1989). A 1990s nationwide ad campaign supported by the National Commission on Nursing Implementation Project produced radio and television ads that said "If caring were enough, anyone could be a nurse." In 1990 Nurses of America (NOA), an advocate organization sponsored by the National League for Nursing (NLN), implemented a very successful program directed toward improving the image of nursing as depicted on television, on radio, in print, and on lecture circuits. Consultants were contracted to work with executives, politicians, and celebrities on presenting nursing in a positive manner. This approach reinforced the image of the modern-day professional nurse as having decision-making and problem-solving skills.

Media Watch, a national newsletter, began addressing the image of nursing in the Spring of 1990. This publication of NOA was sponsored by the Tri-council, comprising the American Nurses Association (ANA), American Organization of Nurse Executives (AONE), and the NLN for the purpose of informing the public about the role that the modern nurse has in healthcare delivery (Wallace, 1990). NOA welcomes the reactions of professional nurses to the way they perceive nursing is portrayed in the media. Remember, the so-called television comedy, "Nightingales"? Because of the outcry from professional nurses and the public against the negative way in which this program presented nurses, Lee Iacocca withdrew Chrysler's advertising support. Shortly thereafter, the program was canceled. The newsletter may be obtained by writing to *Media Watch*, 350 Hudson Street, New York, NY 10014.

It is time the public viewed the nurse as someone other than an overweight, mean, disciplinarian, or a sex-crazed broad jumping into dark utility rooms with doctors. The journey toward attaining a professional image is, has been, and will continue to be challenging. Journalist and author Suzanne Gordon (1991) stated in an interview with Leah Binder, editor of *Media Watch*:

> We need a Nurses, "Caring" or "Liberation" Movement to make society look at the largest profession and to see what extraordinary things nurses are doing . . . Nursing is moving in the right direction, but nurses need to be much more assertive, much less humble about what they do.

And this is happening now! In *Megatrends for Women*, Aburdene and Naisbitt (1992) examine the current impact nurses are having on healthcare. Nursing stereotypes are dissolving as nurses take leadership roles in effecting change. In a landmark study done in 1986 at George Washington University, nurses were credited with decreasing the mortality rate in critical care areas. A second study in 1989 indicated that physicians rated nursing expertise as the primary feature that determined excellent hospital care. These studies demonstrate that the image of nursing improves as nurses assume increasingly influential positions in healthcare (Aburdene and Naisbitt, 1992).

What Constitutes a Profession?

There are many ways to describe a "professional." What meaning does the word have for you as a graduate professional nurse? Controversy over the definition of the term *professional* as it relates to nursing is not a new issue. Strauss (1966), a noted sociologist, found the word professional used in reference to nursing in a magazine article published in 1892 entitled "Nursing, a New Profession for Women." The 1990s nurse owes a lot to Isabel Adams Hampton (later Isabel Hampton Robb) for her visionary focus of the late 1800s. She was an outstanding advocate for the professionalization of nursing. In her textbook *Nursing Ethics* (1901) she wrote:

> The trained nurse, then, is no longer to be regarded as a better trained, more useful, higher class servant, but as one who has knowledge and is worthy of respect, consideration and due recompense . . . She is also essentially an instructor; part of her duties have to do with the prevention of disease and sickness, as well as the relief of suffering humanity . . .

> These are some of the essentials in nursing by which it has become to be regarded as a profession, but there still remains much to be desired, much to work for, in order to add to its dignity and usefulness. As the standard of education and requirements become a higher character and the training more efficient, the trained nurse will draw nearer to science and its demands and take a greater share as a social factor in solving the world's needs.

Much analysis of the term has occurred in the literature since the early 1900s and continues through the current decade.

The classic work of Abraham Flexner, written in 1915, was used initially by the medical profession to begin to form its identity and redefine itself as a profession. As a sociologist, Flexner began examining his own profession. This was at a time when occupations such as medicine, social work, and nursing were moving away from their occupational focus and toward redefinition and professionalization. Modern socialists continue to address the question "What are the characteristics of a profession?" Flexner's criteria continue to be cited in today's definition of a profession. His criteria, as cited by Becker (1970), include the following:

1. Professional activity is basically intellectual with great personal responsibility.
2. It is based on great knowledge, not routine activities.
3. It is practical rather than theoretical.
4. It has a technique that can be taught which is the basis for professional education.
5. It is organized internally.

6. It is motivated by altruism, with members working for some aspect of the good of society.

In the 1950s, Caplow defined several steps in the process of "becoming professional." He identified the importance of forming an association that defined a special membership. He suggested that making a name change to clarify an area of work or practice would subsequently produce a new role. With the creation of this new role the group would then establish a code of ethics along with legal components for licensure to practice and educational control of the profession (Caplow, 1954). The process of becoming professional as described by Caplow was taking place in nursing in 1897 with the establishment of the ANA. Other aspects of professionalization were also beginning to develop. For example, the Nursing Code of Ethics was suggested as early as 1926, although it wasn't written or published by the ANA until the early 1950s. Revisions were made in 1956, 1960, and 1968, with the last revision in 1976 including interpretative statements.

Nursing education began shifting very slowly from a three-year diploma program to the two-year associate degree program and four-year baccalaureate program. Inconsistency in nursing education continues to be a point of criticism when the question "Is nursing a profession or a semi-profession" is addressed.

Fifty years after Flexner's criteria and twenty years after Caplow's work, Pavalko (1971) described eight dimensions of a profession. We'll examine Pavalko's dimensions of a profession and their specific application to nursing in more detail in the next section. Nursing continues to apply these dimensions in an ongoing effort to move nursing out of the realm of a mere occupation.

Responding to the questions in Box 3–1, which presents the fourth model of professionalism, Levenstein's model, will help you identify common themes in describing a profession. What are your thoughts about the nursing profession using his criteria?

Others have written about professions and their development, but these four sociological models present some logical characteristics for you to use to examine professionalism. According to Henshaw, a noted nursing leader and Director of the Nursing Research Institute, a profession includes self-regulation and autonomy with ultimate loyalty and accountability to the professional group (Talotta, 1990). Nursing is a dynamic profession and continues to strive to enhance a professional image—which leads us to the next question.

Is Nursing a Profession?

Eunice Cole, past President of the ANA, describes nursing as a dynamic profession that has established a code of ethics and standards of nursing practice, education, nursing service, and research components. The standards for both the professional and practical dimensions of nursing are continually reviewed and updated. Nurses, strong in numbers and yet splintered professionally in

---

BOX 3–1

Levenstein's Characteristics of a Profession

What Do You Think About . . .

◆ The Element of Altruism

   How do you define caring in your clinical practice?

◆ Code of Ethics

   Are you familiar with the ANA Code of Ethics?

◆ Collaboration with Groups and Individuals for Benefit of the Client

   What other groups do you work with in your clinical setting that effect the health needs of the client and family?

◆ Colleagueship Demonstrated By:

   An Organization for Licensing—

   What is the role of the State Board of Nursing?

   A Group that Helps Insure Quality—

   Are you aware of the role of the NLN in accreditation of nursing programs?

   Peer Evaluators of Practitioners—

   What is the role of job evaluations in terms of professional growth?

◆ Accountability for Conduct and Responsibility for Practice Decisions

   Who monitors professional conduct issues from a legal and ethical point of view?
   Does shared governance reflect more control of one's nursing practice?

◆ Strong Research Program

   Are you aware that a national center for nursing research is now operating in Washington, D.C.?

many ways, represent the largest group of healthcare providers in the United States; there are 2.1 million registered nurses, with 80% of that number employed in nursing. Using Pavalko's eight dimensions to describe a profession, let's examine nursing and issues that challenge the collective whole.

1. **A profession has relevance to social values.**

   Does nursing exist to serve self or others? Nursing historically had its roots in true altruism with lifelong service to others. Nursing defined itself in the ANA's *Social Policy Statement* (1980) as the "diagnosis and treatment of *human responses* to actual or potential health problems." As nurses, we focus not only on the treatment component of patient care but also on wellness and health promotion issues as a part of our nursing practice. The goal is to shift the focus of healthcare so that primary prevention becomes more "valued." As it does, nurses will be increasingly important because of their ability to be teachers of health promotion activities and managers of wellness, activities that have an impact on social values.

2. **A profession training or educational period.**

   According to Florence Nightingale, a nurse's education should involve not only a theory component, but also practice. More recently, Kibbee (1988) stated that an emerging profession such as nursing should have a rigorous and systematic education program for those who wish to enter the field. This perspective has stimulated questions regarding the level at which one enters nursing such as:

   ◆ Is a two-year program able to provide an adequate educational basis for the professional?

   ◆ Is the nurse prepared for "modern-day" nursing functions if educated at the diploma level?

   ◆ Is it necessary to complete a four-year Bachelor of Science in Nursing (BSN) program in order to handle the challenges of the healthcare environment and client or family needs?

   These questions have been discussed back and forth since the publication in 1965 of an ANA position paper that charged the profession with the goal of establishing nursing education at the baccalaureate level within twenty-five years. Twenty-five years have come and gone, and this issue continues to divide the profession. The inability of nursing organizations and educational systems at all levels to come to agreement on this issue has affected the solidarity of the profession. Only a few states have eliminated diploma programs and only one state, North Dakota, has legally mandated the BSN as the degree for entry into practice. Will the turn of the century see unity of educational trends? Let's hope so. Beyond this generic degree controversy are the issues associated with specialization: should the Master of Science (MSN) degree be the entry-level degree, or a doctorate (PhD) in nursing be required to enter into specialty nursing practice? The last decade has not resolved the issue. Will the year 2000?

3. **Elements of self-motivation address the way in which the profession serves the client or family and large social system.**

In 1990 the Tri-council of Nursing along with the American Association of Colleges of Nursing designed a "Nursing Agenda for Health Care Reform" to collectively express the views of nurses concerning healthcare. Endorsed by thirty-nine major specialty nursing organizations, this document, summarized in Table 3–1, presents a plan to change a healthcare system that currently focuses on treatment of illness to one that focuses on primary healthcare services along with the promotion, restoration, and maintenance of health. The nursing healthcare reform encourages consumers to be more responsible for their health while supporting a "partnership" between consumers and providers. The document also suggests that new community sites for healthcare delivery be built in a more cost-effective and efficient manner to meet consumer needs (Nursing Agenda for Health Care Reform, 1991).

Political activity is a way of translating social values into action. Nursing is presented with special challenges when, for example, nurses must "strike" for pay and benefits or demonstrate a united front to gain federal funding rather than continuing a passive role in such issues. The concept

TABLE 3–1 *Summary of "Nursing's Agenda for Healthcare Reform"*

The following points represent what nursing believes to be the "core of care," essential healthcare services that should be available to all people in the United States.

The basic components of nursing's "core of care" include:
◆ A restructured healthcare system which:
—Enhances consumer access to services by delivering primary healthcare in community-based settings.
—Fosters consumer responsibility for personal health, self-care, and informed decision making in selecting healthcare services.
—Facilitates utilization of the most cost-effective providers and therapeutic options in the most appropriate settings.

◆ A federally defined standard package of essential healthcare services available to all citizens and residents of the United States, provided and financed through an integration of public and private plans and sources:
—A public plan, based on federal guidelines and eligibility requirements, will provide coverage for the poor and create the opportunity for small businesses and individuals, particularly those at risk because of preexisting conditions and those potentially medically indigent, to buy into the plan.
—A private plan will offer, at a minimum, the nationally standardized package of essential services. This standard package could be enriched as a benefit of em-

Table continued on following page

TABLE 3–1   *Summary of "Nursing's Agenda for Healthcare Reform"*
Continued

ployment or individuals could purchase additional services if they so choose. If employers do not offer private coverage, they must pay into the public plan for their employees.

◆ A phase-in of essential services, in order to be fiscally responsible:
—Coverage of pregnant women and children is critical. This first step represents a cost-effective investment in the future health and prosperity of the nation.
—One early step will be to design services specifically to assist vulnerable populations who have had limited access to our nation's healthcare system. A "Healthstart Plan" is proposed to improve the health status of these individuals.

◆ Planned change to anticipate health service needs that correlate with changing national demographics.

◆ Steps to reduce healthcare costs include:
—Required usage of managed care in the public plan and encouraged in private plans.
—Incentives for consumers and providers to utilize managed care arrangements.
—Controlled growth of the healthcare system through planning and prudent resource allocation.
—Incentives for consumers and providers to be more cost efficient in exercising healthcare options.
—Development of healthcare policies based on effectiveness and outcomes research.
—Assurance of direct access to a full range of qualified providers.
—Elimination of unnecessary bureaucratic controls and administrative procedures.

◆ Provisions for long-term care, which include:
—Public and private funding for services of short duration to prevent personal impoverishment.
—Public funding for extended care if consumer resources are exhausted.
—Emphasis on the consumers' responsibility to financially plan for their long-term care needs.

◆ Insurance reforms to assure improved access to coverage, including affordable premium, reinsurance pools for catastrophic coverage, and other steps to protect both insurers and individuals against excessive costs.

◆ Access to services assured by no payment at the point of service and elimination of balance billing in both public and private plans.

◆ Establishment of public/private sector review—operating under federal guidelines and including payers, providers, and consumers—to determine resource allocation, cost reduction approaches, allowable insurance premiums, and fair and consistent reimbursement levels for providers. This review would progress in a climate sensitive to ethical issues.

of nursing as truly altruistic may conflict with the concept of a future generation of nurses who may view nursing as a job rather than a profession. As a graduate nurse, you are also a new professional who will help effect many changes in the healthcare arena. Healthcare costs are escalating, and it is predicted that without a major system change healthcare spending will reach $2.1 to $2.7 trillion by the year 2000.

4. **A profession has a code of ethics.**

Nursing, like other professions, has ethical dimensions. The ANA published the Nursing Code of Ethics in 1950 and revised it with interpretative statements in 1976. Key points of the Code are given in Table 3–2. The Code of Ethics is discussed in more detail in Chapter 12.

TABLE 3–2   *Nursing's Code of Ethics*

1. The nurse provides services with respect for human dignity and the uniqueness of the client unrestricted by considerations of social or economic status, personal attributes, or the nature of health problems.

2. The nurse safeguards the client's right to privacy by judiciously protecting information of a confidential nature.

3. The nurse acts to safeguard the client and the public when healthcare and safety are affected by the incompetent, unethical, or illegal practice of any person.

4. The nurse assumes responsibility and accountability for individual nursing judgments and actions.

5. The nurse maintains competence in nursing.

6. The nurse exercises informed judgment and uses individual competence and qualifications as criteria in seeking consultation, accepting responsibilities, and delegating nursing activities to others.

7. The nurse participates in activities that contribute to the ongoing development of the profession's body of knowledge.

8. The nurse participates in the profession's efforts to implement and improve standards of nursing.

9. The nurse participates in the profession's efforts to establish and maintain conditions of employment conducive to high-quality nursing care.

10. The nurse participates in the profession's efforts to protect the public from misinformation and misrepresentation and to maintain the integrity of nursing.

11. The nurse collaborates with members of the health professions and other citizens in promoting community and national efforts to meet the health needs of the public.

Reprinted with permission from the American Nurses Association, Kansas City, MO.

5. **A professional has a commitment to life-long work.**

   By this Pavalko means that a professional sees his or her career as more than just a stepping stone to another area of work or as an intermittent job. Nursing, however, is a female-dominated profession; role conflicts exist as the nurse is challenged with changing jobs and accepting part-time work to accommodate family or personal needs. One study indicates that 78 to 80% of nurses are employed, one third of whom on a part-time basis (Aiken and Millinix, 1987). Some people have described the nurse working part-time as an "appliance nurse," implying that she is working for the "next television" or "new refrigerator," rather than viewing nursing as a life-long career. It is the professional commitment nurses have and how much they value the professional role that adds quality to the career, not the hours that are worked in a given period of time. Nursing as a career brings not only financial rewards, but also the opportunity for continued education, and when there is involvement and commitment to the profession, reflects the values of the individual.

6. **Members control their profession.**

   Nurses are not entirely autonomous. While nurses work under professional control, they are under legislative control as well. One of these controls is the State Board of Nursing, which controls the scope of nursing practice within the state and professional practice standards that are supported at both local and national levels. The ANA developed Standards of Nursing Practice in the late 1960s and continues to refine this document. Developing professional practice standards indicates to the larger social system that nursing can define and control its quality of practice. These national standards are incorporated into institutional standards to help guide nursing practice. Because nurses practice in such varied settings, the nurse who is in the "ideal setting for autonomy" may be the nurse who is in private practice, e.g., nurse midwives or psychiatric-mental health specialists. The majority of nurses in this country work within a structured setting. Trends in those settings are slowly changing to give nurses a stronger voice. For example, nursing care delivery systems that use case management and shared governance reflect more progressive and autonomous environments. Does nursing truly control its scope of practice through professional organizations and State Boards? Does nursing have more autonomy in the area of practice roles? Jean Steele, past President of the ANA's Cabinet on Nursing Practice and a nursing leader relates that the most precious hallmark of a profession is self-regulation (Stelle, 1985).

7. **A profession has a theoretical framework on which professional practice is based.**

   Nursing continues to be based in the sciences and humanities, but a nursing *theory* is evolving. It was not until the 1950s that nursing theory was "born."

Dr. Hildegard Peplau in 1952 published a nursing model that described the importance of the "therapeutic relationship" in health and wellness (Peplau, 1952). Since then other nursing theorists such as Rogers, Roy, Orem, and Neuman have contributed to our evolving theory-based nursing science.

8. **Members of a profession have a common identity and distinctive subculture.**

The "outward" image of nursing has changed remarkably within the past fifty years. Nurses were once identified by how they looked rather than by what they did. The nursing cap and pin reflected the nurse's school and educational background. The modern-day trend emphasizes that it's not what is worn but what is done that reflects one's role in the nursing profession. The struggle to shift out of rigid dress codes was a major issue in the 1960s. Clothing and other symbols do identify a subculture, and changes in that identification process occur slowly. How many nurses do you know who wear their nursing cap in daily nursing practice? Does your school have a special nursing cap?

Nursing colleagues provide a source of attitudes and values about the profession. The desire to affiliate with fellow members of the subculture of nursing and model one's behavior on theirs has a significant role in an individual's nursing socialization process.

Another way of encouraging cohesive group dynamics and a sense of belonging is through membership in alumni associations and professional associations. Many schools of nursing have alumni associations, student nurse associations, and/or nursing honor societies (e.g., Sigma Theta Tau). These groups provide social interaction during the nursing education years and are great ways to build colleagueship.

There is great diversity in attitudes of nurses toward belonging to a professional organization. The ANA is considered the official voice of nursing and yet only about 10% of the total nursing population of 2.1 million nurses belong. Is this small percentage because many nurses choose to join a specialty organization with which they identify?

When evaluating nursing using Pavalko eight dimensions it would seem at first that nursing fits his criteria of a profession. However, the lack of consistency in all areas support the term *emerging profession* as one that describes nursing most appropriately. As a new graduate nurse, do you perceive nursing as an "emerging profession"?

Professionalism is a social process, and perhaps by the year 2000 nursing will have moved toward professional solidarity. Will the turn of the century resolve the conflicts on educational preparation? Will we see further refinement and application of nursing theories? Will nurses have more control of nursing practice regardless of the clinical setting? Will there be an increase in the percentage of nurses who are committed to a career focused on nursing? Will nursing "come together" and become not only a true profession, but the largest and most powerful of all the healthcare professional groups?

These are the kinds of questions that you, the graduate nurse, will be challenged with as you enter the real world of nursing. Some writers have likened nurses to "sleeping beauties" who close their eyes to anything unpleasant or innovative (Spitzer and Davier, 1988). We can't afford to be sleeping; nurses need to be involved with changing their own destiny. Nursing is at one of the most exciting crossroads in its history; there are opportunities to redefine the image of the professional nurse and to become a powerful force in healthcare!

NURSING ORGANIZATIONS

What Should I Know About Professional Organizations?

Nursing organizations have significant roles in empowering nurses in their "emerging professionalism." Yet, many nurses do not belong to a national organization like the ANA or the NLN, or even to specialty focused groups like American Association of Critical Care Nurses (AACN) or the National Nurses Society on Addictions (NNSA). The issue of belonging to a professional organization has been examined by researchers over the past years with no conclusive findings as to why or how nurses choose nursing organizations. Some have suggested that organizations that represent nursing as a whole such as the ANA and the NLN do not meet the needs of the individual nurse practicing in today's changing healthcare environment.

In the early 1950s, belonging to a professional nursing group was popular. By the 1980s, membership in both the ANA and the NLN declined by 10 to 15% while the nursing population increased by 150%. During this same period of time, specialty organizations such as the Association of Operating Room Nurses (AORN) and the Oncology Nursing Society (ONS) experienced an increase in their membership. Does this shift in affiliation reflect a shift in practice settings from the generalist area to the specialty areas, and that nurses are selecting a specialty organization that represents their current practice? Affiliation with a nursing organization and networking with colleagues is valuable and meaningful. The literature suggests that the nurse will associate with a professional organization that addresses the welfare of its members (Orsolitis, 1983). As a new graduate, you will need to examine your options for joining a professional group and then demonstrate your professional commitment by active involvement.

The question should be "Which one(s) should I join?" rather than "Should I even join an organization?" Some organizations give discount memberships

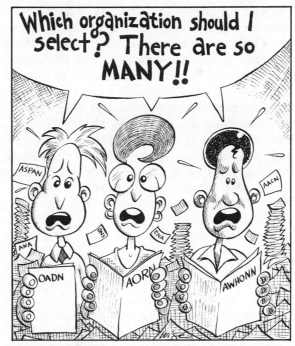

FIGURE 3–1   *Cartoon of nurses shopping for organizations.*

© Copyright 1994 W.B. SAUNDERS COMPANY

to new graduates the first 6 to 12 months following graduation and provide payment options (Fig. 3–1). Trying to understand the alphabet soup of nursing acronyms and their respective organizations can be frustrating and confusing at best. Let's look at a selected profile of the various organizations with some historical notes to assist in making the best choice as you begin your nursing career. A directory of nursing organizations can be found in Appendix B. A more detailed listing can be found in the Spring issue of the *American Journal of Nursing*.

What Organizations Are Available to the New Graduate?

AMERICAN NURSES ASSOCIATION. The ANA is identified as the professional association for registered nurses. It was through the early efforts of Isabel Hampton Robb and others that the Nurses Associated Alumnae of the United States and Canada was formed. A group of fifteen nursing "leaders" began discussion about forming a professional association at the World's Fair in 1890. Six years later, alumnae from the training schools organized the professional association now called the ANA. Canadian members split off from the original group in

1911 and formed its own professional association. The ANA's organizational structure has undergone many changes over the years.

Currently when an individual joins the ANA, they join not only their state organization, but also become part of the larger national organization. Usually within the state there are separate groups called districts or chapters with which the individual can affiliate. This method geographically groups smaller clusters of members together according to their special practice interests. The ANA's current membership comprises about 11% of the nurses in the United States. This percentage has remained constant over the past four years. The ANA publishes a booklet every four to five years called *Facts on Nursing*. This document presents a composite of nursing demographics and statistical information that helps to describe the current state of nursing.

In 1974, an amendment to the Taft-Hartley Act allowed professional nursing organizations to be considered labor unions. Following this significant event, some nursing administrators and managers withdrew their memberships in ANA because of the potential conflict of interest between professional affiliation and the workplace. However, this change generated another major nursing organization, the Association of Nurse Executives (AONE).

The ANA has been at the forefront of policy issues and represents nursing in legislative activities. The ANA's Cabinets and Councils have provided Standards of Practice for both the generalist and the specialist. The Scope of Nursing Practice document defines nursing practice. Another part of the organization provides credentialing services and certifies nurses in twenty-two different practice areas. The ANA's continuing education component provides credibility to workshops and educational programs.

NATIONAL STUDENT NURSES ASSOCIATION.   The National Student Nurses Association (NSNA) is often affiliated with the ANA, however, it is a fully independent organization and publishes its own quarterly journal, *Imprint*. It was formed in 1952 for students enrolled in nursing programs. Becoming a member of the NSNA may be viewed as a way to begin the "professional" socialization process. Often members of the NSNA serve on selected committees of the ANA and speak to the House of Delegates regarding student-related issues.

AMERICAN NURSES FOUNDATION (ANF) AND THE AMERICAN ACADEMY OF NURSING (AAN).   Two other organizations often associated with ANA are the American Nurses Foundation and the American Academy of Nursing. Briefly described, these organizations serve special purposes in support of research and recognition of nursing colleagues. The ANF was established as a tax-exempt corporation to receive monies for nursing research. With the establishment of the National Nursing Research Institute, the focus has changed to one of support in the areas of policy making as well as research or educational activities. The AAN was established as an honorary association for nurses who have made significant professional contributions to the profession. When a nurse is elected to the AAN, the person is called a Fellow and the credentials following the individuals name are FAAN. The official publication of this organization is *Nursing Outlook.*

NATIONAL LEAGUE FOR NURSING.   The NLN, established in 1952, can be traced to the 1893 organization of the American Society of Superintendents of Training Schools for Nurses of the United States and Canada (ASSTS). Between the late 1800s and the early 1900s, seven nursing organizations formed and joined under the collective name and function of the NLN. One of the unique features of the NLN is that both individuals and agencies are members. The NLN's objective is to foster the development and improvement of all nursing services and nursing education. Therefore, non-nurses can join the NLN to fulfill its purpose of promoting the consumer's voice in some nursing policies. Having graduated from nursing school, the new graduate may be most familiar with the NLN's function as an accrediting body in nursing education.

Is your school an NLN-accredited nursing program? Some of the NLN's activities include:

◆ Maintaining a testing division.
◆ Accrediting schools of nursing at all levels of education.
◆ Working with specialty organizations as their testing agency for certification.
◆ Providing consultation.

The NLN publishes a journal, *Nursing and Health Care* (prior to 1979, the journal was called *Nursing Outlook*).

INTERNATIONAL COUNCIL OF NURSES.   The International Council of Nurses (ICN), established in 1899, is the international organization representing professional nurses. The ANA, NLN, and many other nursing organizations are constituent members of the ICN. The focus of this nursing organization is on worldwide healthcare issues as well as nursing issues. This organization meets every four years and has a membership of ninety-eight nursing organizations. The headquarters for the ICN is in Geneva, Switzerland.

NATIONAL FEDERATION FOR SPECIALTY NURSING ORGANIZATIONS.   The National Federation for Specialty Nursing Organizations (NFSNO) collectively represents the largest numbers of nurses practicing in the United States. Its purpose is to foster excellence in specialty practice. The NFSNO began in the 1970s and meets two times a year as a forum for communication among specialty nursing organizations. Approximately thirty-nine organizations are members and are each represented by two leaders, along with representatives from the ANA and NLN.

SPECIALTY PRACTICE ORGANIZATIONS.   The past fifteen years have demonstrated significant growth in specialty practice in nursing. There are over forty specialty nursing organizations, approximately thirty-three which provide certification in their specialty areas. In the 1980s these organizations met annually as the National Specialty Nursing Certifying Organization (NSNCO) to discuss issues in certification and nursing practice.

In 1988 a group of national nursing leaders and nursing leaders from organizations in NSNCO came together through the support of the Josia Macy, Jr. Foundation for several strategic planning meetings. These sessions focused on the issues of the nursing shortage, quality of nursing specialty practice, and nursing certification. An outcome of the discussion was the possibility of forming an organization made up of all nursing organizations that certify individuals for specialty nursing practice. It was proposed that one organization would serve as a central authority to coordinate and advance the certification process for nurse specialists. The purpose of this new organization would be to standardize certification programs and educate consumers about professional nursing certification. It was in the fall of 1991 that the American Board of Nursing Specialties (ABNS) was incorporated, with eight nursing organizations as charter members. The ABNS's primary objective is to increase consumer awareness of the meaning and value of specialty nursing certification (ABNS, 1991). The ABNS has implemented an application process for all nursing specialty organizations. There are twelve standards that an organization needs to address to become a part of ABNS.

For a variety of reasons the majority of certifying specialty nursing organizations have remained in the NSNCO. Some organizations may not choose to meet the twelve standards that ABNS asks the nursing organization to address in its application. For example, one of the controversies that challenges nursing in the movement toward the "Board concept" is the question of what level of education the candidate should obtain before being considered for certification. The ANA has moved toward requiring a baccalaureate degree for candidate eligibility. As a member of the ABNS the member organization must require by the year 2000 a minimum of a baccalaureate degree for their respective candidates who sit for certification. A grandfather clause (a clause creating an exemption based on circumstances previously existing) would exempt any nurse certified prior to this time. As painful as the change process is to most individuals, the intent of these national trends is to continue nursing's progress toward professionalism.

▼

As a new graduate, how do these changes in specialty nursing practice effect you? How do you anticipate them affecting your practice setting in five years?

▲

OTHER HEALTH-RELATED ORGANIZATIONS.   The American Red Cross is part of about 120 Red Cross organizations from around the world. Nurses of the American Red Cross pioneered public health nursing in the early 1900s. Since the 1950s its focus has been more toward volunteer efforts and the establishment of home health nursing courses, disaster nursing, and organizing volunteers to assist in hospitals and nursing homes (Kozier and Erb, 1991).

In summary, the role that professional organizations have in enhancing the image of nursing is significant. Their impact is seen in both educational and practice issues for both generalist and specialist nurse roles. Organizations provide nursing a voice in policy issues and serve to unite nurses as a group of professionals. Ultimately, it may be nursing organizations that will serve as the catalyst for change in the healthcare system, and their impact will be felt in the next century.

CREDENTIALING: LICENSURE and CERTIFICATION

What Is Credentialing?

In the early days of nursing before the Nightingale era, anyone could say they were a nurse and practice their "trade" as they wished. It was only within this century that nursing became a credentialed profession. A credential can be something as simple as a written document of an individual's qualifications. A high school diploma is a credential that indicates a certain level of education has been attained. A credential can also signify a person's performance. The attainment of a title (e.g., FAAN) signifies excellence in performance; a postgraduate degree from an institution of higher learning (PhD or EdD) indicates success in terms of academic achievement.

In nursing the educational credentials that an individual holds indicate not only academic achievements, but also that a minimum level of competency in nursing skills has been attained. Academic achievement is represented by an associate degree in nursing (ADN), a diploma in nursing, or a baccalaureate degree in nursing (BSN, BS). This academic preparation leads to credentialing as a registered nurse (RN). Additional nursing credentials may reflect areas of specialty practice, such as Critical Care Registered Nurse (CCRN) and Certified Addictions Registered Nurse (CARN). Figure 3–2 summarizes how professional and legal regulation impact the individual, the institution, and the public.

What Is Registration and Licensure?

Licensure affords a protection to the public by requiring the individual to demonstrate minimum competency by examination. In 1923 all forty-eight states had some form of nursing licensure in place. Nursing licensure is a process by which

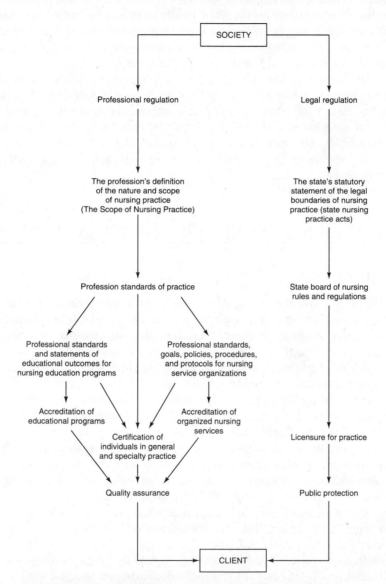

FIGURE 3–2   *Flow chart on professional and legal regulation of practice.*

(American Nurses Association: The Scope of Nursing. Kansas City, Mo., 1987.)

a governmental agency grants permission to an individual to practice nursing. This accountability is maintained through a governmental agency responsible for the licensing and registration process. The state boards of nursing are the governmental agencies responsible for this process. Each board of nursing varies in structure and design based on the nurse practice act within each state. The state boards of nursing also exercise legal control over schools of nursing within their respective states. In 1978 all boards of nursing formed a national council, the National Council of State Boards of Nursing (NCSBN), to present a more collective front on nursing education and licensure.

All schools of nursing submit curricula for evaluation and approval by their state board of nursing. The board of nursing within each state enforces the legal regulatory functions through the nurse practice act of that state. These regulatory functions are designed to delineate the scope of nursing practice and to "protect the public."

In order to practice nursing in the United States the graduate nurse must successfully complete the National Council Licensure Examination for Registered Nurses (NCLEX-RN). After successful completion of the NCLEX-RN, the graduate nurse may use the title registered nurse and the initials R.N. after her name. The NCSBN also controls the practice of vocational/practical nursing. It is the responsibility of the graduate nurse to be aware of the provision of the nurse practice act in the state in which they are working. There are variations between states in what is required to obtain and maintain the nursing license. Some states may require continuing education credits to renew yearly licenses, while other states may consider continuing education as optional for professional growth. (Appendix A is a complete listing of the state boards of nursing and their respective addresses.)

How Do I Obtain a License?

Basically, there are two different procedures for obtaining a license, *licensure by examination* (applying for an initial license) and *licensure by endorsement* (applying for a license in a state or jurisdiction when already licensed in another state). As a new graduate you will be applying for licensure by examination. What's involved in this process?

LICENSURE BY EXAMINATION.   First, you must have graduated from an approved educational program and be able to speak English. Most states require that the applicant be of "good moral character" and some require "good physical and mental health" (LaBar, 1984). Second, all states require that the applicant pass the NCLEX-RN examination and submit appropriate fees. There are usually several fees: one to the state for the license application, one to the company that prepares and scores the examination, and another for an interim work permit.

▼

Be prepared during your last semester to save approximately $100 for both the NCLEX-RN and the license application fee.

▲

$

If you plan on working in another state and want to take the examination in that state, be sure to write early for their application information. (Detailed information on the NCLEX-RN can be found at the end of this book.)

LICENSURE BY ENDORSEMENT.   Endorsement means granting the license without having to take the examination again. Is endorsement the same as reciprocity? No, *reciprocity* is the acceptance of a license by one state only if the other state does likewise. With regard to the licensure of nursing, there are no uniform or reciprocal agreements between states at this time. Each applicant is considered individually based on the rules and regulations of the particular state board of nursing. Because licensing laws are uniform throughout the United States, licensure by endorsement (not reciprocity) readily facilitates a nurse's transition when moving to another state.

Currently there is only one state, North Dakota, where licensure by endorsement is not available to registered nurses from other states. To be licensed as a registered nurse in North Dakota, you must have a baccalaureate degree, and to practice as a practical nurse you must have an associate degree. At the time this regulation went into effect, the State Board of Nursing of North Dakota "grandfathered" all nurses then licensed in North Dakota, regardless of their educational preparation, but did not include nurses licensed in another state.

What Is Certification?

Certification is a voluntary process by which a nongovernmental agency or association certifies that an *individual* licensed to practice a profession has met certain predetermined standards specified by that profession for specialty practice (ANA, 1978). Certification is a credential beyond licensure, but has a variety of interpretations for both the nursing profession and the public. In some states, the Nurse Practice Act requires that one be certified to qualify for expanded practice in a specialized role, such as a nurse practitioner, nurse midwife, or clinical nurse specialist.

The movement toward certification in nursing practice areas has experienced the most growth within the past forty years. It was in 1946 that credentialing was first required for entry into practice as a nurse anesthetist (i.e., Certified Registered Nurse Anesthetist or CRNA). Twenty-five years later, the Nurse Midwives followed suit by requiring certification through the American College of Nurse Midwives as an entry-level credential. In the early 1970s the ANA began programs to certify nurses at both the generalist and specialist levels. As the nursing license is recognized as indicating minimum competency, the certification credential indicates preparation beyond the minimum level.

At What Point Is Certification Obtained, At the Generalist or the Specialist Level?

According to the ANA, generalist nurses may practice in a specialty area of nursing, but are called specialists if they have an advanced degree (MS or PhD prepared) (ANA, 1990). Since the ANA began their certification activities in the 1970s, 72,000 nurses in nineteen different specialty areas have been credentialed (Markway, 1990). This number represents the majority of the generalists as well as specialists. In 1992 the ANA certified 3,300 nurses in twenty-two areas of nursing practice (American Nurse, 1992). Other organizations that represent specialty practice have had tremendous growth in membership and credentialing activities. Outside of the ANA, over thirty-three organizations now certify nurses nationally, with the number of nurses certified totaling over 150,000 (Collins, 1987).

Specialty nursing organizations are among the largest nursing organizations in the nation. The majority of these groups offer certification at various levels of educational preparation. Because of the growth in areas of specialty practice and certification, the American Board for Nursing Specialty (ABNS) was incorporated in the early 1990s to address the issues of standardization among nursing certification organizations. The intention of the ABNS is to:

◆ Regulate and standardize all nursing certification programs.

◆ Establish minimum educational requirements for certification.

◆ Define what constitutes a nursing specialty.

◆ Require collaboration between the certifying organization and specialty association (ABNS, 1991).

Certification is gaining increased recognition by employers and consumers. In one large East Coast hospital, nurses certified in their area of specialty received a salary increase of $10,000/year (Markaway, 1990). This type of recognition is another advantage of certification.

The *American Journal of Nursing* publishes a directory that lists addresses and phone numbers of nursing organizations that provide certification. This information is frequently found in the Spring issue of the journal. Appendix B also lists organizations and their mailing addresses.

What Is Accreditation?

Accreditation is often confused with credentialing. It is defined as a process by which a voluntary, nongovernmental agency or organization approves and grants status to *institutions* or *programs* (not individuals) that meet predetermined standards or outcomes. The accreditation of nursing programs by the NLN is an activity with which you, the new graduate, may be most familiar. The NLN has been accrediting nursing programs since 1949 with the purpose of improving the quality of nursing education. This peer review process is a voluntary mechanism utilized by nursing programs and serves to review and evaluate all program aspects. Using published criteria and guidelines, each school or agency prepares a rather involved self-study. After the self-study is completed, the school is visited by representatives (usually two) of the NLN. The visitors present their report of the program along with the self-study to members of the NLN Board of Review. The NLN Board of Review votes on whether or not to accredit the nursing program. By the end of 1991, there were more than 1,550 nurse educational programs that were NLN accredited, which is about 75% of all basic programs nationwide (Kelly, 1992). A list of NLN-accredited programs is published each year in Nursing and Health Care. Hospitals are also accredited by the Joint Commission on Accreditation of Health Organizations (JCAHO) as a way of ensuring quality healthcare.

What Nursing Journals or Literature Are Available?

Nursing journals were first published as a way of maintaining communication with other nursing organizations. At the turn of the century, two nursing journals existed in the United States: *The Nightingale*, a monthly publication started by Sarah Post, and *The Trained Nurse* (later called *Nursing World*), started by Mary Francis. The oldest nursing journal, *The American Journal of Nursing*, was first published in *1900* by the ANA, and is still in publication today. *Nursing 93* and *RN* are two other widely read nursing journals, but they are not affiliated with any professional organizations.

Because of the changing healthcare environment and the proliferation of knowledge in healthcare, what is taught in a nursing education program today may be out of date in about five years. Naisbitt (1984) talks about this issue in *Megatrends* and concludes that we have moved from the Industrial Age to the Information Processing Age, with nursing in the role as information giver. Nursing journals continue to be a major link between nursing organizations and professionals in this age of information explosion.

As a new graduate, what type of journals do you subscribe to and read? It is important to keep up with new information to maintain practice skills and a current knowledge base. You may consider subscribing to a professional nursing journal before graduation; many offer discount subscriptions to new graduates.

CONTROVERSIAL ISSUES: ENTRY INTO PRACTICE AND THE NURSING SHORTAGE

Florence Nightingale once described nursing as a "progressive art in which to stand still is to step backward." Her thoughts from over a hundred years ago still hold true today with regard to the education and nursing shortage issues, the two areas that can move nursing forward in terms of influence and power as a profession and also affect the profession's ability to impact on healthcare trends.

What Is "Entry into Practice" and Where Is It Going?

The issue of entry into practice began in 1965 with the ANA position paper that advocated the baccalaureate level as the entry level for professional nursing. At that time the ANA targeted 1985 to be the year to achieve this goal. Since then it has been a highly emotionally charged issue within the ranks of professional nursing and nursing education. It is not the intention of this book to endorse one position or another, but rather to present a historical accounting of the events and the positions of selected professional organizations, along with the pros and cons of the issue (Table 3-3).

The following is a summary of the two sides (pro and con) of the entry into practice issue:

ARGUMENTS IN SUPPORT OF CHANGING THE ENTRY LEVEL REQUIREMENT

1. Raising the level of entry will promote the professional status of nursing.
   - Most professions have the baccalaureate degree as a minimum level of education for entrance into the profession. No other recognized profession has achieved professional status without the baccalaureate degree.
   - The leadership in nursing needs to reflect professional values, advanced education, research, and theory development.
2. The increasing and expanding scientific and technical knowledge base requires the nurse to have a baccalaureate education to assume the new roles.
   - There is a higher level of acuity in the hospitalized client.
   - There has been a rapid increase in healthcare technology, requiring more advanced skills and knowledge.
   - With these changes in the healthcare system there will be an increased need for coordination and collaboration with other healthcare professionals.
3. With increased educational requirements there will be improved client care.

TABLE 3–3   *Chronological Progression of the "Entry into Practice" Issue*

1965—ANA
- *Position Paper on Educational Preparation for Nurse Practitioners and Assistants to Nurses*—minimum preparation for beginning professional nursing at the baccalaureate level

1983—ANA
- Board of Directors commits $500,000 over a five-year period to support outcomes of *Position Paper*

1984—ANA
- Established goal to have the BSN recognized as the educational base for nursing in 50% of the states by 1992 and in 100% by 1995

1985—ANA House of Delegates accepts the following:
- BS in nursing as minimum educational requirement to practice professional nursing and to retain the legal title of Registered Nurse
- ADN as the educational requirement for licensure to practice technical nursing and that the title of Associate Nurse as the legal title for the person licensed to practice technical nursing

1985—National Association for the Advancement of Associate Degree Nursing (NOAADN)
- Establishment of a national organization to represent ADN education and practice

1985—NLN
- Adoption of position in support of two levels of nursing practice: professional and associate

1987—NLN
- NLN Board discusses titling and licensure issues
- Title of Associate Nurse be designated for graduates of associate degree and diploma programs and the title Professional Nurse be designated for graduates of baccalaureate programs; both will retain title of Registered Nurse (RN) upon successful completion of the NCLEX-RN

- The broader the knowledge background, the broader the scope of practice.
- Nurses will be able to function more independently in their expanded roles in the future.

4. Some studies indicate that nursing administrators prefer to hire baccalaureate nurses.

5. Decreased public confusion with only one type of educational requirement for licensure.

6. It is more cost effective to employ baccalaureate nurses, as they can function in a wider variety of healthcare settings.

ARGUMENTS AGAINST CHANGING THE ENTRY LEVEL REQUIREMENT.

1. There will be a significant increase in the cost of education and healthcare if the entry level requirement is changed.
   ◆ A baccalaureate degree is more expensive and takes longer to obtain.
   ◆ Currently there are not enough baccalaureate nursing programs to provide the number of registered nurses needed, therefore, additional funding would be required for expansion and development of programs.
   ◆ It is anticipated that healthcare and education costs will continue to rise and that there will be a decrease in funding for nursing education. Where will the difference be made up?

2. There has been no evidence to support the theory that baccalaureate nurses are more effective than associate degree or diploma graduates.
   ◆ In evaluating the candidates who successfully complete the NCLEX, the percentage of passing grades among the associate degree and diploma graduates has in the past ten years consistently exceeded that of the baccalaureate graduates (National Council Summary, 1992).

▼

Of 11,277 U.S. ADN candidates, 92.7% passed
Of 2,040 U.S. diploma candidates, 91.7% passed
Of 4,429 U.S. BSN candidates, 88.7% passed

▲

   ◆ According to Waters (1981), "Associate degree nursing education has succeeded in preparing a graduate nurse who performs the RN role, and in doing so, has failed to conform to premises that describe a limited scope of practice. The ADN programs have failed by succeeding."

3. Currently the majority of registered nurses are being educated in associate degree programs. A move to the baccalaureate requirement would significantly decrease the number of graduating nurses.

4. Associate degree nursing programs offer access to an educational system that can effectively meet the needs of those who are unable to complete a four-year program in college.

5. The need for registered nurses will continue to increase; it is currently predicted that the number of graduates will have declined by the year 2000.
   ◆ The Omnibus Reconciliation Act of 1987 required licensed nursing staff in nursing homes.

What Is the Status of the Nursing Shortage?

The National Commission Study on Nursing produced new statistics on nursing's impact in the healthcare arena at a time when the healthcare climate was ready for change. In some parts of the country the nursing shortage is still a crisis (Fig. 3–3). It is considered not only a professional resource issue but one that affects financial stability, quality of care, and access to healthcare by consumers (Orsolitis, 1989). Nursing is at the forefront in providing information and assistance in identifying much-needed reform in the current healthcare system (see Appendix 3–4). In 1990, Congress approved the Rural Nursing Incentive Act, whereby nurse specialists could begin receiving direct reimbursement for the services they provide. It has been suggested that "rather than perpetually putting out the fires of the nursing shortage, nursing should begin to think of itself as the architect of a radically new structure of health care delivery." (Hall and Stevens, 1991 p. 2). Some current and projected data regarding the nursing shortage is given in Figure 3–3.

The *Seventh Report to the President and Congress on Health Personnel* indicates that in the United States the nursing supply will decrease as the requirements for nursing increase. Specifically, the report indicates that the number of students

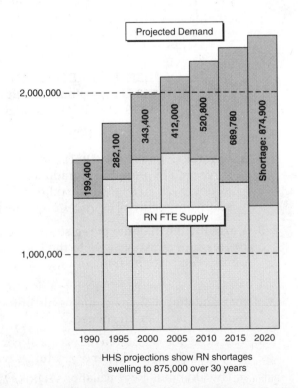

HHS projections show RN shortages
swelling to 875,000 over 30 years

FIGURE 3–3   *Growing shortage seen in HHS projections.*

(*USA Today*, November 1, 1990, p. 7A.)

graduating from nursing programs will peak in the mid-1990s and decline by the year 2000, with further decline by 2020. The Omnibus Budget Reconciliation Act of 1987, which requires nursing staff in nursing homes to be licensed, will create increased demands for RNs. Further data from the Bureau of Labor Statistics projects that jobs in healthcare will increase from 6.8 million in 1986 to more than 10 million in the year 2000.

Will nursing be ready to meet the challenges of the changing healthcare environment? Does nursing reflect professionalism clearly? Is the image positive? Do we need to develop autonomy in practice? Who holds nursing accountable for practice in all areas? Is nursing ready to resolve educational splintering and work cooperatively at different levels of practice? Can nursing become more effective and active on the political front? Will research be used to advance practice at both the generalist and specialist levels? Will the healthcare agenda for the 1990s be a turning point for nursing practice?

The questions go on and on. Answers to these questions will come from nurses in practice, education, and research in a collective fashion. Nurses have debated education issues for 120 years. These issues must be resolved for nursing to move forward in order to make a significant impact on the professional image. As a new graduate you will be a part of this exciting transition as nursing takes control and directs the course of its future.

....

As Winston Churchill said, "If we spend all our time debating the past we shall lose the future."

....

REFERENCES

Aburdene, P., Naisbitt, J. (19920: *Megatrends for Women.* New York, Villard Books.

Aiken, L., Millinix, C. (1987): The nursing shortage: Myth or reality. *N Engl J Med* 317:641.

American Board of Nursing Specialties (1991): *Application for ABNS Approval.* Washington, D.C.

American Nurses Association (1978): *The Study of Credentialing in Nursing: A New Approach.* Vol 1., The report of the committee, Kansas City.

American Nurses Association (1987): *The Scope of Nursing.* Kansas City.

American Nurses Association (1988): *Social Policy Statement.* Kansas City.

American Nurses Association (1990): *The Career Credentials: Professional Certification,* The 1990 certification Catalog, Center for Credentialing Services, Kansas City.

American Nurses Association (1992): *American Nurse.* 24(10):16.

Auttonberry, D. (1988): The emerging role of the masters prepared nurse. *Nurs Manag* 9:9.

Becker, H. (1970): *Sociological Work: Method and Substance.* Chicago, Adline.

Bullough, V., Bullough, B. (1978): *Care of the Sick.* New York, Watson.

Caplow, T. (1954): *The Sociology of Work.* Minneapolis, University of Minnesota Press.

Collins, H. (1987): Certification: Is the payoff worth the price? *RN* 7:36.

Dunbar, S. (1987): Entry into practice: The continuing saga. *Heart Lung* 16:2.

Fickeissen, J. (1985): Getting certified. *AJN* 3:265.

Gordon, S. (1991): Prisoners of men's dreams, *Media Watch: A Publication of Nurses of America* 2:3.

Hall, J., Stevens, P. (1991): Nursing shortage. *Nurs Outlook* 39:2.

Kaler, S. (1989): Stereotypes of professional roles. *Image* 21:2.

Kalish, B., Kalish, P. (1983): Improving the image of nursing. *AJN* 83:48.

Kelly, L.Y. (1992): *The Nursing Experience.* 2nd ed. New York, McGraw Hill, p. 514.

Kibbee, P. (1988): An emerging professional. *J Nurs Admin* 18:4.

Knapp J. (1990): Assuring continuing competency. *Speciality Nurs Forum* 2:2.

Kozier, B. (1989): *Introduction to Nursing.* Menlo Park, CA., Addison-Wesley.

Kozier, B., Erb, C. (1991): *Concepts and Issues in Nursing.* Menlo Park, CA, Addison-Wesley.

LaBar, C. (1984): *Statutory Requirements for Licensing of Nurses.* Kansas City, American Nurses Association.

Lancaster, J. (1990–91): The nursing shortage: Myth or fact. *Helix.*

Leddy, S., Pepper, J. (1985): *Conceptual Bases of Professional Nursing.* Philadelphia, JB Lippincott.

Levenstein, A. (1985): The road to professional growth. *Nurs Manag* 15:7.

Licardo, L. (1991): New hope for an old soap-General Hospital. *Media Watch: A Publication of Nurses of America* 2:6.

Markway, P. (1990): How to become certified. *Am Nurse,* 22(6): 4–8.

Martin, C. (1990): Response from an educational perspective. *Nurs Clin North Am* 25:3.

Naisbitt, J. (1984): *Megatrends.* New York, Warner Books.

Naisbitt, J. (1989): Report on the American nurse shortage. *Nurse Educ* 14:5.

Naisbitt, J. (1989): Nursing news and notes. *Nurse Educ* 14:5.

Naisbitt, J., Aburdene, P. (1990): *Megatrends 2000.* New York, William Morrow.

Orsolitis, M. (1983): New knowledge about attitudes toward professional nursing organizations. *J Ne Y State Nurses Assoc* 14:4.

Orsolitis, M. (1989): Reorganizing nursing for the future: Nursing commission's recommendations and research implications. *J Appl Res* 2:2.

Pavalko, R. (1971): *Sociology of Occupations and Professions.* Itasca, IL, Peacock Publishers.

Peplau, H. (1952): *Interpersonal Relationships in Nursing.* New York, Putnam Press.

Robb, IH. (1901): *Nursing Ethics.* Cleveland, J.B. Savage, pp. 35–35. Cited in Dolan, JA, Fitzpatrick, ML, Herrmann, EK (1983): *Nursing in Society: A Historical Perspective.* 15th ed., Philadelphia, W.B. Saunders, p. 210.

Schaffer, K. (1989): Research: Future impact on image and retention. *Dimens Crit Care Nurs* 8:1.

Spitzer, R, Davier, M. (1988): New patterns of professional relationships internal to the organization. *Ser Nurs Manag* 1:5.

Strauss, A. (1966): The structure and idealogy of American nursing: An interpretation, in *The Nursing Profession.* New York, Wiley.

Talotta, D. (1990): Role conceptions and professional role discrepancy among baccalaureate nursing students. *Image* 22:2.

USA Today, November 1, 1990, p. 7A.

Waite, R. (1990): Update on the activities on the National Commission on Nursing implementation project. *Aspens Advisor for Nurse Executives* 5:6.

Wallace, B (1990): Greetings from the executive director. *Media Watch: A Publication of Nurses of America* 1:1.

4

Nursing Education

Gayle P. Varnell, Ph.D., R.N., C.P.N.P.

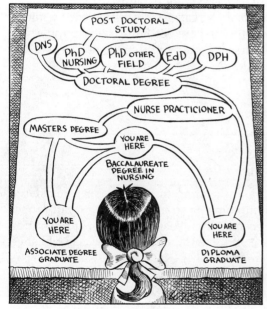

Pathways to Career Goals.

Education should not be a destination—but a path we travel all the days of our lives.

—Anonymous

Education is the ability to listen to almost anything without losing your temper or your self-confidence.

—Robert Frost

After completing this chapter, you should be able to:

◆ Compare and contrast the three basic types of educational preparation for nursing: diploma, associate degree, and baccalaureate degree program.

◆ Describe the educational preparation for a graduate degree.

◆ Compare and contrast the alternative options provided by the career ladder, external degree, BSN Completion Programs, and the University Without Walls programs.

◆ Describe the purpose of nursing program accreditation.

◆ Discuss the future of nursing education.

After struggling to complete your basic educational preparation for nursing, you are probably looking forward to that first paycheck as a registered nurse and the last thing on your mind is returning to school for more education! It is not the purpose of this chapter to discuss the issue of entry into practice or to debate which type of program is better. The purpose of this chapter is to help you look at where you are educationally, and to offer directions for you in regard to educational opportunities to enhance your career goals. Before looking down the path at the variety of educational offerings available to you to meet those career goals, let's look at the variety of pathways that lead to the basic educational preparation for a registered nurse.

Which path did you travel? There are five paths that lead to one licensing examination, the National Council Licensure Examination for Registered Nursing (NCLEX-RN). The first three paths (diploma, associate degree, and baccalaureate) are the most common and usually require a high school diploma or the equivalent for admission. The other less common paths are the master's degree and doctoral degree, which both accept college graduates with a liberal arts major into their programs. Other paths that are becoming more popular are the ladder programs (from practical nurse to associate degree nurse) and the two-plus-two program (from associate degree to baccalaureate nurse).

PATH OF DIPLOMA EDUCATION

What Is the History of Diploma Nursing?

The oldest form of educational preparation leading to licensure as a registered nurse (RN) in the United States is the diploma program. The majority of nurses practicing in the United States today received their basic educational preparation in a diploma program (Fig. 4–1). The first nurse training school was established at the New England Hospital for Women in 1872 (Kalisch and Kalisch, 1986). From that initial program, the number of diploma schools quickly rose, from 15 in 1890 to 432 in 1900 (Bullough et al., 1983). By the 1920s there were almost 2,300 programs. During the Great Depression, many of the hospital schools of nursing went bankrupt and had to close (Fitzpatrick, 1983).

In the beginning, nursing education consisted of on-the-job training based mainly on the specific needs of the particular hospital in which the school of nursing was housed, not on the learning needs of the individual student. In other words, nursing students provided cheap or free labor.

These apprenticeship programs differed in quality and length. The size of the hospital also influenced the experience of the nursing student. Larger hospitals offered more exposure to a variety of clinical experiences. Standardization of nursing programs was not considered until the National League for Nursing (NLN) (earlier known as the National League of Nursing Education) and the

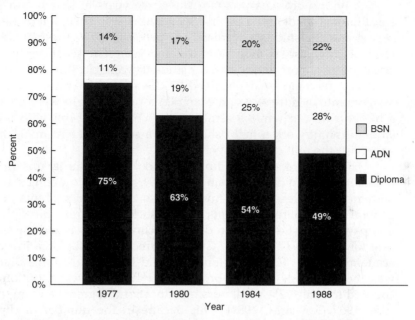

FIGURE 4–1 *Percentage of RNs in the United States, by type of basic nursing education, 1988.*

(Reprinted with permission from NLN (1991): *Nursing Data Review.* Publication No. 19-2419. New York, NLN.)

Winslow-Goldmark study in 1923. Standardization did not occur until the 1940s.

The theory classes in these early nursing schools were generally laid out in blocks of study that included medical nursing, surgical nursing, psychiatric nursing, obstetrics, pediatrics, operating, and emergency department experience, as well as classes in anatomy, physiology, nutrition, pharmacology, history of nursing, and often a course called "professional adjustments." Nursing students would work on a unit in the hospital, attend class for a couple of hours, and then return to work some additional hours on a unit. A typical day could be twelve or more hours in length. Nursing students covered all three hospital shifts.

In the early diploma schools, a typical student was a single woman who lived in a dormitory with other nursing students. There were strict codes of conduct that had to be followed, as well as rigid dress codes. Anyone who did not follow these rules was subject to expulsion from the program. As an example, married students were not allowed in the program. If a student married, she had to hide her marriage. If her marriage was discovered, she was subject to expulsion from the program. In many of the diploma schools, these strict rules and regulations were not relaxed until the 1960s.

A typical diploma program was three years in length and had four classifications of students. The first six months was considered the probationary period and the students were called "probies." The students were considered freshmen the last six months of the first year. The second-year students were classified as juniors and third-year students were classified as seniors. The level of a student could be determined by the student's attire and by their clinical assignments or duties. As an example, a probie might wear an apron without a bib and no cap while a senior wore a bib and apron with a cap. A junior student might work a night shift while a senior student might be assigned to supervise the unit on a night shift.

The standardization of diploma school nursing programs brought about in the late 1940s and early 1950s by the NLN saw many nursing schools affiliating with nearby colleges and universities so that their students could meet the general education requirements in areas such as anatomy, physiology, sociology, and psychology. Education in diploma schools emphasized the skills needed to care for the acutely ill client. Graduates received a diploma in nursing, not an academic degree. From 1872 until the mid-1960s the hospital diploma program was the dominant nursing program. In 1980, however, diploma schools accounted for only 22% of all nursing education programs as compared to 80% in 1959–1960 (Rowland, 1984). This decline in the number of diploma schools continues (Table 4–1). Perhaps one of the reasons for the decline in the diploma

TABLE 4–1 *Basic RN Programs and Percentage Change from Previous Year, by Type of Program: 1980 to 1989**

PUBLIC AND PRIVATE NURSING PROGRAMS	NUMBER OF PROGRAMS									
	1980	1981	1982	1983	1984	1985	1986	1987	1988	1989
All Programs	1,385	1,401	1,432	1,466	1,477	1,473	1,469	1,465	1,442	1,457
Public	861	870	902	916	935	942	950	970	979	1,005
Private	524	531	530	550	542	531	519	495	463	449
Baccalaureate	377	383	402	421	427	441	455	467	479	488
Public	198	196	203	210	213	217	227	235	239	245
Private	179	187	199	211	214	224	228	232	240	241
Associate Degree	697	715	742	764	777	776	776	789	792	812
Public	624	638	662	669	684	688	688	698	704	726
Private	73	77	80	95	93	88	88	91	88	85
Diploma	311	303	288	281	273	256	238	209	171	157
Public	39	36	37	37	38	37	35	37	36	34
Private	272	267	251	244	235	219	203	172	135	123

Reprinted with permission from NLN: Nursing Data Review. Publication No. 19-2419. (1991) New York, NLN.

*Excludes American Samoa, Guam, Puerto Rico, and the Virgin Islands.

programs is that the courses offered at the hospital frequently did not confer college credit. Students working on furthering their education in nursing were discouraged at the lack of transfer of college credit from their diploma education. While the majority of current diploma programs are associated with institutions of higher learning where the graduates receive more college credit, the graduate still may not receive college credit for the nursing courses. Some diploma programs have advanced to what is called a "single purpose institution." This type of nursing program has baccalaureate degree granting privileges for nursing only.

What Is the Educational Preparation of the Diploma Graduate?

The current preparation of a diploma nurse varies in length from one to three years and takes place in a hospital school of nursing. This type of program may be under the direction of the hospital or in some instances be independently incorporated. The diploma program may include general education subjects such as biology, physical and social sciences, and nursing theory and practice. The diploma program serves qualified applicants who want an early and ongoing opportunity to be in contact with clients and other healthcare personnel (NLN, 1989c).

Graduates of a diploma program are prepared to function as beginning practitioners in acute, intermediate, long-term, and ambulatory healthcare facilities. Graduates of a diploma program are not prepared for supervisory or administrative type positions.

Standards and competencies for diploma programs are developed and maintained by the NLN Council of Diploma Programs. Minimal competencies of new graduates are as follows (NLN, 1982):

◆ Establishes a nursing data base for individuals with well-defined health needs having predictable and unpredictable outcomes.

◆ Develops individual nursing care plans through use of the nursing data base incorporating principles of organization and management.

◆ Performs independent nursing measures including preventive, habilitative, and rehabilitative measures according to the need demonstrated by individuals and families.

◆ Initiates efforts to improve nursing practice by evaluating the effectiveness of nursing care and taking the appropriate action(s).

Advantages of diploma programs include the fact that their nursing instructors are actively involved in clinical practice. Graduates of diploma schools have the greatest amount of clinical experience in a hospital setting. Since there is a close relationship between the nursing school and the hospital, graduates are well prepared to function upon graduation. Many of the diploma graduates continue to work in the same hospital upon graduation and therefore experience an easier role transition.

In diploma schools, theory and clinical practice are introduced concurrently. Diploma nursing students, according to Hocker, "are offered nursing theory equivalent to that offered in the other RN preparatory schools" (Hocker, 1984, p. 38). Choinski et al. further state that nursing courses in baccalaureate programs usually are "limited to the last two academic years, or approximately 18 months, while diploma schools offer from 24 to 36 months of nursing theory and practice" (Choinski et al., 1978, p. 28).

PATH OF ASSOCIATE DEGREE EDUCATION

What Is the History of Associate Degree Nursing?

The associate degree nursing program has the distinction of being the first and, to date, only educational program for nursing that was developed from planned research and controlled experimentation. Since its beginning in 1951, the associate degree nursing program has grown to over 800 programs in 1993, producing more graduates annually than either diploma or baccalaureate programs. These graduates are employed in hospitals, outpatient departments, nursing homes, and physicians' offices.

In 1951, Mildred Montag published her doctoral dissertation, "The Education of Nursing Technicians," which proposed education for the RN in the community college. Historically, there were several events and trends that influenced the development of the associate degree program. One of these events was World War II. Needing additional nurses to meet the military as well as the homefront needs, the legislature created the Cadet Nurse Corps, which provided financial incentives to nursing schools that could prepare students in less than the traditional three years. The Cadet Nurse Corps proved that qualified nurses could be educated in less time than the traditional three years. After World War II, the number of community colleges increased from 610 in 1940 to 1100 in 1970 (Medsker and Tillery, 1971). During the same time, diploma schools were experiencing an annual decline in enrollment. The community college movement brought to the community many vocational and adult education programs. The "open-door" policy and the low tuition of the community college made the concept of higher education more accessible to all regardless of race, marital status, age, or sex. The Canadian experiment in nursing education was another historical event that had an impact on the founding of the associate degree nursing program. This research investigated alternative models of nursing education, finding that nurses could be equally prepared in two years instead of three when a school had complete control over a program.

It was Dr. Montag's original proposal that the associate degree program was to be a terminal degree to prepare nurses for immediate employment. According to Dr. Montag, there was a need for a new type of nurse, the "nurse technician," whose role was broader than that of a practical nurse, but less than that of the professional nurse. The technical nurse was to function at the "bedside." Her duties, according to Dr. Montag, were to be as follows: (1) to give general nursing care with supervision; (2) to assist in the planning of nursing care for clients; and (3) to assist in the evaluation of the nursing care given (Montag, 1951).

An advisory committee was established in 1952 by the American Association of Junior Colleges. Along with the NLN, this committee was to conduct cooperative research on nursing education in the community college. The goals of the Cooperative Research Project were threefold: (1) to describe the development of the associate degree nursing program; (2) to evaluate the associate degree graduates; and (3) to determine the future implications of the associate degree on nursing. The original project was directed by Dr. Montag at Teachers College of Columbia University and included seven junior colleges and one hospital from each of the six regions of the United States.

In the proposed technical nursing curriculum, there was to be a balance between general education and nursing courses. Unlike the diploma programs, the emphasis was to be on education, not service. At the end of two years, the student was to be awarded an associate degree in nursing and was to be eligible to take the state board examinations for registered nurse licensure. This degree was seen as terminal and not a step toward obtaining a baccalaureate degree (Montag, 1959).

What Is the Educational Preparation of the Associate Degree Graduate?

The current preparation of an associate degree nurse usually begins within a community college, although some programs are based within a senior college or university. The program is eighteen to twenty-one school calendar months in length. The NLN mandates that the program of learning be within the accepted limits of 60 to 72 semester credits (90 to 108 quarter credits) and that there be a balanced distribution of no more than 60% of the total number of credits allocated to nursing courses (NLN, 1991). In some programs, the student must complete the general education and science course requirements prior to beginning the nursing courses. At the end of the program, the student receives an associate degree in nursing.

Associate degree nursing education has helped to bring about a change in the type of student who enrolls in nursing. Traditionally, nursing students have been composed mainly of single, white females below the age of nineteen who are from middle-class families (Kaiser, 1975). Associate degree programs attract a more diverse group of older individuals, minorities, men, and married women.

Students bring with them a variety of educational backgrounds. There is a growing trend for individuals with baccalaureate and higher degrees in other fields to seek admission to associate degree programs (Fitzpatrick, 1983). One of the strengths of the associate degree program is that the students tend to be older and goal-oriented, and have a more realistic perspective of the work setting. Along with their maturity, these students bring with them life experiences that are applicable to nursing. The flexible scheduling patterns of a community college allow students to attend college part-time. Standards and competencies for associate degree programs are developed and maintained by the NLN Council of Associate Degree Programs, and are as follows (NLN, 1990):

◆ Develop, implement, and evaluate individualized plans of care.

◆ Use nursing process as a basis for decision making.

◆ Promote participation of the client, family, significant others, and members of the health care team in the plan of care.

◆ Make decisions and take actions that are consistent with standards for nursing practice and licensing laws.

◆ Manage care for a group of clients in a time and cost-effective manner.

◆ Are accountable for performance of nursing activities delegated to other workers.

◆ Obtain consultation when the situation encountered is beyond the nurses' knowledge and experience.

◆ Promote continuity of client care by utilizing appropriate channels of communication external to the organization.

◆ Participate in evaluation of the client care delivery system.

◆ Foster high standards of nursing practice.

◆ Participate in learning activities to maintain safe practice.

◆ Construct a course of action when confronted with ethical dilemmas in practice.

◆ Seek assistance for colleagues whose behaviors indicate a potential impairment.

◆ Participate in self-evaluation and peer review.

◆ Participate in agency committees and conference.

◆ Participate in professional organizations.

◆ Participate in research conducted in the employing institution.

The three interrelated roles for the graduate are as provider of care, manager of care, and member within the discipline of nursing. The competencies describe the behaviors of associate degree graduates at the time of graduation, as well as expected behaviors (anticipated competencies) six months following graduation (NLN, 1990).

According to the educational outcomes document (NLN, 1990), the goal of associate degree nursing programs is to prepare the graduate for direct client care. The majority of associate degree graduates, although prepared to provide care for clients across the life span, are employed in settings where the focus is on the adult client (NLN, 1990).

Dr. Montag's original proposal for the associate degree program to be a terminal degree is no longer applicable. In 1978, the American Nurses Association (ANA) proposed a resolution regarding associate degree programs, stating that they no longer were to be thought of as terminal but as part of the career upward mobility plan. The associate degree program has provided students with the motivation to further their education and the opportunity for career mobility. Although many nursing students end their nursing education with an associate degree, many enter the associate degree program with all intentions of continuing their education in nursing at the baccalaureate level (Haase, 1990).

PATH OF BACCALAUREATE EDUCATION

In this discussion, only the "generic" baccalaureate programs will be addressed. A generic student is defined as a student who enters a baccalaureate nursing program with no training or education in nursing. A generic program is defined as a program that includes lower division (freshman and sophomore) liberal arts and science courses with upper division (junior and senior) nursing courses. RNs entering baccalaureate programs will be addressed later on in this chapter.

What Is the History of Baccalaureate Nursing?

A few early training schools were affiliated with universities in order to provide some of the science courses. In 1889, Mercy Hospital in Chicago affiliated with Northwestern University. The science courses offered to the nursing students were outside the academic curriculum and did not lead to a degree. Teacher College of Columbia University also played a critical role in the establishment of baccalaureate nursing education by establishing a one-year course in hospital economics in 1899 that was later extended to two years in 1905 (Anderson, 1981).

The University of Minnesota is credited with establishing the first nursing program within a university setting in 1909. In the beginning, this program was not a baccalaureate program, but more of a superior diploma program. It was not until 1919 that the University of Minnesota instituted an undergraduate baccalaureate degree in nursing.

The early beginnings of baccalaureate education can be traced back to the

1923 Goldmark Report and to the studies done by the Committee on the Grading of Nursing Schools in 1928 (Kalisch and Kalisch, 1986). These reports both recommended that nursing education be considered a type of higher education. Many of the early nursing leaders, such as Isabel Hampton and Adelaide Nutting, also advocated placing nursing education within a college or university, but like any new idea there was controversy. In opposition to baccalaureate education were the majority of nurses and the diploma schools. Physicians were also in strong opposition, stating that nurses were already overtrained.

The early baccalaureate nursing programs were usually five years in length and consisted of the basic three-year diploma program in addition to two years of liberal arts. In 1919, there were eight baccalaureate programs.

What Is the Educational Preparation of the Baccalaureate Graduate?

The current preparation of a baccalaureate nurse is four to five years in length (120 to 140 credits) and emphasizes courses in liberal arts, sciences, and humanities. Approximately one half to two thirds of the curriculum comprises non-nursing courses. In order to qualify for a baccalaureate program, the student must first meet all of the college or university's entrance requirements. Usual entrance requirements include college preparation courses in high school (i.e., foreign language, advanced science and math courses) and a high cumulative grade point average. Most colleges also require a college entrance examination such as the Scholastic Aptitude Test (SAT) or American College Test (ACT).

During the first two years of college, the student usually is enrolled in liberal arts and science courses with other non-nursing students. It is not until late in the sophomore or early junior year that nursing courses are introduced. The emphasis in the baccalaureate nursing program is on developing critical decision making skills, on exercising independent nursing judgments, and on beginning research skills.

The graduate of a baccalaureate program must fulfill not only the degree requirements of the nursing program, but also those of the college. Upon completion of the program, the usual degree awarded is a Bachelor of Science in Nursing (BSN).

The graduate of a baccalaureate program is prepared to care for individuals, families, and groups in a variety of institutional and community settings, to prevent illness, and to maintain as well as restore health (Leddy and Pepper, 1985). The NLN lists the following activities for the graduate nurse of a baccalaureate program (NLN, 1987):

◆ Provide professional nursing care, which includes health promotion and maintenance, illness care, restoration, rehabilitation, health counseling, and education based on knowledge derived from theory and research.

- Synthesize theoretical and empirical knowledge from nursing, scientific, and humanistic disciplines with practice.
- Use the nursing process to provide nursing care for individuals, families, groups, and communities.
- Accept responsibility and accountability for the evaluation of the effectiveness of their own nursing practice.
- Enhance the quality of nursing and health practices within practice settings through the use of leadership skill and a knowledge of the political system.
- Evaluate research for the applicability of its findings to nursing practice.
- Participate with other healthcare providers and members of the general public in promoting the health and well-being of people.
- Incorporate professional values as well as ethical, moral, and legal aspects of nursing into practice.
- Participate in the implementation of nursing roles designed to meet emerging health needs of the general public in a changing society.

PATH OF MASTER'S DEGREE EDUCATION

Master's degree (MSN) programs are particularly attractive to the growing number of college graduates who later in their lives decide to become a nurse (Smith, 1989). There are only a few colleges and universities that offer master's degree programs leading to the initial professional degree in nursing. Yale University, the University of Texas at Austin, and the University of Tennessee are a few of the institutions that have such a program. Generally, the program is two years in length. Upon graduation, these students demonstrate the same expected entry level competencies in nursing as those of the baccalaureate degree. Graduates are then eligible to take the licensure exam to become an RN (Schraeder, 1988).

PATH OF DOCTORAL DEGREE EDUCATION

The last path to discuss, and the least common, is the doctoral path leading to the RN licensure examination. This program was begun in 1979 at Case Western Reserve University. Rush University in Chicago initiated a similar type of program in 1988 and the University of Colorado began a nursing doctorate program in 1990 (Forni, 1989).

GRADUATE EDUCATION

What About Graduate School?

Whatever path you chose to become an RN, there is one thing for certain: it wasn't easy. After putting life, liberty, and the pursuit of happiness on the back burner while you worked toward becoming an RN, it may seem like pure insanity to subject yourself to more education!

Graduate education in nursing is pursued after obtaining a BSN degree (or a basic nursing master's degree). It includes specialization and mastery of skills and knowledge in a clinical interest area and competence in research methodology. The goal of graduate education is to prepare nurses who will be capable of improving nursing care through the advancement of nursing theory, science, and clinical practice. Included in graduate education is the development of clinical skills, and preparation in the areas of administration, supervision, and/or teaching (Rowland, 1984).

Graduate education programs are available on either a part-time or full-time basis. Graduate programs require a good grade point average at the undergraduate level. A prerequisite for most graduate programs is satisfactory scores on the Graduate Record Examination (GRE) and/or the Miller Analogies Test. It is strongly recommended that all students, whether they plan on pursuing graduate studies or not, take the GRE after completing their undergraduate studies. The last thing you want to do is take another test, but it is much easier to score higher while the information is current in your mind than to try to take the test later when you decide that you want to continue your education.

What Is the History of Graduate Nursing Education?

Graduate nursing programs in the United States originated during the late 1800s. As more nursing schools sought to strengthen their own programs, there was increased pressure placed on nursing instructors to obtain advanced preparation in education and clinical nursing specialties.

The Catholic University of America in Washington, D.C. offered one of the early graduate programs for nurses. It began offering courses in nursing education in 1932 and began conferring a master's degree in nursing education in 1935.

Historical data before the mid-1950s are difficult to obtain because initially the accreditation procedures grouped all postdiploma programs into the category of postgraduate education. The curriculum varied widely between programs. Some of the courses were the same for both undergraduates and graduates, which further complicated the issue.

The NLN's Subcommittee on Graduate Education first published guidelines for organization, administration, curriculum, and testing in 1957. These guidelines have been revised throughout the years and reflect the focus in master's education on research and clinical specialization.

Until the 1950s, the majority of collegiate nursing schools were located in the northeastern part of the United States. Seventy-five percent of the master's-prepared nurses obtained their degree at Teachers College (Fitzpatrick, 1983). With the establishment of the Southern Regional Educational Board and the Western Interstate Commission on Higher Education, the number of master's programs in the South and West has increased dramatically.

Why Do I Want a Master's Degree?

▼

You've got to be kidding! More school?

▲

Sure, maybe right now an advanced degree may not be in your career plans, but later on after you have been practicing nursing, you may change your mind. Master's programs vary from institution to institution, as do the admission and course requirements and costs. The majority of programs are at least one full year in length, with many programs being expanded to two years. There are the more traditional models in which the student takes the required courses for the degree and then may or may not have to write a thesis. There are also nontraditional models that include outreach programs; summers-only programs; RN-to-MSN tracks for RNs who do not have an undergraduate degree; as well as RNs who hold a bachelor's degree in another field. In the future, we will see even more types of programs being designed to meet the needs of the returning graduate student.

How Do I Know What Master's Program Is Right for Me?

In choosing a program for graduate studies, one of the best sources of information is the NLN's *Graduate Education: Route to Opportunities in Contemporary Nursing* (NLN, 1989d). The NLN also publishes a list of NLN-accredited programs in nursing education at the doctoral, master's, baccalaureate, associate, and diploma levels as well as information on scholarships and loans for nursing education.

Your career goals and interests will help you to determine what choice is best for you. Keep in mind that one way to expand your nursing base is to attend a graduate school in a different area of the country from where you obtained your undergraduate education. A person's knowledge base is thought to be more "marketable" if they are not "in-bred," which means that they don't have all of their degrees from one institution. If this is not a possibility for you, then you have to choose the next best route to obtaining your career goals. The important thing is that you have considered all the options. After all, if you are going to expend the time, energy, and finances to obtain a graduate degree, you want to get the most from it.

Why Do I Want a Doctoral Degree?

Power, authority, and professional status are usually associated with a doctoral degree. Doctoral-prepared nurses provide important leadership in the improvement of nursing practice, in the development of research, and programs of nursing education. There is a growing need for doctoral-prepared nurses. More nurses today are seeking doctoral education than ever before.

There are two basic models of doctoral degrees in nursing. There is the academic degree, or Doctor of Philosophy (PhD), and the professional degree, or the Doctor of Nursing Science (DNS, also DSN, or DNSc). At the end of 1989, there were 47 doctoral programs in nursing with 36 programs awarding the PhD (Forni, 1989). The PhD continues to be the most highly esteemed degree in higher education. Nurses also have other doctoral degree options available to them such as the Doctor of Education (EdD), the Doctor of Public Health (DPH), the Doctor of Philosophy in another discipline besides nursing, and the non-traditional external-degree doctorate.

It is important to remember that the doctorate in nursing is basically a new concept. Before 1965, the most common doctoral degree earned by nurses was the Doctor of Education (EdD). It was not until the establishment of the federally supported Nurse Scientist Training Program in 1962 that there began a shift toward obtaining a PhD. The DNS has been awarded since the early 1960s (Rowland, 1984).

How Do I Know What Doctoral Program Is Right for Me?

As with the master's degree, it is important to look at your career goals before deciding what doctoral program is best for you. To help you with that task, look at the NLN publications specific to doctoral education. Ask yourself how much time can you devote to obtaining a doctorate degree? The average time it takes to complete a doctorate degree once being admitted to the doctoral program is 4.5 years (Rowland, 1984). Can you be a fulltime student or must you continue to work? What do you plan to do with the degree once you get it?

"Today, a doctorate in nursing should be the first choice for nurses seeking doctoral education" (Allen, 1990). Is this a realistic goal? Is there an institution available to you that offers a doctorate in nursing or would you have to consider moving? What are your career and professional goals? Do you want to teach? The PhD is considered the research degree. It prepares an individual for a lifetime of intellectual inquiry and has an increased emphasis on postdoctoral study. On the other hand, the DNS is viewed as the practical degree. The goal of this program is to prepare an advanced practitioner for the application of knowledge with an emphasis on research. The original intent of the DNS was to prepare nurses to do clinical research. Deans of nursing programs state that they prefer a PhD in nursing over those with a PhD in another discipline or a DNS (Allen, 1990).

OTHER TYPES OF NURSING EDUCATION

What Are the Other Available Educational Options?

In the 1960s, baccalaureate programs made it very difficult for the RN to return to school to earn a baccalaureate in nursing. Most of the time, these nurses found themselves receiving no credit for their past education or experience. A resolution passed in 1978 by the ANA that urged the creation of quality career mobility programs with flexibility to assist those individuals desiring academic degrees in nursing helped to change this philosophy. There are several basic patterns to achieve upward mobility in nursing, and within these basic patterns there are many variations. Career ladder programs, BSN completion programs, external degree programs, and university without walls programs are the basic patterns that will be addressed in this section. In assessing the educational options that are available, one source of information is the Directory of Career Mobility Programs in Nursing Education published by the NLN. This directory presents a current listing covering the United States and its jurisdictions of nursing programs that offer mobility to students to advance their careers by offering varying degrees of credit for relevant education and experience. Along with this resource, the potential student should also contact the individual schools for additional information regarding their particular programs. Their addresses can be found in this directory.

What Is a Career Ladder Program?

The career ladder concept focuses on the articulation of educational programs permitting advanced placement without loss of credit or repetition. There are many variations of this type of program. Multiple-exit programs provide opportunities for students to enter the educational system and exit at various designated times having gained specific education and skills. An example is a program that goes from practical nurse to registered nurse at the associate, baccalaureate, master's, and doctoral levels. A student in such a program may decide to leave the educational system at the completion of a specific level and be eligible to take the licensure examination applicable to that educational level. Upon termination, the student may choose to work for a while and later return for more education at the next level without having to repeat courses on previously acquired knowledge or skills.

One such program is project LINC (Ladders in Nursing Careers), which was developed in New York City for the purpose of providing educational advancement opportunities for individuals who are in entry or mid-level jobs in nursing. It is a collaborative effort involving over forty hospitals and long-term care facilities in the New York City area and serves as a state and national model of educational mobility.

A growing number of basic nursing education programs within the community college setting are beginning to offer career ladder-type programs, affiliating themselves with upper division colleges in the area. A student can enter the community college to spend one year studying to become a practical or vocational nurse. After a year, the student can decide to stop and take the practical nurse licensure examination or continue and complete the associate degree in nursing. At the end of the second year, the student is eligible to take the RN licensure examination and may choose to either exit as an associate-degree nurse or continue on at an affiliated upper-division college and obtain a baccalaureate degree.

What Is a BSN Completion Program?

A BSN completion program is a baccalaureate program designed for students who already possess either a diploma or an associate degree in nursing and hold a current license to practice as an RN. Depending on the part of the country, these programs may also be known as registered nurse baccalaureate (RNB) programs, baccalaureate registered nurse (BRN) programs, two-plus-two, or capstone programs. In the majority of programs, nurses receive transfer credit in basic education courses taken at other institutions plus either some transfer credit for their previous nursing courses or the opportunity to receive nursing credit by passing a nursing challenge exam. The usual length of these programs is two years depending on the number of course requirements completed at the time of admission to the program. In an effort to meet the needs of the returning student, many BSN completion programs offer flexible class scheduling, which allows the student to continue working while going to school. Another innovation being implemented to address the needs of individuals seeking baccalaureate degrees in outlying geographic areas is telecommunications studies.

What Is an External Degree Program?

The external degree program is a program that gives credit for an individual's knowledge, regardless of how that knowledge was acquired. The external degree program is a nontraditional program that allows a student to obtain a degree from a degree-granting institution by fulfilling the requirements of the program. This type of program allows the student to gain credit and meet external degree requirements without attending classes. Two examples of external degree programs for RN education are the New York Board of Regents External Degree Programs (REX) for ADN and BSN education. Both of these programs are designed to allow an individual to obtain a degree in nursing without leaving their jobs or their communities. These programs are NLN accredited. In these programs, all students are required to pass specific college-level tests and performance examinations in two components: general education and nursing. Tests are administered in several cities throughout the United States. Upon completion of the external degree program, students are eligible in most states to take RN licensure examination. There are also external degree programs in which a person can earn a doctoral degree.

What Is a University Without Walls?

The University without walls concept is a program that allows an RN to obtain a baccalaureate degree by taking courses at a local college or community college instead of taking the courses on the university campus that will confer the degree. The student is usually assigned an on-campus advisor who helps plan the course of study in order to meet the college requirements. Past education and work experiences are taken into consideration. Instead of the traditional grading system and recording of credit hours, a file is kept by the individual participant and routinely reviewed with the on-campus advisor. When all the requirements are successfully met, a bachelor of arts degree is awarded.

Michigan State University School of Nursing and Skidmore College in Saratoga Springs New York offer university without walls programs. Advantages of this type of program include the following:

- ◆ Ability of an individual to remain employed while working on continuing education.
- ◆ Flexibility of course design that gives credit for experience.
- ◆ The elimination of travel costs.
- ◆ The opportunity to apply newly acquired knowledge to the work setting.
- ◆ Older students do not feel out of place as they might returning to a regular college campus-type setting.

In summary, there are five different educational paths that all lead to the same destination: the opportunity to take the licensure examination to become an RN. The diploma, associate degree, and baccalaureate programs are the three most common paths while the master's and doctoral programs are the less common paths. The similarities of the programs are that the students all take the same licensing exam (NCLEX-RN), that the schools all must meet certain state board standards, and that the schools all have the option of voluntary national accreditation through the NLN.

There are many other educational options, both traditional and nontraditional, available to the RN seeking more advanced educational preparation. Although there continues to be controversy over educational preparation for entry into practice, there is a general consensus that nursing education needs to work towards greater educational mobility for registered nurses in order to meet the future needs of nursing.

ACCREDITATION

Why should you be concerned whether the nursing program you are attending, or thinking about attending, is accredited? Accreditation assures you, the student, and the public that educational standards over and above the legal requirements of the state have been achieved. It guarantees the student the opportunity to obtain a quality education. Accreditation is strictly a voluntary process. The U.S. Department of Education and the Council on Postsecondary Accreditation has designated the NLN as the accrediting body for all nursing programs. Currently, the NLN accredits over 1500 educational programs. The NLN publishes specific guidelines outlining policies and procedures for accreditation of each level of nursing education.

In order to be eligible for accreditation, a nursing education program must meet the specific conditions set forth by the NLN. One of these criteria is that the institution offering the nursing program be also accredited by an appropriate state accrediting agency. Schools of nursing meeting this criterion are then eligible to initiate the accreditation process and must pay a fee for this service. The nursing program conducts an extensive self-study that addresses certain criteria set forth by the NLN and submits this document for review. Besides the written self-study, there is an accreditation visit. The accreditation visit is conducted by site visitors from the NLN. These visitors are peers employed in programs like the one they are evaluating. The purpose of the site visit is to verify, clarify, and amplify the written self-study report and document congruency between the report and the actual practices of the institution and the nursing program. The board of review for each NLN council then evaluates the self-study report and the site visitor's report and makes recommendations to faculty and administrators regarding any needed improvements to the program. Based on these findings, the nursing program is granted or denied accreditation.

Some graduate nursing programs require completing an NLN-approved undergraduate program as a prerequisite for admission to their master's or doctoral program. The NLN publishes an official and complete list of NLN-accredited programs annually.

NURSING EDUCATION: FUTURE TRENDS

Education is a life-long process and an empowering force that enables an individual to achieve higher goals. Student access to educational opportunities is paramount to nursing education. A chapter on nursing education would not be complete without taking a look at the future.

The Changing Student Profile

Future nursing programs will need to be flexible in order to meet the learning needs of a changing student population. It has been previously stated that there is a growing population of nontraditional students—individuals who are making mid-life career changes due in part to job displacement or job dissatisfaction. The student population tends to be older, married, and with families. More poor, minority, and foreign students are looking toward nursing education for career opportunities.

These changes will mean that nurse educators will need to further address the needs of the adult learner. There will need to be more programs that permit parttime study and allow students to work while attending school. One option may be for more night or weekend course offerings. There will continue to be a need for more emphasis on remedial education such as developmental courses in math, English, and English as a second language. The diversity in student population means diversity in learning rates, which might be addressed with more self-paced learning modules.

Educational Mobility

Educational mobility will need to be further addressed. There is a growing number of individuals in healthcare seeking more education. The issue is not one of entry into practice, but rather of how to best facilitate these individuals returning to nursing school for educational advancement. The states of Arkansas, California, Colorado, Florida, Hawaii, Maryland, Minnesota, Missouri, New Mexico, North Dakota, Texas, and Utah have already established statewide articulation programs in order to offer greater career mobility in nursing (McHugh, 1991). Additional states are currently studying articulation programs.

A Shortage of Qualified Nursing Faculty

According to the U.S. Department of Health and Human Service's Seventh Report to the President and Congress (1988), the most severe shortage will be among baccalaureate and higher degree nurses. Student access to educational opportunities will depend on the availability of qualified instructors. There will need to be federal government financial assistance to help increase the supply of nurses with master's and doctoral degrees.

Technology and Education

Educational learning will continue to change with technological advancements in telecommunications and computer-assisted instruction. Nurses and nurse educators will need the education necessary to implement these advancements into the curriculum and into nursing practice. As with cable television, which has extended the boundaries of the classroom, these new technologies will facilitate the offering of outreach programs.

Shift Away From Acute Care Settings

There has been a major shift from inpatient to outpatient nursing services. Society is now developing a variety of new healthcare settings. Are nurses educated for these new roles? What will be the role of the advanced practitioner? Will there be enough nurses educationally prepared to meet these new challenges?

The Aging Population

There is a growing aging population. By 2030, people over the age of 65 will represent 21 percent of the population (NLN, 1987). According to Naisbitt and Aburdene (1990), "If business and society can master the challenge of daycare, we will be one step closer to confronting the next great care-giving task of the 1990s—eldercare." Already, there are well over 2,000 adult daycare centers in the United States. Nursing needs to address the provision of healthcare to the elderly and include it in their curriculum.

▼

What great opportunities in nursing!!

▲

The future of nursing looks bright and exciting. With the technological advances and the shift away from acute care settings, nurses have the opportunity to chart their own destiny.

REFERENCES

Allen, J. (1990): Consumers Guide to Doctoral Degree Programs in Nursing. NLN Publication No. 15-2293. New York, NLN.

American Nurses Association (1974): Standards for Continuing Education for Nursing. Kansas City, ANA.

American Nurses Association (1978): First Position Paper on Education for Nursing. *Am J Nurs* 1231.

Anderson, N.E. (1978): The historical development of American nursing education. *J Nurs Educ* 20(1):18.

Bell, J.G., Simons, F.A., Norris, J. (1983): An alternate pathway to a BSN . . . accelerated programs. *Nurs Educator* 8(4):34.

Brainard, N.S. (1983): From RN to BSN (anecdote). *Am J Nurs* 83(3):490.

Braude, J.M. (1959): *New Treasury of Stories For Speaking and Writing Occasions.* Englewood Cliffs, NJ, Prentice-Hall.

Brower, H.T. (1982): Potential advantages and hazards of nontraditional education for nurses. *Nurs Health Care* 3:268.

Bullough, B., Bullough, V., Soukup, M. (1983): Nursing Issues and Strategies for the Eighties. New York, Springer.

Callin, M. (1983): Going back of school: An open letter to a nurse thinking of returning for further education. *J Contin Educ Nurs* 14(4):21.

Choinski, C., Hammer C., Hamm, S., et al. (1978): Playing with the entry requirement: A game we can't afford. *RN* 41(12):27.

Conway-Rutkowski, B. (1982): Future trends in post-basic nursing education. *J Nurs Educ* 21:5.

Deleruye'lle, L., Challey, P. (1983): Credit where credit is due . . . RNs who are returning to school. *Am J Nurs* 4(7):105.

Department of Health and Human Services (1988): Seventh Report to the President and Congress on the Status of Health Personnel in the United States. Washington D.C., Bureau of Health Professions, Health Resources and Services Administration, Department of Health and Human Services.

Deering-Flory, R., Neighbors, M. (1992): NLN competencies for the associate degree nurse. *Nurs Health Care* 12(9):474.

Feldman, H., Jordet, C. (1991): On the fast track. *Nurs Health Care* 10(9):491.

Fitzpatrick, M. (1983): Prologue to Professionalism. Bowie, MD, Robert J. Brady Co.

Forni, P.R. (1987): Nursing's diverse master's programs: The state of the art. *Nurs Health Care* 8(2):770.

Forni, P.R. (1989): Models for doctoral programs: First professional degree or terminal degree? *Nurs Health Care* 10(8):429.

Freda, M.C. (1985): Better ways to the BSN? You bet! The 'Salit' approach to the BSN debate. *RN* 46(6):59.

Haase, P.T. (1990): The Origins and Rise of Associate Degree Education. Durham, NC, Duke University Press.

Hawken, P. L. (1987): NLN perspective: News from the President. *Nurs Health Care* 8(2):770.

Hocker, B.B. (1984): Reflections of the Characteristics of Diploma Programs and Competencies of the Graduates in the Curriculum. National League for Nursing Publication no. 16-1953. New York, NLN, p. 26.

Kaiser, J.E. (1975): A Comparison of Students in Practical Nursing Programs and in Associate Degree Nursing Programs. National League for Nursing Pub. no. 23-1592. New York, NLN.

Kalisch, P.A., Kalisch, B.J. (1986): The Advance of American Nursing. 2nd ed. Boston, Little, Brown & Co, 1986.

Lalor, L. (1983): Better ways to the BSN? You bet! Doing a two-step to the BSN. *RN* 46(6):59.

Leddy, S., Pepper, J. (1985): Conceptual Bases of Professional Nursing. Philadelphia, J.B. Lippincott.

Lenburg, C.B. (1984): Preparation for professionalism through regents external degrees. *Nurs Health Care* 5(6):319.

Lenburg, C., Johnson, W., Vahey, J. (1973): Directory of Career Mobility Opportunities in Nursing. New York, NLN.

Mahdi, E. (1987): Learning needs in a changing world. *The Futurist* 21:60.

McHugh, M. (1991): Direct articulation of AD nursing students into an RN-to-BSN completion program: A research study. *J Nurs Educ* 30(7):293.

Medsker, L.H., Tillery, D. (1971): Breaking the Access Barriers: A Profile of Two Year Colleges. New York, McGraw-Hill.

Montag, M.L. (1951): The Education of Nursing Technicians. New York, G.P. Putnam's Sons.

Montag, M.L. (1959): Community College Education for Nursing. New York, McGraw-Hill.

Montag, M.L. (1982): The external degree. *Imprint* 29(4):25.

Murphy, J.G. (1981): Doctoral education in, of, and for nursing: An historical analysis. *Nurs Outlook* 29:645.

Naisbitt, J., Aburdene, P. (1990): Megatrends 2000. New York, William Morrow and Co.

National League for Nursing (1973): Characteristics of Associate Degree Education in Nursing. Publication No. 23-1500, Council of Associate Degree Programs. New York, NLN.

National League for Nursing (1978): Patterns in Nursing: Strategic Planning for Nursing Education. Publication No. 15-2179. New York, NLN.

National League for Nursing (1982): Criteria for the Evaluation of Diploma Programs in Nursing. 6th ed. New York, NLN.

National League for Nursing (1983): Education for Nursing: The Diploma Way 1983-84. Information About NLN Accredited Diploma Programs in Nursing. National League for Nursing Publication. No. 16-1314, Council Diploma Programs. New York, NLN, p. 1.

National League for Nursing (1987): Characteristics of Baccalaureate Education in Nursing. Publication No. 15-1758, Council on Baccalaureate and Higher Degree Programs. New York, NLN.

National League for Nursing (1989a): Associate Degree Education for Nursing 1989-1990. Publication No. 23-1309. New York, NLN.

National League for Nursing (1989b): Baccalaureate Education in Nursing: Key to a Professional Career in Nursing 1989-1990. Publication No. 15-1311. New York, NLN.

National League for Nursing (1989c): Education for Nursing: The Diploma Way 1989-1990. Publication No. 16-1314. New York, NLN, 1989.

National League for Nursing (1989d): Graduate Education in Nursing: Route to Opportunities in Contemporary Nursing 1989-1990. Publication No. 15-2221. New York, NLN.

National League for Nursing (1990): Educational Outcomes of Associate Degree Nursing Programs: Roles and Competencies. Publication No. 23-2348, Council of Associate Degree Programs. New York, NLN.

National League for Nursing (1991): Criteria and Guidelines for Accreditation of Associate Degree Program. 7th ed. Publication No. 23-2439, Council of Associate Degree Programs. New York, NLN.

Nayer, D. (1983): Back to school. *Nurs Times* 79(31):61.

Rawlins, T., Riordan, J., Delamaide, G., Kilian, G. (1991): Student nurse recruitment: determinants for choosing a nursing program. *J Nurs Educ* 30(5):197.

Rowland, H. (1984): *The Nurse's Almanac*. 2nd ed. Rockville, MD, Aspen Publications.

Sallee, K. (1987): Final story on grandfathering. *Current Concepts Nurs* 1(2):10.

Schraeder, B.D. (1988): Entry-level graduate education in nursing: Master of science programs, in *Perspectives in Nursing* 1987-1989. New York, NLN.

Smith, P. (1989): Nonurse College Graduates in a specialty Master's Program: A Success Story. *Nurs Health Care* 10(9):495.

Smullen, B.B. (1982): Second-step education for RNs: the quiet revolution. *Nurs Health Care* 3:369.

Swenson, R.S. (1983): Associate degree nursing education at thirty years. Associate degree nursing: The gift of thirty years. Publication no. 23-1948. Council of Associate Degree Programs. New York, NLN, p. 1.

UNIT III

SKILLS

IN

NURSING

MANAGEMENT

5

Challenges of Nursing Management

Carol Singer, Ed.D., R.N.

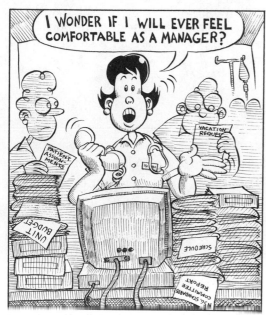

Nursing management can be challenging.

What you do speaks so loudly I can't hear what you say.

—Unknown

After completing this chapter, you should be able to:

◆ Differentiate between management and leadership.

◆ Describe various types of management.

◆ List characteristics of a good leader.

◆ Compare and contrast different leadership styles.

◆ Distinguish between power and authority.

◆ Apply problem-solving strategies to clinical management situations.

◆ Use the decision making process in clinical situations.

◆ Define the task and maintenance roles that group members assume to ensure effective group functioning.

◆ Identify the characteristics of effective work groups.

A s you get *closer* to meeting your goal of being a "real" nurse, it is important to consider the role of the nurse as a leader and manager.

I don't want to be a manager, I'm a new graduate!
I want to take care of patients, not be a paper pusher!

Not so!! Nursing in any role is a "people business," and dealing with people is what management is. When you accept your first position as a graduate nurse, you must realize that you are entering a work group that spends at least one third of the day interacting with each other. Nurses must use interpersonal, leadership and management skills to be effective in their roles.

Management requires different levels of functioning depending on what role the individual nurse is in. For instance, as a new graduate, you will have primary management responsibility for the patients you are assigned to care for. This may include planning and coordinating the care with other nursing personnel, such as nursing assistants. It also may require working with other members of the health team to meet patient needs. With more experience, you may be put in a position as a team leader or charge nurse with responsibility for managing a group of staff members who provide care for a larger number of patients, perhaps even an entire unit.

MANAGEMENT vs. LEADERSHIP

What Is the Difference Between Leadership and Management?

Although the terms *management* and *leadership* are frequently interchanged, they do not have the same meaning. A leader selects and assumes the role; a manager is assigned or appointed to the role. Managers have responsibility toward organizational goals and perform organizational tasks, such as budget preparation and scheduling. Although it is desirable for managers also to be good leaders to be effective in influencing others, there are "leaders" who are not "managers" and, more frequently, "managers" who are not "leaders!" So let's discuss in more detail what the actual differences are.

Management is a problem-oriented process with similarities to the nursing process. Management is needed whenever two or more individuals work together toward a common goal. The manager coordinates the activities of the group to maintain balance and direction. There are generally four functions which the manager performs. These functions are *planning* (what is to be done), *organizing* (how it is to be done), *directing* (who is to do it), and *controlling* (when and how it is done). All of these activities go on continually and simultaneously, with the percentage of time spent on each varying with the level of the manager and the characteristics of the group being managed. Managers must be attentive to *both* of the dimensions of their job, the mission and goals of the organization, and the interpersonal relationships with the staff. The successful manager is one who respects the people of the organization as individuals, *and* who cares how well the tasks are done.

Leadership, on the other hand, is a way of behaving, an interpersonal ability to cause others to respond, not because they have to, but because they want to. Leadership, as well as management, is needed for effective group functioning, but in a different manner. The manager determines the agenda, sets time limits, and facilitates group functioning. The leader serves to influence the activities of a group toward identifying goals and carrying out the activities needed to reach those goals.

▼

Florence Nightingale was certainly a leader, but how did she manage other nurses?

▲

What Is Meant By a Management Style?

There are a variety of different management styles that you may come across in your nursing practice, but they basically fall on a continuum between autocratic and laissez-faire styles (Fig. 5–1).

The *autocractic manager* uses an authoritarian approach to direct the activities of others. This individual makes most of the decisions alone without input from other staff members. Under this style of management, the emphasis is on the tasks to be done, with little concern shown for the individual staff members who perform the tasks. The autocratic manager may be most effective in crisis situations, where structure and control are critical to success, as, for instance, during a cardiac arrest or code.

On the other end of the continuum is the *laissez-faire manager* who maintains a permissive climate with little direction or control exerted. This manager allows staff members to make decisions and implement them independently and relinquishes all power and responsibility to them. Although this style of management may function effectively in highly motivated groups, it is not usually effective in the bureaucratic healthcare setting that requires many different individuals and groups to interact with each other.

In the middle of the continuum is the *democratic manager*. This individual is people-oriented and places the major focus on effective group functioning. The goals of the group are identified and the manager is perceived as a member of the group who is the organizer and who keeps the group headed in the right direction. The environment is open and communication goes both ways. However, the democratic manager, while encouraging participation in decision making, recognizes that there are situations in which it may not be appropriate and is willing to assume the responsibility for decision making when it is necessary.

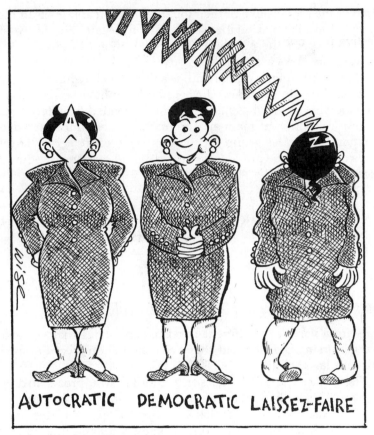

FIGURE 5–1   *Management styles.*

▼

Time to use your brain now and look at managers who may fit into these categories.

▲

What Are the Characteristics of a Good Leader?

There have been many attempts to define what makes a good leader, resulting in a variety of concepts proposed. Researchers have tried to identify what characteristics or traits are necessary to be a good leader. Several of these studies defined the concept of a "born leader," which implies that the desired traits were inherited. Later research indicated that the situation itself had a significant influence on the effectiveness of the leader. It became clear that desired traits could be learned through education and experience. It also became clear that the most effective leadership style for one situation was not necessarily the most effective for another. Today, leaders must have a variety of skills and possess the ability to select the best style of leadership needed for each situation. The concept of *contingency leadership* is sometimes used to refer to this flexible approach. The leader's style varies *contingent* on the situation. Although this may sound complicated, it can easily be compared to your approach to patient care. That is, you individualize a care plan based on the needs of a particular patient, then you implement the care using available resources. The good leader uses the same flexible approach in individual situations.

There are two major areas related to leadership abilities. These areas are identified as job-centered behavior and employee-centered behavior. A leader's behavior may emphasize both areas, may be limited in both areas, or be high in one area and low in the other. The leader who is high in both job-centered and employee-centered behaviors cares equally for the needs and feelings of the employee and getting the job done effectively and efficiently. This individual uses democratic concepts in management and views the tasks to be accomplished as a team member. At the other extreme would be the leader who has little concern for either the employee or the task to be accomplished. You would expect this individual to approach management with a laissez-faire attitude.

Alternatively, a leader who uses the autocratic style of management is probably high in job-centered behavior and low in employee-centered behavior. The leader who is high in employee-centered behavior and low in job-centered behavior would fall between the democratic and laissez-faire manager on the continuum. Let's look at a few examples:

*Tom is a **high employee-centered and high job-centered democratic** leader. He is a person who cares equally about the employee as a person and getting the job done efficiently and effectively. Another type of leader is Jean who is **high job-centered and low employee-centered.** She is a person who focuses on the job to be done with little concern for the needs or feelings of her employees. A great deal of work is accomplished with her autocratic style of management. Randy, on the other hand, cares more for his employees and an individual's feelings and needs than getting the job done. He is a **high employee-centered and low job-centered** leader. Finally, the laissez-faire leader, Laura, is the kind of person who just doesn't seem to care for either her employee's needs and feelings or the need to get the job done. She would be considered a **low employee-centered and low job-centered** leader.*

While most agree that an individual leans toward one of these four possible combinations, it has been found that fluctuations from one combination to another occur depending on the particular situation. In the healthcare setting, good leaders carefully balance job-centered and employee-centered behaviors to effectively meet both staff and patient needs.

Can you think about individuals you know whom you consider to be good leaders? What personality traits do they possess?

A good leader works toward established goals and has a sense of purpose and direction (Box 5–1). Rather than *push* staff members off in many directions, this leader uses personal attributes to organize the activities and *pull* the staff toward the goals. Remember it is easier to pull than to push!

Let's take a moment now to summarize the main concepts of leadership that we discussed.

◆ Leadership can be learned.

◆ Leaders are developers of people.

◆ One's style of leadership is dependent on one's basic personality and the particular situation in which the individual is functioning.

◆ The demands of the situation in which a leader is to function influence the qualities, characteristics, knowledge, and skills necessary for successful leadership.

◆ The degree to which the leader is knowledgeable and competent directly influences the subordinates' feelings of security and their ability to cooperate toward goals.

POWER AND AUTHORITY IN NURSING MANAGEMENT

Do You Know the Difference Between Power and Authority?

Power is having the ability to affect change and influence others toward meeting identified goals. *Authority* relates to a specific position and the responsibility associated with it. The individual has the authority or the right to act in situations in which one is held responsible for within the institutional hierarchy. Today, there is much discussion in nursing about the importance of power and the concept of *empowerment*. To empower nurses is to provide them with more autonomy in their roles. The concept of power directly relates to administrative willingness to allocate it and nurses willingness to accept it together with the accompanying responsibility.

▼

Remember, power and responsibility always go hand in hand!

▲

BOX 5–1

Leadership Characteristics

First, write in the person's name on the left and then list the characteristics in the spaces on the right. See if you can identify two different individuals you know who have somewhat different characteristics, but are both good leaders!

◆ Name   ◆ Leadership Characteristics

1. _____   _____

    _____

    _____

    _____

    _____

    _____

2. _____   _____

    _____

    _____

    _____

    _____

Now, see if you can take those characteristics that you identified and fill in the blanks below!

A good leader has: e _ _ _ _ _ _ _ sm

se _ _ -c _ _ _ _ _ _ d _ _ ce

mat _ _ _ _ _ _

a concern for _ _ _ _ _ _

dec _ _ _ _ _ -m _ _ _ _ _ ab _ _ _ _ y

a s _ _ _ _ of _ _ _ or.

A good leader also is: s _ _ _ ere

ta _ _ _ _ _

acc _ _ _ _ _ _ e

appr _ _ _ _ _ _ l _

What Are the Different Types of Power?

There are many different types of power so let's discuss the most common. *Legitimate power* is power connected to a position of authority. The individual has power as a result of their position. The head nurse has legitimate power, as well as authority, as a result of her position. *Referent power* refers to power that is given as a result of personal characteristics, often called charisma. Many successful leaders have referent power in that they are liked and admired by others as individuals first. *Reward power* is closely linked with legitimate power in that it comes about because the individual has the power to provide or withhold rewards. If your supervisor has the power to authorize salary increases or scheduling benefits, then they have reward power. *Expert power* is based on specialized knowledge, skills, or abilities that are recognized by others and respected. The individual is perceived as an expert in an area and has power in that area because of it. For instance, the enterostomal therapist has expertise in the care of individuals who have had ostomies. Therefore, staff nurses seek out the therapist as a resource and use the expert's knowledge to guide the care of these patients. *Information power* is possessed by individuals who have knowledge that is needed by others to function effectively in their roles. This type of power is perhaps the most abused power! The phrase "knowledge is power" often is used to relate to an individual who withholds information from subordinates to maintain power. The leader who gives directions without needed rationale or known constraints is abusing information power. *Coercive power* is that which is derived from fear of consequences. It is easy to see how a parent would have coercive power over children based on the threat of punishment. This type of power also can be present in dealing with staff members with whom unfavorable assignments can be used as "punishment."

It is important for leaders and managers to understand the concept of power and how it can be used and abused in working with others. Nurses as a whole need to identify ways to increase their power within the health team. Graduates need to be aware of and implement methods and resources to increase their personal power. Staff nurses can develop expert power by increasing competency in their roles and in clinical skills. Refining interpersonal skills to enhance the ability to work with others can expand many types of power. This includes communicating clearly and completely what people need to know and delegating to those who know how to accomplish a task. Demonstrating a willingness to give and receive feedback and being positive in communicating also are important. All of these are ways that individuals can develop and enhance power in working with others. It is also important to recognize those things that can detract from power. Appearing disorganized, either in personal appearance or in the work environment; engaging in petty criticism or rumor spreading; and being unable to say "no" without qualification are some of the behaviors that can detract from power.

MANAGEMENT PROBLEM SOLVING

What About Using Problem Solving Strategies in Management?

Management is a problem-oriented process. The effective manager analyzes problems and makes decisions throughout all the planning, organizing, directing and controlling functions of management. Problem solving can be readily compared with the nursing process (Table 5–1). The two are essentially the same processes. If we compare the steps of one to the other you will see the similarity.

As with the nursing process, problem solving does not always flow in an orderly manner from one step to the other. Throughout the process, feedback is sought, which may indicate a need for altering the plan to reach the desired objective. The most critical step in either process is identifying the problem (identified as *nursing diagnosis* in the nursing process). Frequently, what was originally identified as "the problem" may be too broad or unclear. Only the symptoms of the problem may be seen initially or there may be several problems overlapping. If an approach is used to relieve only the symptoms, the problem will still exist. The good manager will guide the process of identifying the problem by asking questions such as "What is happening?", "What is being done about it?", "Who is doing what?", and "Why?" It is important to differentiate between facts and opinions and to attempt to break down the information to its simplest terms. Think of it as being a Detective, looking for every clue!

Once the problem is clearly identified, the group should "brainstorm" all possible solutions. Often, the first few alternatives are not the best or most practical. Identifying a number of viable alternatives usually provides more flexibility and creativity. All possible solutions must fall within the constraints that are present, such as staff abilities, available resources, and institutional policies. The more complex the problem, the more judgment is required. In some cases, the problem may extend beyond the manager's scope of responsibility and authority and it may be necessary to seek "outside" help.

Once all the alternatives are identified, each must be evaluated in relation to changes that would be required in existing policies, procedures, staffing, etc.,

TABLE 5–1   *Nursing Process vs. Problem Solving*

NURSING PROCESS	PROBLEM SOLVING
Assessment	Data gathering
Analysis/Nursing diagnosis	Definition of problem
Development of a plan	Identification of alternative solutions
Implementation of plan	Implementation of plan
Evaluation/Reassessment	Evaluation of solution

and what effect these changes would have. Ask "What would happen if . . . " questions to clarify short- and long-term implications of each alternative. Always keep in mind that the "perfect solution" is not possible in most situations.

Problem solving represents a choice made between possible alternatives that is thought to be the *best* solution to be taken for a particular situation. At its best, problem solving should involve ample discussion of the possible solutions by those who are affected by the situation and who possess the knowledge and power to support the possible solution. Once an alternative has been selected, it should be implemented unless new data or perspectives warrant a change. Feedback should be sought continuously to provide ongoing evaluation of the effectiveness of the solution. Remember, simply choosing the best alternative does not automatically ensure its acceptance by those who work with it!

Frequently, implementing the "solution" to a problem causes several other problems to arise. If that happens, don't let the new problems distract from the implementation, but rather pause and consider each individually, solve it, and then return to the original plan. After a period of trial, evaluate the progress that has been made. A complete solution may not have been reached, but progress should be visible. If not, a slight modification in the approach may be necessary, or a completely new alternative is needed. The old adage "If at first you don't succeed, try, try again" is most appropriate when applying the problem-solving process! Remain positive, confident, and flexible! Eventually a possible solution will work! Let's apply the process to an actual problem.

> *You are the head nurse on a busy medical-surgical unit with thirty-two patients. Staff have complained to you that too much time is being spent during morning change of shift report. After asking questions and seeking out additional information, you determine that a more clear definition of the problem is that the night charge nurse does not give a clear, concise report. Involving the night charge nurse in the problem-solving process helps to define the problem, as the nurse does not have adequate knowledge of how to give a change of shift report.*

Can you see how once the problem has actually been clarified, it seems much more amenable to an acceptable, perhaps even easy, solution?

How Do We Relate Problem Solving and Decision Making?

By definition, the two are almost the same process with *one very notable difference.* Decision making requires the definition of a clear objective to guide the process. A comparison of the steps of each will illustrate this difference (Table 5–2). While both problem solving and decision making are usually initiated by the presence of a problem, in decision making the objective may not be to solve the problem, but to deal only with the results of the problem. It also is important to distinguish between a "good decision" and a "good outcome." A *good outcome* is what is desired, while a *good decision* is one made systematically that reaches the desired

TABLE 5–2   *Problem Solving vs. Decision Making*

PROBLEM SOLVING	DECISION MAKING
Define problem	Set objective
Identification of alternative solutions	Identify and evaluate alternative decisions
Select solution and implement	Make decision and implement
Evaluate outcome	Evaluate outcome

objective. A good decision may or may not result in a good outcome. While it is desirable to have both good decisions and good outcomes, the good decision maker is willing to take the necessary risk even if the outcome is not positive.

> Susan is the evening charge nurse on a medical unit that has a census of twenty-four patients. One of the patients is terminally ill and seems to be having a particularly difficult evening. The patient requires basic comfort measures but little complex care. Susan has a choice of assigning the patient to another RN or to a nurse aide. If she assigns the RN, the workload for the other staff will be heavier and she, herself, will have to administer medications. She decides to assign the RN to offer emotional as well as physical support for the patient. During the shift, the RN spends time sitting with the patient. Close to the end of the shift, the patient dies. Was this a good decision with a bad outcome or a good decision with a good outcome?

Decision making is value based while problem solving is a more scientific process. Nurses make decisions based on personal values, life experiences, perceptions of the situation, knowledge of risks associated with possible decisions and their individual ways of thinking. Because of this, it is possible, even probable, that two individuals given the same information and using the same decision making process, would come up with different decisions.

In today's ever-changing healthcare environment, it is important for nurses and nurse managers to be effective in both problem solving and decision making. The quality of patient care is dependent on the ability of the nurse to effectively combine problem solving with decision making. To do so, nurses must be attuned to their individual value systems and understand the effect it has on thinking and perceiving. The values associated with a particular situation will limit the alternatives generated and the final choice of a decision. For this reason, the fact that nurses typically work in groups is beneficial to the decision-making process. Although the process is the same, generally groups offer the benefits of a broader knowledge base for defining objectives and more creativity in identifying alternatives. The effectiveness of the group decision-making process is dependent on the dynamics of the group. It is, therefore, important for nurses to understand and maximize the group process by understanding the roles of individuals within the group and the dynamics involved in working in groups.

GROUP DYNAMICS

What Is Meant By Group Dynamics?

Can you remember previous discussions in nursing school about group dynamics as they related to your peer group? How about in relation to therapeutic groups? The concepts are the same when talking about work groups!

Members of the nursing and health teams are interdependent in meeting patient needs. This interdependency involves continual interaction between and among members of different groups. If the staff forms a cohesive group, each member benefits through group participation by increasing his or her understanding and the ability to give care. In addition, this cohesiveness will benefit groups which include patients and family members.

All groups go through phases, whether the group meets for a single time, once a year, or once a day. These phases are called the *initiation, working,* and *termination* phases. During the *initiation* phase, the goals and purposes of the group are defined, leadership evolves, and individual roles are determined. An important aspect of this phase is building rapport and trust among group members. The *working* phase begins once the initiation phase has been accomplished and the dynamics of the group are tentatively established. This phase deals with problem solving and the achievement of the goals of the group. Once the task is completed and problems resolved, the *termination* phase begins and the group attempts to bring closure to its activities. At this point, it is important to summarize the accomplishments of the group to make members feel good about themselves and the work that has been done.

What Types of Roles Are Needed to Promote Group Functioning?

There are two different types of roles that group members perform. They are identified as *task* roles and *maintenance* roles. *Task* roles are generally defined as follows:

- **Initiating:** introductory activities, such as making suggestions and providing new ideas for group functioning.

- **Seeking information:** gathering facts and data, seeking advice and opinions, and asking questions.

- **Giving information:** offering information from other resources and sharing suggestions and ideas that support the group activity.

- **Clarifying:** rephrasing ideas, giving examples to explain suggestions, and tracking progress being made.

- **Coordinating:** reviewing group activities and demonstrating relationships between group activities and other groups.

- **Summarizing:** recording consensus of group, summarizing actions taken, and reviewing group process.

Group maintenance roles are defined as follows:

- **Supporting:** showing concern for group members and being responsive to them.

- **Mediating:** trying to maintain harmony by seeking compromises and reducing differences between group members.

- **Gate-keeping:** encouraging participation from all group members.

- **Following:** compromising self when consensus of group supports another idea and promoting group harmony.

- **Tension-reducing:** using humor or calling for breaks in activities to decrease tense and possibly disruptive situations.

- **Standard setting:** relating current group activity to standards already established by the group and guiding decision making to avoid conflict with the standards.

Both task and maintenance roles are necessary for the group process to be effective. Individual members generally assume one or more roles within the group based on their personality and value system, as well as their position and status within the group. Each group will have a different dynamic as a result of these factors, even if the same members function in other groups as well.

What Effect Does the Leader Have on the Group?

The leader's philosophy, personality, self concept, and interpersonal skills all influence the functioning of the group. A leader is most effective if members are respected as individuals who have unique contributions to be made to the group process. Can you remember our previous discussion of the characteristics of a good leader? The ability to influence and motivate others is particularly important in the group process.

Whenever the combination of people in a group is altered, the dynamics are changed. If the group is in the working phase, it will revert to the initiating phase when a new person or persons are added and will remain there until they have been assimilated into the group and a new dynamic formulated. The most effective groups are those that have had consistent membership and are highly developed. These groups will demonstrate friendly and trusting relationships; the ability to work toward goals of varying difficulty; flexible, stable, and reliable participation of members; and productive, high-quality output. Leadership within these groups is democratic and the members feel positive about their participation and the outcomes of the group process. Now let's apply these principles to a real situation!

When you graduate and accept a nursing position, you will become a new nurse to the work group, causing it to regress to the initiating phase.

You must convince the members of the group that you are worthy of being included in the group. (If this is your first nursing position, you must also convince the group that you are worthy of entering the nursing profession!) To accomplish this task, you should anticipate the feelings of loneliness, isolation, and distance that accompany the initiating phase. Expect to feel that you are being excluded and understand that it is part of the process. Instead, put your energy into forming supportive professional relationships, including their social aspects. Seek and use feedback, and ask for help in areas that are not as familiar to you, such as priority setting. As you contribute your individual talents to the group, you will move from being a dependent new person to full group membership. It is important that you do not underestimate the length of time that may be needed to accomplish this task! Group processes proceed very slowly in most cases, and it may be six months or more before you are accepted as a full member of the work group. Don't be discouraged!

Remember, management skills come with experience in nursing. So, don't be too hard on yourself during the transition phase. Identify nurse managers who have the skills you would like to incorporate into your management style. Look at the positive side of working for various nursing managers as a means to assist you in the development of your personal management style.

REFERENCES

Baillie, V.K., Trygstod, L., Cordone, T.I. (1989): *Effective Nursing Leadership: A Practical Approach.* Rockville, MD, Aspen Publishers.

Chopra, A. (1973): Motivation in task-oriented groups. *J Nurs Admin* 3(1):55.

Curtain, L. (1990): Attitude: A new posture for the nineties. *Nurs Manag* 21(11):7.

Curtain, L. (1991): Leaders: The organization's pacemakers. *Nurs Manag* 22(3):6.

Ellis, J.R., Hartley, C.L. (1991): *Managing and Coordinating Nursing Care.* Philadelphia, J.B. Lippincott.

Hamilton, J.M., Kiefer, M.E. (1986): *Survival Skills for the New Nurse.* Philadelphia, J.B. Lippincott.

Hein, E.C., Nicholson, M.J. (1990): *Contemporary Leadership Behavior.* Glenview, IL, Scott Foresman/Little Brown Higher Education.

Lindquist, K.D. (1990): Teamwork: Joining hands to meet organizational goals. *Health Care Trends Traditions* 1(4):22.

Manthey, M. (1990): From mama management to team spirit. *Nurs Manag* 21(1):20.

Manthey, M. (1990): Three simple rules. *Nurs Manag* 21(12):19.

Marquis, B.L., Huston, C.J. (1987): *Management Decision Making for Nurses.* Philadelphia, J.B. Lippincott.

Moore, W.M. (1991): Corporate culture: Modern day rites and rituals. *Healthcare Trends Traditions* 2(4):16.

Sullivan, E.J, Decker, P.J. (1988): *Effective Management in Nursing.* Menlo Park, CA, Addison-Wesley.

Viau, J. (1990): Theory Z: A new posture for the nineties. *Nurs Manag* 21(12):34.

6

Nursing Service and Healthcare Delivery

Karlene Kerfoot, Ph.D., R.N., C.N.A.A., F.A.A.N.

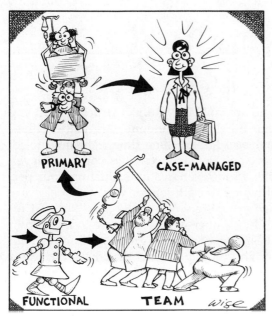

Evolving patterns of nursing care delivery.

> *A person's mind is like a parachute. To work, it first has to be open.*
>
> —J.J. Smith

After completing this chapter, you should be able to:

♦ Identify components to assess in a hospital's organizational structure.

♦ Differentiate between a centralized and decentralized organizational structure.

♦ Discuss various other models of hospital organization.

♦ Discuss patterns of nursing care delivery systems.

To be successful in your career, you should find a setting in which you can agree with the values of the organization, and one that can support your ambitions and future plans. In order to make this very important assessment of where you will fit best, there are several things you should consider. First, you should understand yourself well enough to know what kind of structure you are comfortable with and the kind of people with whom you can work best. Second, you will need to access the organization and determine if the organization fits you. The concept of "job fit" means that certain people fit certain jobs and not others. You need to know which ones you can fit into harmoniously and which ones you cannot. It is not that you are a good or bad person, or that the facility is good or bad. Each person in every organization has certain unique and distinctive peculiarities. You must match your traits with others in the most productive way so that you and the organization are both winners and, consequently, the clients will be well cared for. You can develop a high level of synergy with people in the institution in which you work, which will lead to a happy and productive career when the fit is right.

THE ORGANIZATION OF THE HOSPITAL

So How Do I Go About Assessing the Organization?

Well, first of all, look at yourself. Who are you? Do you like structure? Do you feel better without structure? Are you highly independent? Are you creative? Are you a take-charge person or laid back? Take some time right now to jot down the kind of personality you have and the characteristics you have developed over the years. Refer to Chapter 15 for exercises in evaluating your personality characteristics and for identifying the right job for you.

Now describe the kind of situation where you feel the most support for you and the kind of person you are. Remember when you were in a group or organization in which you did your best. Somehow, this group produced a high level of performance from you although you did not feel that the work was a burden. Instead, you were in harmony with everyone and felt a sense of synergy with the people. Think about the kind of place that allows fullest development and greatest potential for growth.

Now think specifically about the kind of healthcare facility that will help you do your best. Will it be a facility with a religious affiliation? Would you feel more comfortable in a for-profit healthcare institution rather than in a not-for-profit facility? What about current plans in relationship to the facility in which you will first work? Do you plan a career that takes place all in one place or is this first job just a stopping-off place to obtain experience so you can return to school or transfer to another facility? How much of a commitment are you willing to make to the unit and the facility?

People and facilities have a value system that drives them. Sometimes these values are very apparent and well articulated. Sometimes these values are not apparent, but can be inferred from people's behavior and the kind of activities the facility does and does not support. In the best of circumstances, you have values similar to those that are evident in the work setting. In the worst of working circumstances, your value system is not shared with others in the work setting because of the diferent system of values. When values are not shared, there is constant turmoil and struggle, and patient care suffers. Think back to your experience with the different kind of organizations with which you have been associated. What kind of values did they demonstrate? What kind of values were the most important to you in your work setting? What are the values that motivate you? Below, on the left hand side, list the values that drive you, and on the right hand side, the correlating values you will look for in an organization. Take some more time to think through who you are and the kind of settings in which you work best. Think about how the values influence your future.

Your values will drive your career direction. As hospitals develop their mission from their values, people also develop their missions in life and their career path from the values that drive them.

....

At the end of your life, what would have happened to make you say, "It was great. I did what I wanted to do and I developed the kind of career I wanted. I have no regrets."

....

You can plan a career that will create this kind of outcome by knowing what is important to you. For example, do you value close, intimate contact with patients and their peers? Do you feel more fulfilled working with ideas and

---

BOX 6–1

Think About . . .

Values That Drive My Behavior	Values That Drive a Good Organization
1. _____	1. _____
2. _____	2. _____
3. _____	3. _____
4. _____	4. _____
5. _____	5. _____

plans? Is material success important to you? What is the direction of your personal life and how does it correlate with your career goals? These and other similar questions will help you with the following exercise, which is to complete the mission statement listed below. The point of these exercises is to help clarify who you are, where you are going, and the kind of setting you need to realize your greatest potential.

▼

A successful life is not a one-way street.

▲

The organization and the profession do for you, but you must also do for the profession in order to actualize a high level of satisfaction. Hopefully, you see yourself as a positive participant in the life of your colleagues in the facility in which you work. And, hopefully, you realize that to achieve your greatest potential, you must do your best and achieve a level of excellence in all you do. Judith Bardwick (1991), in her book, *Danger in the Comfort Zone,* discusses the

---

BOX 6–2

Think About . . .

My mission statement When I have completed my life and look back and say I have been happy and successful in my career, I will have accomplished the following mission:

_____

_____

_____

_____

_____

_____

_____

_____

_____

_____

_____

concept of *entitlement*. It is Bardwick's view that people who believe they are entitled to happiness and entitled to a career never achieve their full potential. Feeling entitled only brings the feeling of never having had it all and never having had enough. That is not the goal of a successful person.

What Do I Need to Know to Assess the Organization?

Now that you have described yourself and have thought about the kind of setting in which you work best, continue these exercises on a consistent basis. This ongoing analysis will help you make decisions about the kind of organization that is best for you.

You are now in a position to determine what kind of organization fits you. How do you go about assessing an organization to find what you want? Well, one obvious answer is to ask the people who work in that organization. When you interview for a position, you can interview people who work in the specific work setting in which you are interested. Ask questions that will provide them with an opportunity to respond about certain situations. Think of scenarios to present to people to determine their reactions to situations. How people handle these questions will give you great insight into the way the organization works. If they feel uncomfortable with your novel approach, you will know that this kind of approach is not usual for them. If they rise to the occasion and very openly and candidly discuss their reactions, this will give you a different perspective on their viewpoints. Take some time to think about questions and situations you would like to present when you talk to people in various facilities. Further discussion with regard to interviewing will be found in Chapter 16.

Organizations also present themselves to you through their written documents. When organizations send recruitment materials to you, they are communicating to you and telling you the things they want you to know about them. Organizations spend a great amount of time and money on material that they believe presents their philosophy and attitude toward patients and employees. What an organization chooses to tell you about, tells you about the organization. Carefully analyze the materials presented to you. This is another way of determining the kind of values the organization lives by and deems important. All of these materials are intended to make a statement to you about who they are.

There are also other written documents to examine. For example, a specific nursing unit might have a "mission statement" that tells you who they are and what they are about. The department of nursing will have a philosophy statement that should be the organizing framework around which they structure themselves in delivering nursing care. In some organizations, people know what this mission statement says and how it provides direction to them. In other organizations, people will be unfamiliar with the statement of philosophy. All of these written materials should send a message to you about the organization.

Organizations are guided by people at the top and take on the characteristics these people support. What do you know about the chief executive officer? This person sets the stage and the direction for the organization. You can gather information about the chief executive officer by asking people on interview what this person is like. People in the community will also be familiar with this person and will give you insight into the values and characteristics this person represents. If there has been stability in the top-level executive team over a period of years, that tells you one thing. If there has been constant change with people continually leaving, that tells you another thing about the organization. The same can be said for the chief nursing officer. This person sets the direction for the nursing organization, either by active design or benign neglect, and sets into motion an organization that structures the beliefs about patients, staff, and nursing. It is very important to do a careful analysis of this person and to ask questions about how people feel about him or her. Has he or she had a successful tenure? Is this person well respected? Can people point to a strategic direction and philosophy this person has given to the organization?

Some nursing divisions organize themselves around a nursing theorist or a philosophy of care. Orem's Self Care Theory, Neuman's, and King's Theories, are examples of organizing frameworks that nursing organizations have adopted. If an organization does not have a nursing theorist, it often adopts a philosophy or model according to which it operates. The adoption of an organizing framework will determine how the organization is developed. From the organizing framework will come the goals and objectives of the department of nursing. These goals and objectives will provide you with a long-range view of the direction of this organization. Individual nursing units also occasionally have such an organizing framework on which to base their direction of care. It is appropriate to find out information like this in order to know if you can agree with its direction/philosophy.

TYPES OF ORGANIZATIONS

The way an organization designs itself determines what the organization will be like. There are many different kinds of organizational designs, any of which will indicate how your job will be structured as you develop and deliver patient care. There are certain structures that you will be comfortable with and others you will not be comfortable with. The structure can range from highly centralized to highly decentralized. To determine if an organization is centralized or decentralized, one must know where the majority of the decisions are made and how much flexibility and autonomy people in various parts of the organization have. In highly decentralized organizations, the responsibility of power and authority has been delegated to much lower levels in the organization. In the centralized organization, the decision making remains at the top level of the organization.

What Is a Decentralized Organization?

In a decentralized organization, subordinates are given a wide range of authority that involves decision making and even policy formulation. At the bedside, the nurse is charged with responsibility to make decisions about patient care and to develop the highest quality of care possible. In less decentralized organizations, this responsibility lies with the nurse manager. In the highly centralized ones, it rests with the chief nursing officer.

The trend in the last few years has been toward decentralized structures. Much research has shown that when people are given more responsibility and accountability, their involvement in the work increases as does their motivation and job satisfaction. However, not everyone is ready for decentralized structures. Some nurses are not interested in taking on additional accountability and authority. They prefer to work in a setting where there is less personal responsibility and accountability and where they can be positively directed by nurse managers or other supervisors in the setting. As nursing has become more of an autonomous profession, the move toward decentralized structures has been a natural outgrowth of that movement. However, not all nurses are willing to move in a more autonomous, empowered mode. Not all organizations are moving in this direction either, so there are options available in choosing the kind of organization that fits you best.

What Is Meant By a Centralized Organization?

In centralized organizations, the control of financial management, changes regarding nursing care, and innovations come from a central authority. In the most centralized structure, this activity comes from the chief nursing officer. Centralized structures are common in small organizations. As organizations move to become more decentralized, activities are transferred from the chief nursing officer to the nurse manager or supervisor. Nursing structures have evolved from a history of very centralized organizations. Because nursing was perceived as a practice that needed much "managing," we have many historical legacies of this centralized management style.

Are There Other Models of Organization?

There are many other variations of the concept of centralization/decentralization. New models have entered healthcare that reflect principals of business applied to healthcare. For example, many hospitals are organized around product line or service line, in effect a hospital within a hospital. Small, unique, autonomous units are developed that can concentrate their interest on a specific kind of patient and kind of care. For example, a women's health center, a children's hospital, a sports medicine center, and an oncology center are all examples of organizing around a certain kind of patient and kind of care. A women's center can be organized within a hospital so as to bring together all the services women can potentially use under one administrator. Obstetrics and gynecology services, as well as psychiatric/psychosocial services, plastic surgery, osteoporosis care, exercise groups, and educational classes might all be coordinated under the accountability of one administrator. A definite marketing plan to attract potential patients/clients to this unit will be in place. In this kind of structure, nurses can either work for the administrator (product/service line manager), who may or may not be a nurse, or can report to the nursing division. Or, the nursing staff can be responsible both to the product line manager and to someone in the nursing division. When people have more than one boss, this concept is described as "matrix management." In the situation where the nursing staff is accountable both to the product line/service line manager and the chief nursing officer, these two people will have clearly defined experience and will set the individual expectations for the performance of the nursing staff.

As organizations design themselves, the organization determines the priorities and how people work within that organization. The role of the nurse in a centralized structure is much different than in a decentralized or matrix structure. There is no right answer to the kind of organization design that is best. All organizations work well in specific situations. However, not all people work well in all types of organizations. Some people do not like the abstract matrix model while others find great freedom in this model. Some nurses are flexible enough to work in any model. Depending on your beliefs and your needs, you will find an organizational structure that fits you best and meets with your long-range goals.

Organizational charts are useful in analyzing the organization. Organizational charts are maps that determine who reports to whom. Some organizational charts will show many managers between the chief nursing officer and the staff nurse. These charts will be pyramidal in design. Other organizational charts will be more "flattened" and will show fewer people between the chief nursing officer and the nurse at the bedside (Figs. 6–1 and 6–2). Some of this is dependent on the size of the organization but is also dependent on the style of governance. An organizational chart will tell you your relationship to the chief nursing officer and chief executive officer and will also identify patterns of formal communication. Five types of communication networks are illustrated in Figure 6–3. These five types are the circle, all-channel, Y, Wheel, and Chain. Most of these basic communication patterns are found in large organizations. As you can see by the structure, the Y organization shows a situation in which two employees report directly to a supervisor within a continuing chain of command. If you have to deal with complex tasks, they are more easily done in less centralized, formal communication networks such as the all-channel, whereas simple tasks are handled most efficiently in centralized networks, such as the Wheel. It also would stand to reason that it might be very difficult to accomplish a complex task in an organization that is like the chain (Schutz et al., 1988).

Committees also provide a clue to the running of the organization. In some organizations, the committee structure is very important and very powerful.

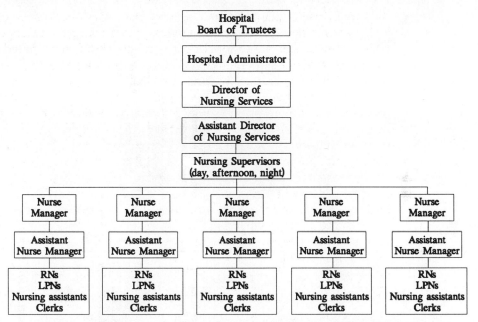

FIGURE 6–1   *Centralized Organizational Structure.*

Some committees, such as task forces or councils, actually make decisions autonomously. In other organizations they are merely advisory, and in some organizations they do not exist. If you have an interest in working within the organization in addition to providing direct patient care, knowledge of the organizational chart would be of importance to you. If you are not interested in anything other than direct patient care, your interest in participating in the governance of the unit/division would not be as great. By analyzing the structure of the organization, you are really asking questions about how the work of the organization gets done. In a centralized structure, obviously, the work gets done by direction from the very top level of the executive structure.

Another way organizations get work done is through participation. *Participative management* is a term for allowing the staff nurse to participate in and provide advice about issues, but not to make actual decisions about the management of the unit or facility. *Shared governance*, which is a step beyond participative management, has come into being in the last few years as a way of sharing certain aspects of the management of the unit or department of nursing with the staff nurse. Over time, staff nurses take on more responsibility and accountability for things such as self-scheduling, the quality improvement program, the recruitment/retention program, and other aspects of managing the unit/department.

An advanced form of the shared governance model is the *self-governed model*,

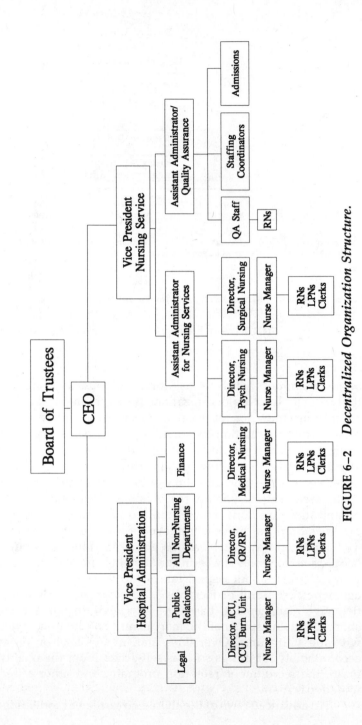

FIGURE 6–2 *Decentralized Organization Structure.*

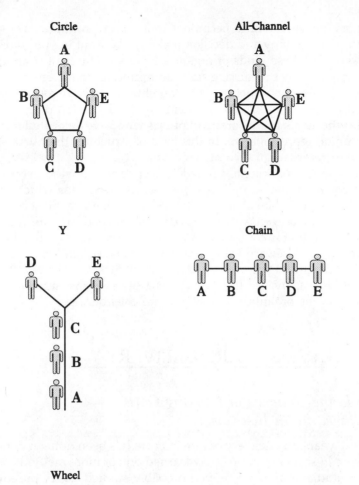

FIGURE 6-3 *Types of Communication Networks.*

in which staff nurses take on all the major accountability of running a unit. A chairperson is usually elected for a defined term to lead the group. This person coordinates the work of the unit over time as others take on accountability for different aspects of the unit such as financial management and quality. Self-governed units are not very common as yet, but shared governance and participatory management is becoming much more common. Depending on the amount of autonomy and decision making you want in your work life, you will choose one of these kinds of organizational structures over another.

Another way the nursing staff communicates to the organization is through a union. In a union structure, the staff chooses to have a union speak for them instead of speaking directly for themselves. The union designates a person or people who speak for the group of nurses who have delegated that responsibility to the union representative. In this kind of structure, the nurse speaks through the union representative to management.

Nursing departments and facilities choose to reward people in a variety of ways. For example, some units have a clinical ladder which rewards clinical expertise or professional accomplishments. Other organizations do not reward individual differences with merit pay and instead provide monetary rewards based on the union contract or an across the board, "cost of living" raise. Organizations also reward informally by various recognition programs and celebrations. Depending on your needs, you will fit with one reward structure better than another. Consider the "perks" and benefits that motivate you; are these available in the organization that you are considering?

PATTERNS OF NURSING CARE DELIVERY

How Is the Delivery of Nursing Care Organized in an Institution?

Over the years, the delivery of nursing care has been done in many ways. While you were in school, you probably learned one or more methods of delivery care. As you studied nursing care, you probably studied a very pure form and probably had the opportunity to practice the kind of nursing care delivery system that was being studied. In the real world, you seldom find the pure forms of delivery systems. People individualize the nursing delivery systems to meet the needs of patients and their staff. Consequently, you must be prepared to work in a system that is not as pure as you learned about in school. One system is not better or worse than another. Various systems are tailor made to meet the individual needs of the people in the organization.

Originally, nursing was organized around the *private duty* model. Registered nurses (RNs) were hired by the patient and provided private duty nursing to one person. The hospital was staffed by student nurses. RNs worked as special duty nurses or in the community doing home care.

The movement to utilize RNs as employees of hospitals came with the advent of World War II. As nurses were required to work more in hospitals, the terrific shortage of nurses during the war effort forced organizations to develop models of nursing. Aids and licensed practical/vocational nurses (LVNs or LPNs) came into being and in some states were allowed to perform functions such as

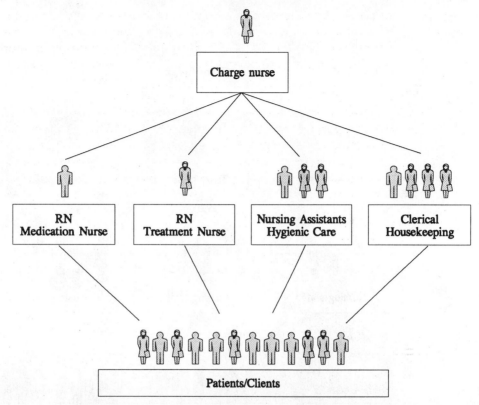

FIGURE 6–4   *Lines of Authority: Functional Nursing.*

administration of medication and treatments. This *functional* kind of nursing, which broke nursing care into a series of tasks performed by many people, resulted in a fragmented, impersonal kind of care (Fig. 6–4).

In the 1950s, *team nursing* evolved. In this type of nursing, groups of patients are assigned to a team headed by a team leader, usually an RN, who coordinates the care for a designated group of patients (Fig. 6–5). The team leader determines work assignments for the team based on the acuity level of the group of patients as well as the ability of the individual team members. A team may be composed of the following:

◆ An RN who is team leader.
◆ Two LVNs/LPNs assigned to patient care.
◆ Two nursing assistants or patient care aides.

Good communication is essential between the team members and the team leader. The team conference is a vital part of team nursing. The purpose of the

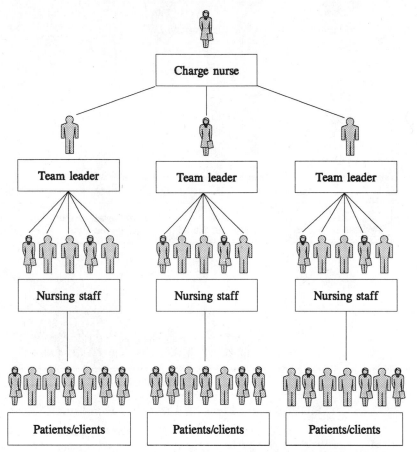

FIGURE 6–5   *Lines of Authority: Team Nursing.*

conference is to assess the needs of the group of patients and to develop and or revise their individual plans of care. It is imperative that the team leader continuously evaluate and communicate to the team members changes in a patient's plan of care. This role often requires the RN to be available at the nurses' station throughout the shift, thus limiting his or her delivery of bedside care. Even though team nursing evolved in the 1950s, there are components of it that remain in current healthcare delivery systems today.

In the 1960s and 1970s, *primary nursing* evolved. In this system, a nurse plans and directs the care of a patient over a twenty-four hour time period. The fragmentation between shifts and nurses is eliminated because one nurse is accountable for planning the care of the patient around the clock. Progress reports, referrals, and discharge planning are usually the responsibility of the primary nurse. When the primary nurse is "off duty," an associate nurse con-

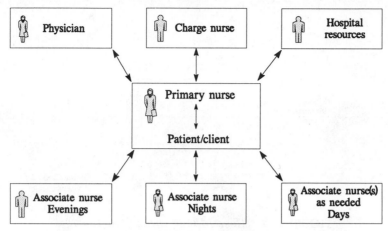

FIGURE 6–6   *Lines of Authority: Primary Care Nursing.*

tinues the plan of care. An RN may be the primary nurse to some of the assigned patients and an associate nurse to others. Some forms of primary nursing evolved into an all-RN staff (Fig. 6–6). Currently, we find primary nursing being mixed and modified with nurse extenders such as paired partners, or partners in care, who are highly trained care assistants who work in a synergistic manner with the RN. While team nursing took the RN away from the bedside, primary and modified primary care have put the nurse back into closer contact with the patient.

One of the most recent models to evolve has been the *case manager model* of nursing care delivery. With the arrival of prospective reimbursement in the form of diagnosis related groups (DRGs) (see Chapter 10 for a detailed discussion) the case managed type of nursing care delivery has become more popular in the acute care facility. Managed care is based on previously identified patient outcomes to be achieved within a specific timeframe while maximizing the utilization of available resources. In this model, a nurse manages a "case load" of patients for which he or she is responsible from preadmission to postdischarge (Fig. 6–7). Figure 6–8 is an example of an abbreviated version of a case management plan that takes into account the number of days allocated by the patient's diagnosis as well as information for teaching and discharge.

Ideally this person has graduate level preparation or is at an advanced level of nursing practice. The case manager role not only requires advanced nursing skills, but also advanced managerial and communication skills. This person may or may not deliver direct patient care. Other care givers (RNs, LPNs/ LVNs, aides, psychiatric techs, patient care attendants, etc.) work under the direction of the case manager. The goal of this organizational structure is to look at the quality and cost of care throughout the patient's episode of illness and

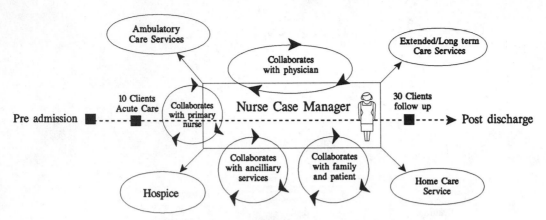

FIGURE 6–7   *Case Management Structure.*

develop ways to treat the patient better by seeing the total picture and continually working to improve the care.

For all of these models, there has been a big push for quality and fiscal responsibility over the past few years. As there are fewer dollars for the health-care system, we must find new models to provide care that will allow patients the high level of care they expect, but within a fiscally constrained environment.

You will probably find in the reality of practice that the expectations for your assignment will be more than what you experienced in school. You will be held accountable not only for the quality of patient care but also the cost. As the healthcare environment becomes more financially constrained, more and more models will look at more cost-effective use of the RN's time. You will also be held accountable for the supplies and resources you consume in delivering patient care. You will be confronted with new initiatives that will experiment with better and more fiscally accountable ways of delivering high-quality care.

How Are Work Assignments Determined?

How your work assignment is determined will vary with individual institutions. A real problem for a healthcare institution is the fact that patient acuity fluctuates dramatically from day to day and from season to season. For example, over the Christmas holidays there is often a significant decrease in the number of elective surgeries, therefore some hospitals may close units. By contrast, in the middle of the flu season, the hospital will be full and might be "short staffed." The amount of staff assigned must reflect the needs of the patient. When there are more patients and sicker patients, more staff is needed. When the patients are not as acutely ill and there are fewer of them, less staff is required.

Facilities determine their staffing needs in a variety of ways. Commonly, the facility has some kind of system to classify patient care needs in order to

NEW ENGLAND MEDICAL CENTER HOSPITALS
DEPARTMENT OF NURSING
CRANIOTOMY-TUMOR REMOVAL CRITICAL PATH
Should apply to 75% of patient population

Patient Name _____
MD _____
PN (ICU) _____
PN (FLR) _____
Date Critical Path _____
Reviewed by MD _____

Address _____
Phone # _____
Case Type Craniotomy Tumor Removal
DRG _____
Expected LOS 7 Days
Farns 5

	PRE-ADM DAY	DAY 1 ICU-5	DAY 2	DAY 3	DAY 4	DAY 5	DAY 6	DAY 7
	> .... OR		F5					
Consult	Anesthesia	Need for Rehab & Social Services			Neuro-ophthalmology Heme-Onc XRT			
Tests	EKG CXR / LBC CBC / Anticonvulsant Level / CT Scan / ABG	LBC / CBC / CT-F/U	Redraw Anti-convulsant level					
Activity		HOB 30-40° Bedrest	Activity as tolerated / Out of bed to chair	Assist with amb.				
Treatments	Call night before Admission [	Neuro VS. q1-2 / Dsg / Jackson Pratt / Venodyne boots / A-Line / Foley / IV	Neuro VS q4-8 → / Dsg .... D/C / Jackson Pratt ..... D/C / A-Line .... D/C / Foley .... D/C / IV ..... D/C IV-when taking adequate PO		check with H.O. how much mobility after D/C / Wash hair, staple out	Dsg off →		
Meds		Anticonvulsant—change to PO / IV Decadron—change to PO / IV Oxacillin × 4 doses / Tylenol/Codeine / ? MS	Anticonvulsant—change to PO .... / IV Decadron—change to PO .... Taper / IV Oxacillin .... D/C	Taper →	Decadron →			
Diet		NPO	Clear Liquid	Reg. Diet				
Discharge Planning			Begin discharge planning-VNA			Confirm discharge date with MD	Discharge orders	Discharge at Noon
Teaching Plans		Pulmonary Toilet	Discharge Teaching (3pg NCR) / Family Teaching →				Reinforce discharge / Family teaching →	

Pre-Op []
Intro to ICU []
Primary Nursing []

Admission Date _____ Discharge Date _____ Discharge Time _____
Days in ICU _____ Variations from standard (record on back) Days in Routine Bed _____

FIGURE 6-8 Managed Care Critical Care Pathway: Craniotomy-Tumor Removal.

(Reprinted with permission of the Department of Nursing, New England Medical Center Hospitals, 1991.)

help in decision making about the number of staff needed as well as the level of expertise required. However, patient classification systems do not measure all the needs of patients. They work on averages and attempt to describe patient needs based on measuring some of the more time-consuming tasks. Patient classification systems are always considered only a guide. There are patients who will consistently require less care than the patient classification system indicates and others who will require more. Patient classification systems are useful in developing the budget for the department because one can look at the historical usage of nursing time to predict future usage. Patient classification systems are also useful as a guide for day to day staffing but can never be used as absolute formula because there are too many variables they do not measure.

Hospital accreditation standards require some kind of acuity system to make sure patients are getting the required nursing hours. Almost all organizations will have some form of an acuity system. This can range from a system they have purchased from a national vendor, to one the organization has developed internally. The most accurate way of determining optimal staffing is through the judgment of a well-experienced nurse who is knowledgeable about quality and fiscal management. This nurse must also use the patient classification system as a guide to determine the exact needs of the patient. In reality, frequently the needs of the patients do not match the number of nurses available. Consistently, there will be more or less nurses than are necessary. The alert, creative nurse can work well in these different situations and will see them as a challenge and opportunity to deliver care more creatively. We can see situations that do not meet the ordinary circumstances as a challenging opportunity to be more creative or we can let them get us down. It is much more fun to see problems as opportunities.

Some nurses have gone so far in their quest for professional stature that they work under a salary model rather than an hourly model. It is difficult to be classified as a professional and work under the hourly wage system. In some organizations, the entire nursing department or separate units have converted to an all-salary model. The advantage of this model is that the nurse receives a given salary regardless of the number of patients and amount of care given. When there are more patients, they work harder but do not receive overtime pay. When there are fewer patients, they work less but do not suffer a loss of income because they are not sent home without pay or forced to take vacation time. In a salary model, which is really a professional model, the nurse works until the job gets done. Some days this might take four hours, some days it might take twelve hours. Over a period of months, the nurses track their overtime and develop a fair, equitable system of sharing the overtime and also the time off when there are too few patients. In reality, many other positions in the hospital are paid this way. Traditionally, billing clerks and admitting clerks are paid a set salary and are not sent home when the census fluctuates. Other professionals, such as social workers and pharmacists, are paid on a salary model. In these salary models, the nursing staff works among themselves to determine the work schedule. Obviously, to go to a salary model, working relationships must be very good.

In addition to determining how the work of the department gets done, you must analyze the work of the unit to determine if this does or does not fit with your perceptions. In some units, portions of the work of the nurse manager are delegated to councils or committees and individual nurses. For example, there will be a council on recruitment and retention, a financial management council or a peer review/practice council. In other organizations, the work of the unit gets done solely through the work of head nurse/nurse manager. In some units there will be active nurse/physician collaboration councils and physicians will be seen as partners in practice. In other units, physicians will talk primarily with the nurse manager and the individual staff nurse will not interact with the physician.

What About Quality Patient Care?

Over time, the way we have looked at quality in nursing has changed. Much of what has been done to control quality has been directed by the accreditation bodies, such as the Joint Commission for Accreditation of Healthcare Organizations (JCAHO), and by professional practice standards. When we looked at the quality of care it was to retrospectively examine the care provided and then to determine if we did, or did not, do a good job. The problem with that approach is that many mistakes happen along the way that are not caught until a retrospective look at the care is done. We have also tried to improve quality by looking at problems and identifying the area that, by our changing, would result in the greatest benefit.

Now the watchword is *continuous quality improvement.* This means that we are constantly and continually looking for opportunities to improve. Even if we think we are doing a good job, we are relentless in our pursuit to do better. We look not only at what the nurse does in the pursuit of quality, but we also look at how the systems of the unit in the hospital can be improved to provide better care at lower cost.

The responsibility for the delivery of quality care used to be vested in the quality assurance department of a hospital. Now it rests with the individual nurse providing direct patient care. As nursing has become more of an autonomous profession, the accountability for quality care has been shifted to the individual practitioner. Therefore, a big part of your practice will be to do a better job than you did yesterday. The organization of quality monitoring is now at the unit level. People who work in various units are responsible for validating quality care, with each unit determining how to measure the quality of care in its own way.

Quality is also measured against the standards of those who consume the care. It does us no good to provide our own idea of excellent nursing care if it does not meet the expectations of our patients, families, and the people who pay for the care. Therefore, the perception of quality as measured by patients, physicians, other departments, and other professionals is becoming much more important. Patients expect certain things from their visit, and if we do not know what their expectations are and do not meet their standards, they perceive that we deliver poor quality of care. In addition to providing excellence in terms of professional nursing care, you will also be charged with the responsibility of delivering care that meets the expectations of all the consumers.

Of course, we cannot talk about delivering nursing care without also considering how much it costs. Today nurses are being challenged to provide excellent care with fewer dollars. To do so, we must take on increased responsibility for the cost of healthcare.

There is no single entity to blame for the rising cost of healthcare. We cannot blame the cost on hospitals, insurance companies, or physicians alone. However, healthcare professionals can make choices that determine how much or how little society will pay for their services. Nurses can help to reduce these costs by becoming more knowledgeable about the cost of equipment (intravenous tubing, syringes, incontinence pads, etc.) they use. Our choice of supplies can have an effect on whether the cost of care will be exorbitant or minimal. Nurses can also help reduce costs by developing and carrying out programs in preventive healthcare. Educating healthcare consumers, whether at bedside or in community settings, is another way to reduce costs.

Such interventions will lead to less medication consumption preoperatively and postoperatively and fewer admissions if the patient truly comes to understand and manage his illness. The cost of nursing care will be a big part of your practice and will be grounds for much discussion as you evolve.

New models are being developed in which we look at the desired outcome and manage backwards to achieve the outcome with the shortest length of stay and the most reduction of expenses. Many payers, through health maintenance organizations and other models, are developing new ways of paying for healthcare. It is common for payers to pay a certain amount (such as with the Medicare program) regardless of the course of the patient's illness. Prospective payments provide us with the same number of dollars no matter how quickly the patient leaves the hospital or how much longer they have to stay because of complications. This is certainly a trend in the future. We will be challenged to develop more innovative and creative ways of attaining excellence in patient care with limited dollars. We can do that. Nurses have always been very cost conscious and cost aware. We are now being provided with more opportunities for that challenge.

The department of nursing is organized in various ways and has a variety of different goals. You will be able to work best in a situation that has a shared system of values with what you believe is important.

▼

The greatest gains in terms of quality and finance will come when people work synergistically and have a shared vision of how healthcare can be improved.

▲

REFERENCES

American Nurses Association (1988): Case management: a challenge for nurses (draft). Kansas City, MO, ANA.

Bardwick J (1991): *Danger in the Comfort Zone.* New York, AMACOM Books.

Schutz C., Decker, P.J., Sullivan, E.J. (1988): *Nursing Management: An Experimental/Skill Building Workbook,* 2nd Ed., Menlo Park, CA, Addison-Wesley.

Zander, K. (1988): Nursing case management: Resolving the DRG paradox, *Nurs Clin North Am* 23(3):503.

7

Effective Communication

Lynette Jack, Ph.D., R.N., C.A.R.N.

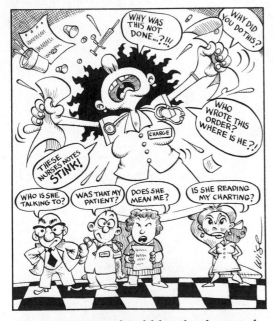

Communication should be clearly stated and directed to the appropriate responsible individual.

Nurse: *What seems to be the trouble?*
Patient: *I keep thinking no one can hear me.*
Nurse: *What seems to be the trouble?*

After completing this chapter, you should be able to:

◆ Describe the basic components of communication.

◆ Identify effective ways of communicating with other healthcare workers.

◆ Describe an assertive communication style.

◆ Apply effective communication skills in common nursing activities.

You are probably wondering why there is a chapter in this book about communicating. After all, you've been talking with people for many years, and things seem to be going OK. Well, you're right—you do already have some communication skills. There, doesn't that feel good? Pat yourself on the back for what you've already learned. This chapter will help you apply what you do well to situations in the workplace that require effective communication skills. This chapter may also help you learn new ways of handling complex situations that commonly happen in nursing. So, if you're ready to proceed, let's review briefly some basic concepts about communication.

THE COMMUNICATION PROCESS

What Are the Parts of the Communication Process?

Communication begins with a person who creates a message, based on her own perception of a situation. This person is the sender, who transmits the message, using words, actions, body language, tone of voice, and facial expressions. The message goes to a receiver, who has to interpret and evaluate the message, including all the signals and the words. When the receiver sends a message back to the sender to let her know what she heard or saw, that is called feedback. So, communication is basically the giving and receiving of information.

Much of the skill involved in effective communication has to do with how clear the message is. The actual words that are used are known as the message's content. Sometimes the words used are very clear and the message is easily understood. But at other times, the words used might mean different things to different people. And the way in which the words are said may change how they are interpreted. Check Box 7–1 to see how many different ways this information can be interpreted.

We all know that the words said make up what we call verbal communication. When we add body movements, facial expressions, and tone of voice to the parts of the message being communicated, we are adding nonverbal communication. An angry voice and crossed arms can change a message from a friendly, supportive one to a hostile and critical message. The way we choose to communicate is known as process. The process may clarify the message or confuse the receiver. Consider this one-act play as an example:

....

SCENE ONE:

Susan has been working on a very busy surgical unit for six weeks since she graduated from nursing school. She is approached by the dietician, who says to her "I was so relieved when I got to the unit and saw that you had

---

BOX 7–1

Try This . . .

1. How many different ways can you communicate this sentence to change its meaning?

   "I don't care how you've done that procedure before; do it my way now."

   _____

   _____

   _____

2. When the instructor says to you:

   "Come to my office at 2:00. There's something I want to talk to you about."

   What are some possible interpretations of the message?

   _____

   _____

   _____

   _____

---

already requested a dietary modification for Mr. Smith following his surgery. Imagine that; I didn't even have to tell you to do it."

SCENE TWO:

Susan: *"Can you believe the arrogance of that dietician? Just because she's been here forever and I'm new, does that give her the right to treat me like I'm a stupid third grader?"*

Nancy (another new graduate): *"How do you know that's what she meant?"*

Susan: *"I could just tell by the frustration in her voice and how she moved away from me so quickly. It was as if she couldn't stand to talk to me anymore."*

SCENE THREE (THE NEXT DAY ON THE UNIT):

Dietician: *"Susan, I wanted to thank you again for your initiative yesterday with Mr. Smith. I was having a particularly stressful day and the thought of having to do one more task just seemed to overwhelm me. You really helped me out."*

    Susan: *"I'm glad you said something about it. I wasn't sure what you meant then, and I feel much better."*

Grensing (1990) suggests several reasons why communication fails to be effective, which can be applied to our one-act play. Nonverbal signals may mean different things to different people and can be easily misinterpreted. So can the words we use. In addition, if we are short of time, it is hard to hear clearly and remember pieces of important information. And finally, the personalities of the sender and the receiver may create a bias or distortion of the message.

What Are Basic Principles of Effective Communication?

Here are some suggestions for improving our communication with others.

1. Communication is a process involving interaction between at least two people. Merely giving information is not communication, unless the opportunity for a response is given.

2. The message sender has a responsibility to make the message as clear as possible. You can verify what has been received by asking "Would you share with me how you interpreted what I just said?"

3. Whenever possible, use the simplest, most precise words you can. Your words must be understood by the listener.

4. Encourage the receiver of your message to provide feedback in order to verify that the message has been interpreted in the way it was intended. The receiver might say "So what you're saying is . . . " or "Let me make sure I understand you . . . ".

5. Remember that nonverbal behavior communicates a message, even when words are not used. Try to match your nonverbal behaviors to the feeling or tone of the message you want to send to others.

6. Your reputation and credibility will make it easier for you to communicate during difficult situations. When you are trustworthy, reliable, and competent, people will listen more carefully and be more likely to interpret your messages in a positive way.

7. Since communication is an interactive process, it is much more successful within the context of a sound relationship. To create and maintain that positive relationship with others, you need to acknowledge the needs, feelings, and contributions of others. This helps create a climate more open to communication.

8. Whenever possible, communicate directly with the person you want to

receive your message. This allows for immediate feedback and verification, and can reduce the chances of misunderstanding.

9. Concentrate on the communication happening in the present. Avoid the temptation to daydream or plan ahead what you might say or do next.

10. Be aware of your personal values and biases and try to keep them from interfering with your ability to communicate.

What Are Facilitative Messages?

Strayhorn (1977) divides messages into two types: facilitative and obstructive. Table 7–1 describes some examples of facilitative messages. These create a positive outcome, where the people communicating with each other feel good about their interactions. It may take some self-awareness and some practice to send facilitative messages, but it is worth it. Your relationships with other healthcare

TABLE 7–1 *Facilitative Messages*

TYPE	DEFINITION	EXAMPLE	EFFECT
1. I want statements	Asks for a specific behavior	"I want you to let me practice this skill by myself, and then check me in three days."	Simplest way to communicate what you want within a relationship
2. I feel statements	Shares your feeling when the other person did a specific behavior	"I felt irritated just then when you told me to clean the nurses' station."	Allows you to get in touch with and share your feelings in a way undistorted by assumptions
3. I like and I don't like statements	Indicates your pleasure or displeasure with a specific behavior	"I liked it when you told me I did a good job with that patient." "I didn't like it when you yelled at me in front of other nurses."	Helps define what would make you happier; positive reinforcement most effective in changing another's behavior
4. Reflection	Tells the other person what you think you heard so he can verify or deny your interpretation	"Sounds like that really upset you."	Helps increase listening skills, reduces distorted messages, acknowledges feelings
5. Open-ended statements	Indicate general area of interest, but leaves specific to other person	"Tell me your reactions to the new medication cart."	Offers attention and encourages communication to begin

TABLE 7–1 *Facilitative Messages Continued*

TYPE	DEFINITION	EXAMPLE	EFFECT
6. Agreeing with part of a criticism or argument	Refuses to argue by agreeing or sympathizing with some part of the other's statement	The head nurse has just said to you, "You don't have any sense." You say, "It's true that I could be smarter than I am."	Avoids wasting time arguing; allows you to remember that you don't have to be perfect; focuses energy on negotiation of wants
7. Asking for more specific criticism	Allows you to ask what behaviors the critic didn't like, what behavior she would like in the future	The head nurse says, "You're doing that all wrong." You reply, "What would you like me to be doing instead?"	Turns an argument into an opportunity for productive negotiation; keeps anger at a minimum
8. Bargaining	Sender offers to sacrifice for the other if the other will sacrifice for him in return	"OK, I'm hearing that you don't want me to criticize you publicly. If I work on quitting doing that, will you work on asking me for help when you don't know how to do something?"	Offers positive incentives for meeting others' needs
9. Citing specific behaviors and observations	Names specific behaviors and events and describes them without drawing conclusions about meaning	"I noticed during the meeting that you weren't saying much, weren't smiling. I'm wondering what was going on?"	Allows the other person to hear about his behavior and clarify what those specific behaviors meant; reduces misperception
10. Asking for feedback	Asks the other person's reaction to what you have just said	"I'm interested in how you react to that idea."	Allows the sender to be sure the message was received as it was intended; allows further clarification
11. You are good, you did something good, your something is good statements	Conveys something was worthwhile	"You've really grown in your ability to handle complex situations." "That was good."	Draws attention to positive aspects of the other person and makes the other person feel good, appreciated
12. I intend statements	Conveys independent action the person plans to take	"I intend to be more careful about my charting."	Indicates the person accepts responsibility for his behavior
13. Communication postponement	Asks for postponement of a discussion until a more favorable time	"I'm feeling hurt and angry right now and would like some time to think before we talk more."	Allows you to be in emotional control

From *Talking It Out: A Guide to Effective Communication and Problem Solving* (pp. 53-76) by J.M. Strayhorn, Jr., 1977, Champaign, IL: Research Press. Adapted by permission.

TABLE 7–2 *Obstructive Messages*

TYPE	DEFINITION	EXAMPLE	EFFECT
1. Communication cutoffs	Statement or action that cuts off communication in order to avoid unpleasant feelings or to express hostility	"Just forget it—I won't ever bring it up again." "You don't care about me, just like everybody else."	Makes it impossible to negotiate a mutually acceptable solution to needs
2. Put-down questions	Rhetorical question used to communicate a dissatisfied feeling in an indirect way	"What's the use in my doing anything for you when you always screw it up later anyway?"	Creates a need to attack or defend
3. You are bad, you did something bad statement	Conveys a negative value judgment about the other person	"You don't care about anybody but yourself."	Makes the other person feel threatened and less worthy; leads to further attack
4. You should statements	Statements that begin "you should have . . .," or "you shouldn't have", or "you ought to . . ."	"You shouldn't feel so bad." "You should have prepared better for this."	Lessens self-worth and may lead to conflict between guilty feelings and anger
5. Defending oneself	Response to criticism in which person tries to prove what he did was right	"It wasn't my fault that patient started screaming; I was trying to be nice. That doctor sure was rough and uncaring, though."	Creates focus on placing blame, rather than looking for a solution
6. Sarcasm	Making a humorous statement, opposite of what is meant, to express hostility	"Oh **sure,** you're **never** late. We all really believe that."	Promotes attack and defense; allows the sender to avoid responsibility for expressing anger honestly and directly
7. Commanding	Directing another person to do something in an authoritarian voice that implies no choice	"You can't do that sort of thing around here."	Creates a power struggle and resentment
8. Expressing dissatisfaction through a third party	Communication not directed at the person to whom it is intended	Susan says to the head nurse, "You really ought to speak to Mary. She refuses to help any of the rest of us when we are really busy."	Allows attack and avoidance, may also lead to distorted messages

TABLE 7–2 *Obstructive Messages Continued*

TYPE	DEFINITION	EXAMPLE	EFFECT
9. Assuming rather than checking it out	Assume your perception of an ambiguous or nonverbal message was correct without checking it out verbally	Susan sees the head nurse and a doctor in conversation at the door of one of her patient's rooms. The head nurse looks angry and is shaking her head. Susan concluded that they think she gave terrible care to that patient. In reality, they are talking about a hospital policy committee meeting.	Misunderstandings persist without being cleared up, and actions are based on mistaken assumptions
10. Premature advice	Offer advice without first having encouraged the person to freely explore his feelings	Susan: "My head nurse really bothers me. She keeps giving me too much work." Mary: "If I were you, I'd tell her off. She has no right to treat you that way. Don't let her push you around."	Often the advice is not appropriate and closes off exploration of the real issue

From *Talking It Out: A Guide to Effective Communication and Problem Solving* (pp. 53-76) by J.M. Strayhorn, Jr., 1977, Champaign, IL: Research Press. Adapted by permission.

workers will be satisfying and ultimately, the patients you care for will benefit.

Strayhorn (1977, p. 7) summarizes the benefits of learning to use facilitative messages: "If I can avoid antagonizing the other person, make my wishes known, find out the other person's wishes, explore various options, and make decisions accordingly, then I am much better equipped to bring happiness to others and to allow them to bring happiness to me."

What Are Obstructive Messages?

Strayhorn (1977) says that obstructive messages generally make it much more difficult for people to communicate effectively within a positive relationship. Table 7–2 has some examples of obstructive messages. The purpose of recognizing facilitative and obstructive messages is to be more attentive to the process of communication, so that you can be more effective at getting your needs met. Try identifying facilitative and obstructive responses in Box 7–2.

BOX 7–2

Try This . . .

See if you can come up with some facilitative responses and some obstructive responses to these situations.

1. You are trying to finish your assignment and your team leader keeps asking you questions. This is interfering with your work.

   _____

   _____

   _____

2. One of your co-workers repeatedly asks you for money and never pays you back.

   _____

   _____

   _____

3. You need to be off this weekend to take care of a family emergency. Your head nurse tells you that her staffing needs must come first and you will have to work.

   _____

   _____

   _____

   _____

COMMUNICATION IN THE WORKPLACE

Communicating with the Healthcare Team

Sharing information with the members of the healthcare team requires different approaches. This communication on a daily basis may involve delegation of a nursing procedure to an LVN or aide, clarification of a doctor's orders or re-evaluating a patient care assignment of another healthcare team member, and coordinating various hospital departments (Radiology, Dietary, Pharmacy, etc.) to provide nursing care.

How Can I Effectively Communicate With My Boss?

Upward communication with supervisors takes on a formal nature. It is important to learn and then use channels of communication. This means if you are a team member, you share information with your team leader. The team leader shares information with the supervisor, who shares information with the assistant director of nursing, who shares information with the director of nursing, and so on. You can see that there are many levels of nursing between the bedside nurse and the people with major decision-making responsibility.

Do you remember the game you played as a child, where someone started by whispering a secret to the person next to her, and each person repeated the secret down the line until the last person, who spoke the secret aloud? The secret may have started out as "Jenny was out picking berries today so she can bake a pie." By the end of the line, it may have become "Jenny is so allergic to cherries that she breaks out into hives." The point is that messages can get very distorted when they travel through many people in the upward flow of communication. Sullivan and Decker (1988) say it is important in communicating with superiors to state needs clearly, explain the rationale for requests, and suggest benefits to the larger unit. It's also important to listen objectively to the response of the supervisor, since she may have good reasons for granting or not granting the request.

Van Tell (1989) gives these tips for talking to your boss:

1. Use the communication style your boss is most comfortable with. This may be verbal or written, detail-oriented or global, and short-range or long-range.
2. Try not to appear afraid of your boss.
3. Try to be as honest as possible with your boss.
4. Call attention to your achievements.
5. Never talk to your boss when your anger has you out of control.
6. Think through what you want to communicate before you begin.
7. Acknowledge your boss's point of view.
8. Ask for what you need to improve, based on your own self-evaluation.

How Can I Effectively Communicate With Other Nursing Personnel?

When you speak with other professional nurses, you are communicating in a lateral, or horizontal, flow of information. This flow is based on a concept of equality, where no person holds more power than the other. This is best done in a work climate that promotes a sense of trust and respect among colleagues. When nurses work well together, their cohesiveness makes success more likely. This takes work and the deliberate use of facilitative messages.

Ideally, professional nurses should view themselves as communicating laterally, as equals, with members of other healthcare disciplines, even including physicians. At the basis of this is the ability to see yourself as competent and worthy of being an equal to physicians, social workers, dieticians, and others. To gain this self-confidence is a major goal of every new graduate. The use of effective communication, as described and practiced in this chapter, will help.

How Can I Effectively Communicate With Patient Care Assistants?

Even a new graduate will soon be providing direction to nursing assistants and other levels of nursing personnel. It is important to remember that those people have needs for satisfaction and self-esteem too. Directions given do not need to be authoritative commands, unless an emergency demands immediate action in a prescribed way. Sullivan and Decker (1988) suggest that when you provide direction, you need to think through exactly what you want to be done, by whom, and in what timeframe. You need to get the full attention of the other person, so you know she is hearing you accurately. Then give clear, simple instructions in step-by-step order, using a supportive tone of voice. Before the other person goes to do the task, ask for feedback to verify that she has accurately heard your instructions. Finally, follow-up is necessary to make sure your directions were carried out, and to find out what happened, in case something more needs to be done. Involving the other levels of nursing personnel in the planning and evaluation of care will increase their sense of responsibility for the outcomes, and will help you to seem less authoritarian.

What Does My Image Communicate to Others?

▼

Remember that old saying "Don't judge a book by its cover?"

▲

Unfortunately, we know that most people don't follow that suggestion. People do get impressions about us from our image—the way we look, sound, talk, and act. Often, we are less careful about the messages we send with our appearance and behavior than we are when we choose our words. But our image may speak louder than our words. Think about it. Would you feel comfortable accepting nutrition advice from a 300-pound nurse? How would you like it if your instructor criticized your professionalism while wearing dirty shoes, a wrinkled uniform, bright red nail polish, and four earrings in each earlobe?

What would you think about a doctor whose progress notes contain many misspelled words and poor grammar?

Communication is enhanced by your credibility. And people listen more to people they respect. Your image will help you communicate a professional credibility. The place to start projecting a positive image is with the first impression your appearance creates (Hunsaker and Alessandra, 1980). Good personal hygiene is a must. Each day you have to pay attention to your grooming. This means a flattering, neat haircut; clean, well-fitting clothes; reasonable makeup and perfume; minimal jewelry; clean, sensible shoes. Your image is improved greatly if your weight is appropriate for your height and bone structure. Your appearance at work should conform to the norms for professionals in your work setting; save your individuality for your personal time away from work.

Another aspect of your image is your depth and breadth of knowledge. You need to know your particular kind of nursing thoroughly if you want others' respect. But you also need to know something about a wide variety of subjects so you can have conversations with people beyond nursing. This means keeping up with current events, learning things about art or sports, reading books. When people discover common interests, they are more willing to communicate with you.

Flexibility is necessary for effective communication with all different kinds of people. It means that you are willing and able to adapt your behavior in order to relate more comfortably or effectively with others. Flexibility is part of a positive image because it says to people that you are willing to accept responsibility for changing your behavior in order to meet the professional needs or requirements of others.

People who achieve success in their professional careers are enthusiastic. They let others know they are happy to be at work. They work harder, longer, and more accurately. They are pleasant to be around. They are sincere in their efforts to create a professional image that can be trusted.

Take an inventory of your appearance, knowledge, and attitude. If you're not sure what kind of image you are communicating, ask several trusted friends.

What Should I Know About the "Grapevine"?

Informal communication also flows upward, downward, and horizontally, and is known as the "grapevine." Some people think of this kind of communication as gossip, while others say it's the way things really get done. No matter how we describe the grapevine, we know it flourishes in all settings, because people enjoy the satisfaction of the social interaction and the recognition, and it provides information to employees that may not be easily available in any other way. This may be the quickest way to find out what new job openings are coming, or what the supervisor really values.

Deep and Sussman (1988) provide these tips for controlling the grapevine, which can provide much distorted information.

1. Provide factual information to answer questions before they are asked. Few employees get all the information they feel they need.

2. Communicate face-to-face whenever possible. Don't trust the accuracy of messages through a third party.

3. Whenever rumors are running through the grapevine, hold a meeting to provide information and answer questions.

4. Don't spread rumors. Make sure you have all the facts from their source.

5. Enlist the support of respected leaders to spread the truth.

6. Address significant issues as soon as possible with your manager, so negative feelings can be defused.

7. Make sure what is put in writing is clear and accurately understood.

COMPONENTS OF COMMUNICATION

How Can I Learn to Communicate Effectively in Writing?

Communication takes place not only when words are spoken, but also when they are written and then read by someone else. A big part of a nurse's work depends on her ability to write effectively. This may mean developing written treatment plans, progress notes, job descriptions, requests for consultation, referrals, and memos. Some of you may even write chapters for textbooks or articles for nursing journals!

Here are some guidelines for writing. Determine whether you need to write in a formal way. Most upward communication needs to be formal, which means you use proper titles, format, grammar, spelling, and punctuation. Never allow something you have written to be sent without careful proofreading. Nothing creates a negative impression faster than sloppy work, misspelled words, or poor grammar. If you need to, ask someone else to do this proofreading, but be sure it is done well. Take the time to make necessary revisions before sending your written work on.

Your handwriting must be legible. If people can't read what you've written, you're not communicating with them, and you're wasting everyone's time. Decide what your purpose is before you write. This will help you to organize your thoughts, so that everything you put down helps you to meet your purpose. Learn to write exactly what you mean. Choose words that are clear and specific. Often, this means simple, small words. Be careful to use technical words only when you are sure you are choosing the correct words and your reader will understand you. Keep your sentences short and simple, with only one idea in each sentence. Try using the KISS principle—

▼

KISS principle: Keep It Short and Simple.

▲

When you learn to be clear and concise, you will write the essential information without a lot of flowery phrases. Your readers will be very grateful if they can follow your thoughts easily. Make your first sentence in each paragraph identify the key point for that paragraph. The reader shouldn't have to guess what you are trying to say. Use a format that guides the reader. This means that visually on each page, main points are easy to locate, and concepts are identified by headings or titles. Remember, how well you write is a strong influence on how you are evaluated. What you put down on paper makes a lasting impression, and people will make judgments about your credibility and professionalism for a long time after you have actually written the words.

How Can I Learn to Speak Effectively?

From giving report at change-of-shift, to explaining your plans for a new approach on the unit, to the organization's administration, you will have lots of opportunities to make presentations.

▼

The first step in making effective presentations is to develop a positive attitude.
ACCENTUATE the POSITIVE!

▲

Many of us let our anxiety intimidate us. But public speaking can be a great chance to show off our skills, our ability to be creative, our willingness to be a star entertainer. Think of your presentation as a wonderful opportunity to have the attention of others on just you, even if only for a few minutes.

▼

The second guiding principle in making good presentations is practice.
PRACTICE makes PERFECT!

▲

A well-planned rehearsal gives you a chance to see how long it will take you to say what you want, and will help you feel more comfortable saying the words easily. Here are some tips on preparation from Yeomans (1985):

1. Analyze your audience. What do they already know and what do they need to know?

2. Have an objective or two for what you want your audience to get out of your presentation.

3. Do your homework. Know enough about your subject to make your talk clear and believable. Make sure you're able to answer at least a few questions.

4. Plan how you will make the presentation, including an outline of the content, and the teaching strategies you might use. This may involve visual aids or activities to involve the audience in active participation.

5. If the speech or presentation is an important one and fairly formal, you may want to prepare a script. This means you write out exactly what you will say, and have it typed double-spaced, with a wide margin on the left side. Here you can write notes to yourself about when to use your visual aids, or when to pass out materials for the audience.

6. The more active your audience's participation, the longer they will pay attention. Choose at least one presentation strategy that involves them, such as question/answer, role-play, or small-group discussion. Key points you want your audience to remember should be highlighted visually on slides or overhead transparencies.

7. Use an attention grabber at the beginning to make sure your audience is listening. This may be a friendly greeting, a stimulating question, a startling statistic, a relevant story, or a quote by an expert.

8. Then, tell your audience your purpose, and what your presentation will cover, in brief and concise words.

9. Visual aids should keep the presentation focused and organized. They help you hold your audience's attention.

10. In your closing, you review what you've said, the summary of the benefits or implications of what you've said, and any action you want taken.

11. Be sure to be familiar with the room and equipment you will be using. Make sure everything you need is there before you begin.

12. Make sure your visual aids and handouts are spelled correctly.

13. Speak with confidence, energy, and enthusiasm.

14. Make as much eye contact as you can.

15. Use your hands and arms to make dramatic gestures. They add energy and interest.

What Listening Skills Do I Need to Develop?

Listening efffectively is one of the most powerful communication tools you can have. It's more than just hearing the words of others. Listening involves concentrating all your energy on understanding and interpreting the message with the meaning the sender intended. At least half of the communicating activity we do is listening, and the average listener remembers about 50% of a conversation. Within twenty four hours, he can remember only 25% of the conversation he heard (Hunsaker and Alessandra, 1980).

There are reasons why people are not good listeners (Yeomans , 1985). We simply don't pay enough attention; we hear what we want to hear and filter out the rest. Listening requires concentration, and that means doing nothing else at the same time. Some people see listening as a passive behavior; they want to be in control by talking more. We think a lot faster than people speak, so we often think way ahead, or daydream, or think about other things. It may be that there are too many distractions that interfere with listening, such as background noises or movements.

One of the most problematic reasons for ineffective listening is that people allow their emotions to dictate what they hear or don't hear. This means we pay more attention to people we like or respect, and less attention to people or messages that make us feel uncomfortable. If the message is making demands on us to do more, or change what we do, or do better, we may stop listening in order to deal with our own feelings of anger, guilt, or anxiety. We may start planning our own defensive response while the other person is still talking.

....

Think about situations you've been in where you've had difficulty listening, understanding, or remembering what was said. Consider these examples:

◆ *a psychiatric patient, who has been newly admitted, displays acutely psychotic thought processes by talking rapidly in pressured speech, using words and phrases so loosely connected that the whole conversation is disorganized and incomprehensible.*

◆ *a head nurse spends five minutes screaming at her team leader, criticizing everything she has done that day, and then asks the team leader to carry out a very specific and detailed change in the doctor's orders for a patient.*

◆ *another nurse asks you to hang an IV solution for the patient in room 1253, while you are writing some progress notes on a patient's chart. When you finish, you can't remember the room number where you agreed to hang the IV.*

....

It becomes essential to develop effective listening skills. Here are some tips:

1. Make sure you can hear what is being said. Move closer; eliminate distracting noises; and most of all, don't talk. You can't hear someone else when you're talking.

2. Focus your attention on what is being said. Actively concentrate by analyzing the key points as they are being said. Take notes. Don't do anything

else while you are listening except to concentrate on hearing and understanding what is being said.

3. Recognize and control your emotional response to what is being said. Focus on hearing and seeing accurately what is being communicated. You will have time to ask questions and explore feelings after the other person finishes.

4. Decide in the beginning that you will listen and accept the other person's needs and feelings, whatever they are. Improved understanding of the other person is gained through listening, and will help you to be more effective in solving problems and eliminating negative feelings.

5. Pay attention to nonverbal communication as you listen to the words. Much of the meaning comes through in the tone of voice, facial expressions, and body movements. You must listen with your eyes and your ears.

6. Fight off distractions. Don't let the speaker's style of communicating or mannerisms, or phone calls and other interruptions break your concentration.

7. If a lot of factual, important information is being given, take notes. But just jot down key words or numbers, or the note-taking will become a distraction. You may also ask the speaker to put in writing what he has said.

8. Let the speaker tell the whole story. Don't interrupt or assume you know what will be said.

9. Make an effort to respond positively to the feelings being communicated. Empathy and acceptance will make it easier for the communication to continue.

10. React to the message, not the person. Don't allow your feelings or impressions about the speaker to interfere.

11. Seek feedback of your understanding by verifying what you have heard.

12. Try not to be critical of what you are hearing.

13. Maintain a positive attitude about listening. Recognize that listening is necessary for success. Allow yourself to hear all sides of an issue.

Identify the characteristics of your listening skills in Box 7–3.

What Skills Do I Need for Using the Telephone Effectively?

Many nurses spend time on the phone, talking with physicians, patients and their families, and other healthcare workers. Here are some tips for making telephone communication productive. It is always polite to ask the person you are calling if this is a convenient time to talk regarding the purpose of your call. Often you may encounter difficulties with reaching people by phone. If this

---

BOX 7–3

Try This . . .

Role play these situations with your classmates. Try taking turns being in the boss and subordinate roles.

1. The head nurse has asked the team leader and the nurse providing care to Mr. Smith to explain his progress.

   _____

   _____

   _____

   _____

2. You are the team leader, giving report to two nursing assistants and one LPN, who will be working on your team today.

   _____

   _____

   _____

   _____

3. You are discussing the care of a newly diagnosed insulin-dependent diabetic with the dietician and the social worker.

   _____

   _____

   _____

   _____

"telephone tag" problem persists after two attempts, leave a message for them as to when you will be available to talk. If you anticipate your conversation to involve complex information, make notes ahead of time so you can keep your conversation as brief as possible, but focused. With detailed, critical information that is discussed over the telephone, it is wise to follow up a written communication to that person. Important phone calls should also be followed up in writing; this helps to clarify and confirm the information discussed. If your telephone conversation requires a follow-up action, you need to keep a written record. It is difficult to focus on the telephone conversation if you are attempting to do something else. Your communication will be more effective if you do one thing at a time. (How many times have you been irritated by a car driver who is also talking on the telephone?) Once you have finished your discussion, get off the phone, don't chit-chat or gossip once the information has been communicated. Communicating with physicians via the telephone presents a challenge to new graduates. Table 7–3 presents some helpful tips.

GROUP COMMUNICATION

How Can You Improve Communications in a Group Meeting?

Nurses participate in many meetings, from patient care conferences to more formal committee meetings. Communication within a group of people can be an opportunity to influence the quality of care given to clients. When you participate as a member of a group, the following are positive behaviors that will help you to communicate effectively and will also help the group to accomplish its tasks more efficiently:

- Come prepared. Bring all the "stuff" you need.
- Listen. Be open to other viewpoints.
- Keep on track. Don't visit or chit-chat.
- Present your ideas or opinions. Ask other members for theirs.
- State disagreements. Be able to back it up.
- Clarify when needed. Don't assume.

TABLE 7–3   *Tips for Communicating With Physicians on the Phone*

1. Say who you are right away.
2. Don't apologize for phoning.
3. State your business briefly but completely.
4. Ask for specific orders when appropriate.
5. If you want the doctor to assess the patient, say so.
6. If the doctor is coming, ask when to expect him.
7. If you get cut off, call back.
8. Document attempts to reach a doctor.
9. If a doctor is rude or abusive, tell him so.
10. If you can't reach a doctor or get what you need, always tell your manager.

All of us have been to and participated in meetings that were unorganized, confusing, and a waste of time. Box 7–4 will assist you to identify some unpleasant group meeting experiences and give you the opportunity to change future meetings.

BOX 7–4

Try This . . .

Develop a listening action plan.

1. I listen most effectively when

   _____

   _____

   _____

2. I have difficulty listening when

   _____

   _____

   _____

3. My best listening skills are

   _____

   _____

   _____

4. I need to improve on my skills at

   _____

   _____

   _____

5. In order to improve my listening skills, I will

   _____

   _____

   _____

What Are the Responsibilities of a Group Leader?

If you are the leader of a group meeting, you have additional responsibilities. If you are organized and able to communicate effectively, the meeting is much more likely to run smoothly. This is especially important when you and your group members are especially busy. You can't afford to waste time sitting in an unproductive meeting. Nothing is so irritating as time spent arguing with others when you know your work is piling up on your desk. If the irritation continues to build, you and the other group members will be less committed to the goals of the group, and some will even stop coming. The key to effective meetings is the planning and organization that occurs before the meeting is actually held. Planning should allow the leader to think through what the meeting is for, who should be there, and how the meeting should run (Yeomans, 1985). There should be a clear purpose for every meeting and every item on the agenda. Every item should require some action by the group. If the purpose could be achieved in another way, such as making a phone call or sending a memo, there should be no meeting.

It is the leader's responsibility to send out an agenda ahead of time, and to indicate any preparations members need to make, or materials they need to bring to the meeting. The leader must also be concerned with the room where the meeting will be held. If you are making a formal presentation, some audio-visual equipment will be necessary and the chairs need to be arranged so that everyone can see the presenter and the audio-visuals. If the meeting is for discussion and decision-making, a table where everyone can sit face-to-face is more effective. Look at Figure 7–1. This type of note taking clarifies who is responsible for what activities. Ask for a volunteer to keep track of the timeline information. At the conclusion of the meeting, summarize the decisions and identify the plan of action. Review the timeline information for clarity and understanding regarding group member responsibilities. At the end of the meeting, the time should be established for the next meeting. All members should receive a copy of the timeline information.

ASSERTIVE COMMUNICATION

What Is an Assertive Style of Communication?

All of us have a style or way of communicating with others, often based on our own personality and self-concept. In other words, the kind of person we are and the way in which we see ourselves influences the process of communication. This style can be divided into three common types: passive or avoidant, aggressive, and assertive. Here are some characteristics of each style:

What	Who	When	Done
Inservice on glucometer	Janet & Deb	5/24/94	
Revise suction procedure	Sue & Bill	4/22/94	5/18/94
Review charting and report back to next unit meeting	Tom & Amy	5/1/94	5/18/94

FIGURE 7-1 *Action Timeline for Meetings*

◆ Passive or avoidant behavior means a person lets others push him around; doesn't stand up for himself; does what he's told, regardless of how he feels about it; is not able to share his feelings or needs with others; has difficulty asking for help; feels hurt, anxious, angry at others for taking advantage of him.

◆ Aggressive behavior means a person puts his own needs, rights, and feelings first and communicates that in an angry, dominating way; attempts to humiliate or "put down" other people; conveys a righteous, superior attitude; works at controlling or manipulating others; is seen by others as punishing, threatening, demanding, hostile; shows no concern for anyone else's feelings.

◆ Assertive behavior means a person stands up for himself in a way that doesn't violate the basic rights of another person; expresses his true feelings in an honest, direct manner; does not let others take advantage of him; shows respect for others' rights, needs, and feelings; sets goals, acts on those goals in a clear and consistent manner, and takes responsibility for the consequences of those actions; is able to accept compliments and criticism; acts in a way that enhances self-respect.

Here are three examples of communication styles. Using the descriptions you have just read, see if you can match the person with her style.

JANE

Jane is a very shy, quiet senior nursing student who can't think straight when her instructor asks her questions in the clinical area. She wishes she could be more like her classmates, who seem to find it easy to talk about their experiences during clinical conference. During her evaluation, her instructor says she doesn't know enough theory and can't handle the pressures of the clinical unit. Jane says nothing, signs her evaluation, and when she gets back to her room alone, she cries uncontrollably.

SUSAN

Susan is a senior nursing student who is highly verbal with her classmates. She is known to be opinionated and in every conference with her clinical group, finds a chance to criticize someone. She blames the nursing staff on the clinical unit for making her look bad by giving her too much work to do and not enough time or help. When her instructor tells her she has not used enough theory in her written assignments, she says "It's not my fault; you should have told me sooner."

MARY

Mary is a senior nursing student who is described by her clinical group as goal-oriented and confident. She wrote learning objectives for herself at the beginning of this last clinical experience, and brought them with her, along with a self-evaluation, for her final evaluation conference. She listened to her instructor's suggestions, thanked her, and said "I appreciate your concern for the quality of my nursing skills. I'm aware now of what I need to pay attention to in my first few months in my new job."

If you decided that Jane used the passive or avoidant style, Susan used the aggressive style, and Mary used an assertive style, you made the right decisions. Congratulations!

Why Aren't More Nurses Assertive?

It seems as though many nurses do not consistently act or communicate in an assertive style. Clark (1978) suggests that, deep down inside, many nurses do not see themselves as equal to others. Thus, they have a hard time believing in their own rights, feelings, or needs. This difficulty may have gotten its start in childhood, thorugh exposure to many negative statements or experiences. It's important to recognize that communication style is learned and reinforced over time. Within nursing school and work in the nursing profession, additional experiences or comments may reinforce those negative messages about self-worth. It can be very difficult to change behavior, especially when risk-taking is necessary. The first step is to recognize what the barriers are. What is it that prevents you from being more assertive? Is it previously learned behavior or are you afraid of the repercussions of assertive communication? Check the list in Box 7–5—how many do you feel are true and therefore blocking your ability to develop more assertive communication?

BOX 7–5

Try This . . .

Think of particularly **unpleasant** experiences you've had at meetings. You might think about meetings involving your clinical group or your class officers. Develop a list of ideas about what was wrong with those meetings.

_____

_____

_____

_____

_____

_____

_____

Look over this list of barriers to assertive communication and think about yourself. Do any of these explain your feelings? Assertiveness takes self-awareness and practice. It will help you to identify and accept where you are right now with regard to assertiveness, so that you can make a plan to develop more skills.

What Are the Benefits of Assertiveness?

Assertive communication is the most effective way to let other people know what you feel, what you need, and what you are thinking. It helps you to feel good about yourself, and allows you to treat others with respect. Being assertive helps you to avoid feeling guilty, angry, resentful, confused, lonely. You have a greater chance to get your rights acknowledged and your needs met, which leads to a more satisfying life.

What Are My Basic Rights, as a Person and as a Nurse?

As an adult human being, you have some legitimate rights. You may have to do some work to allow yourself to believe in your rights. You may have learned other values that make it difficult to accept the validity of these rights. But belief in your own value as a separate individual, and confidence in the positive concepts associated with assertiveness as a communication style, will help to believe in your rights. Review the list of ten basic rights of nurses in Table 7–4.

Consider the rights and responsibilities of the nurse. The issue of rights can become one sided. When nurses consider rights, responsibilities must also be included. These rights are yours as a registered nurse; acquiring them and holding them are your responsibility (Chenevert, 1983).

TABLE 7–4   *Ten Basic Rights for Nurses*

1. You have the right to be treated with respect.
2. You have the right to a reasonable work load.
3. You have the right to an equitable wage.
4. You have the right to determine your own priorities.
5. You have the right to ask for what you want.
6. You have the right to refuse without making excuses or feeling guilty.
7. You have the right to make mistakes and be responsible for them.
8. You have the right to give and receive information as a professional.
9. You have the right to act in the best interest of the patient.
10. You have the right to be human.

Reprinted with permission from Chenevert, M (1983): *STAT: Special Techniques in Assertiveness Training for Women in the Health Professions*. St. Louis, C.V. Mosby.

Rights	Responsibilities
To speak up	To listen
To take	To give
To have problems	To find solutions
To be comforted	To comfort others
To work	To do your best
To make mistakes	To correct your mistakes
To laugh	To make other happy
To have friends	To be a friend
To criticize	To praise
To have your efforts rewarded	To reward others' efforts
To independence	To be dependable
To cry	To dry tears
To be loved	To love others

Reprinted with permission from Chenevert, M (1983): *STAT: Special Techniques in Assertiveness Training for Women in the Health Professions.* St. Louis, C.V. Mosby.

How Can I Begin to Practice Assertive Communication?

There are a variety of ways to learn to be more assertive in your communication style, but they all involve self-awareness and practice. It may not feel totally comfortable at first, but as you work at it, assertive communication will come more naturally.

▼

Changing one's behavior requires a conscious decision.

▲

You want to practice being assertive in a situation where there is minimal risk to you, so that you can experience success. If sharing your feelings with your instructor or head nurse makes you extremely uncomfortable, set the situation aside. You can work on it after you are more confident. Share your feelings and practice being assertive with someone you are comfortable with, where personal risk is at a minimum.

It is helpful to practice being assertive by yourself at first. Rehearse what you might say by talking to yourself while looking in a mirror. Once you feel more comfortable, ask a friend to help you practice. The two of you can role-play some assertive conversations. You may even want to videotape or audiotape your practice, so you can get an idea of how you look and how you sound. When you are ready, try out your new assertive communication skills in a mildly uncomfortable situation you would like to change. Pay attention to how you feel. Ask for feedback from the other person. You'll then be able to evaluate your progress and decide what other information you want to practice.

What Are the Components of Assertive Communication?

When you communicate assertively, you are able to describe your own feelings and needs, listen and acknowledge the other person's feelings and needs, define the problem clearly and nonjudgmentally, use body language confidently, and negotiate a workable compromise both can accept.

Here are two ways to think about expressing your feelings and needs:

Strategy 1

> I think . . .
>
> I feel . . .
>
> I want . . .

Strategy 2

> I feel . . . about . . . because . . .

Let's look at an example for each of these.

> *I think we've been working every evening for two weeks on that report for the Nursing Office.*
>
> *I feel tired and cranky because I'm not paying enough attention to my family's needs.*
>
> *I want to ask someone else to write a section of the report.*
>
> *I feel hurt and angry about Dr. Jones yelling at me in front of you because I need to feel competent and respected at work.*

These statements can be successful when you maintain direct eye contact, stand up straight, and speak in a clear, audible, firm tone of voice. After expressing your own feelings and needs, it's helpful to seek clarification of the other person's feelings or needs. This can be done with questions such as:

"How do you feel about that?"

"What were you thinking and feeling at that time?"

"How would that affect you?"

With skillful listening and clear communication, the problem can be defined without placing blame or "putting down" the other person. Notice the use of "I" messages. That indicates willingness to accept responsibility for the process of defining the problem and negotiating a workable solution. To find a compromise, you have to be willing to meet the other person halfway. You may agree to try it your way one time and the other person's the next. Or you may both agree to change or give up something. You may do something for her, if she does something else for you. Remember that in the work setting you cannot always have things exactly as you want them. You must be willing to change and compromise.

What Are Some Examples of Situations Where Assertive Communication Would Be Helpful?

Communicating expectations

Supervisor: *"You're being pulled to the orthopedic unit today because they're short-staffed."*

Nurse: *"I expect to be oriented into the unit and the equipment before I give nursing care, because I haven't worked on that unit in over a year."*

Saying no

Doctor: *"Come with me right now. I need some help doing a procedure on Mr. Smith."*

Nurse: *"No, I can't come with you right now. I'm doing a nursing assessment on Mrs. Anderson. I'll be finished in twenty minutes and will help you then.*

Accepting criticism

Head Nurse: *"It seems to me that you aren't very good at doing care plans, and they're never done on time."*

Nurse: *"I have been falling behind on my care plans. I would like to look at some examples of good care plans. Do you think you could help me with that? I'd be willing to spend some time at home reviewing them."*

Accepting compliments

Patient: *"You give really good backrubs. I feel wonderful now."*

Nurse: *"Thank you. Your feedback is important to me."*

Giving criticism

Nurse: *"I want to talk with you about your care of Mrs. Samuelson. I found her sitting in a wheelchair alone in the hallway. It is your responsibility to make sure that she is not left alone, so nothing happens to her."*

Aide: *"I don't think that's my job."*

Nurse: *"We talked about your responsibilities this morning when you got your assignment. I expect you to complete your assignment as directed or ask for help."*

Providing feedback

Head Nurse: *"I wanted to tell you that I have noticed an improvement in your relationship with Dr. Turner. He has not complained about his patients' care for two weeks, and yesterday he told me that he had a satisfying discussion with you about home healthcare options for Mrs. Atkins."*

Nurse: *"Thank you. I have been working very hard at not responding angrily to his sarcastic comments and criticisms."*

Asking for help

Nurse: *"It is hard for me to do this, because I expect myself to care for all patients without difficulty. But I am having a hard time with Mr. Jones. He seems to have a way of pushing my buttons so I get angry."*

Team Leader: *"Are you asking me for something?"*

Nurse: *"Yes. I need help in understanding why I get so angry at him, and I want to know how to handle him in a more positive way."*

Remember that you need to evaluate how your assertive communication feels to you, and you need to seek feedback from other people about how you are being interpreted. You need to know if people perceive you as aggressive, rather than assertive. It may mean modifying your communication to make sure you are standing up for yourself without violating the rights of others.

It should also be noted that some situations will not get resolved just because you communicated assertively. Finding a workable solution is a process involving other people, who must take responsibility for their own feelings and needs. When others are unable to acknowledge their feelings, unable to listen, or unable to negotiate a compromise, your assertive communication will have made you feel better about yourself, but may not have produced an immediate solution. But keep trying. Persistence pays off.

Remember, too, that there are some situations in which you must simply follow orders. You can't always meet your own needs; you must do what the doctors or your head nurse tell you to do. Sometimes you must put aside your own needs in order to meet the needs of the clients you are caring for. However, your judgment will increase as you gain experience, and you will recognize ways to communicate your needs and feelings, with the goal of improving the processes and procedures used in your work setting.

Now that you have learned a lot about communicating effectively, try doing the student exercise in Box 7–6. And happy communicating!

BOX 7–6

Communication Exercise

Directions: Use the following situations to reflect on key points covered in this chapter. Think of a way to communicate effectively in each situation. You may want to consider your own individual solutions, and then role-play or discuss your ideas in a group of your classmates.

1. Develop a list of ten patients who are hospitalized on your unit. Give for each patient some personal information, a diagnosis, and some data about his or her progress during the last twenty-four hours. Use the information you have listed to give a change of shift report to the four staff members who will be caring for these patients during the next eight hours.

_____

_____

_____

_____

_____

_____

_____

_____

_____

_____

2. You have asked to speak to Dr. Sanders about your concerns in caring for one of his patients, who will require much physical care when she goes home from the hospital. Dr. Sanders has a reputation for being cold, aloof, and very sarcastic. You have never spoken directly to him alone before.

_____

_____

_____

_____

_____

Box continued.

BOX 7–6

Communication Exercise Continued

---

3. You are a member of the hospital's procedures committee. After attending the last meeting, you have been given the responsibility for drafting a revision to the procedure used when administering controlled substances. You know that you need more information before you can begin your work. Send a memo to at least three different members of the hospital staff, identifying what information you would like them to provide for you. Do a follow-up phone call to make sure you get all the information you need.

REFERENCES

Chenevert, M. (1983): *STAT: Special Techniques in Assertiveness Training for Women in the Health Professions.* 2nd ed. St. Louis, C.V. Mosby.

Clark, C. (1978): *Assertive Skills for Nurses.* Wakefield, MA: Contemporary Publishing.

Davis, M., Eshelman, E., McKay, M. (1988): *The Relaxation & Stress Reduction Workshop.* 3rd ed. Oakland, CA, New Harbinger Publications.

Deep, S., Sussman, L. (1988): *The Manager's Book of Lists.* Glenshaw, PA, S.D.D. Publishers.

Grensing, L. (1990): A formula to avoid miscommunicating. *Nursing 90* 10(9):122.

Hamilton, J., Kiefer, M. (1986): *Survival Skills for the New Nurse.* Philadelphia, J.B. Lippincott.

Hunsaker, P., Alessandra, A. (1980). *The Art of Managing People.* Englewood Cliffs, NJ, Prentice-Hall.

Lore, A. (1981): *Effective Therapeutic Communications.* Bowie, MD: Robert J. Brady.

Murphy, T. (1990): Improving nurse/doctor communications. *Nursing 90* 10(8):114.

Pearce, C. (1989): Doing something about your listening ability. *Supervisory Manag* p. 29.

Raudsepp, E. (1990): Seven ways to cure communication breakdowns. *Nursing 90* 10(4):132.

Strayhorn, J. (1977): Talking It Out: A Guide to Effective Communication and Problem Solving. Champaign, IL, Research Press.

Sullivan, E., Decker, P. (1988). *Effective Management in Nursing.* Menlo Park, CA, Addison-Wesley Publishing.

Van Tell, T. (1989). Communicating with your employees and boss. *Supervisory Manag* p. 5.

Vestel, K. (1990): *Management Concepts for the New Nurse.* Philadelphia, J.B. Lippincott, p. 33.

Yeomans, W. (1985): *One Thousand Things You Never Learned in Business School: How to Manage Your Fast-Track Career.* New York, Mentor Books.

8

Conflict Management

JoAnn Zerwekh, Ed.D., R.N., C.A.R.N., C.A.D.A.C.

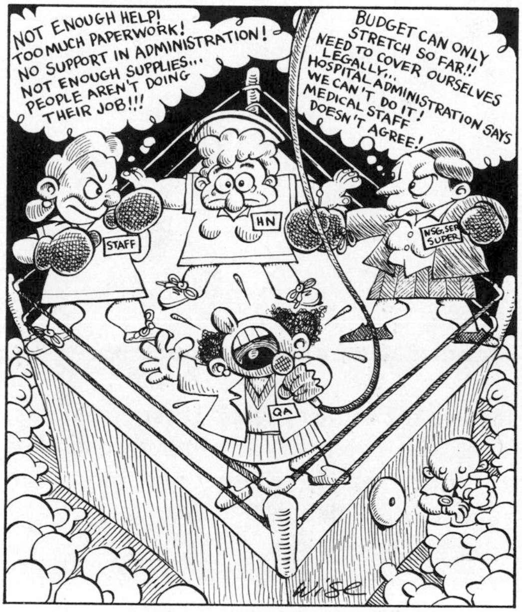

There is a better approach to conflict resolution than fighting it out.

© Copyright 1994 W.B. SAUNDERS COMPANY

Everything that irritates us about others can lead us to an understanding of ourselves.

—Carl Jung

After completing this chapter, you should be able to:

- Identify common factors that lead to conflict.
- Discuss five methods to resolve conflict.
- Discuss techniques to use in dealing with difficult people.
- Discuss solutions and alternatives in dealing with anger.
- Identify situations of sexual harassment in the workplace and discuss possible solutions.

Can you imagine a world without conflict? Why, it would be a world without change! Conflict is inevitable wherever there are people with differing backgrounds, needs, values, and priorities. The presence of conflict in a situation is not necessarily negative, but may in fact have some positive results. As a process, conflict is neutral. Some possible outcomes of conflict might be as follows:

◆ Disturbing issues are brought out into the open, which may avert a more serious conflict.
◆ Group cohesiveness may increase as individuals resolve conflict issues.
◆ New leadership may develop as a consequence of resolution.
◆ The results of conflict can be *constructive*—which occurs when productive outcomes are achieved, or *destructive*—leading to poor communication and creating dissatisfaction.

CONFLICT

What Causes Conflict?

Let's look at some common factors of conflict as they relate to nursing.

Role Conflict.   When two people have the same or related responsibilities with ill-defined or ambiguous boundaries, the potential for conflict exists. For example, a 11PM–7AM shift nurse may be unclear as to whether her shift or the 7AM–3PM shift is responsible for administering enemas till clear on a client scheduled for a barium enema.

Communication Conflict.   Failing to discuss differences with one another can lead to problems with communication. Communication is a two-way process and when one person is not clear, then the process falls apart. A new graduate may find that with a busy schedule, numerous client demands, and a shortage of time she may forget to notify a client's family of a change in visiting hours, only to find the family annoyed that they cannot visit when they arrive.

Goal Conflict.   We all have our own unique goals and objectives for what we hope to achieve in our places of employment. When one nurse places her personal achievement and advancement above everyone else's, conflict can occur.

Personality Conflict.   Wouldn't it be great if we got along with everyone! Of course, we all know that there are just some people whom we just have a difficult time dealing with. The situation is all too familiar, "I'll try and overlook her negative, lousy behavior, after all she doesn't have much of a family life." Trying to change another person's personality is like guaranteeing an unhappy ending to a story.

Ethical or Values Conflict.   During a cardiac arrest, a young graduate nurse has difficulty with the physician's order of "NO CODE," on a young adolescent client. She has difficulty taking care of the adolescent as he reminds her of her younger brother who died tragically in an automobile accident.

Conflicts in nursing may fit into one or more of the above categories. Consider common areas of conflict among nursing staff, including scheduling days off, determining vacation leave, assigning committees, client assignments for care, and performance appraisal, to name just a few.

What Are Common Areas of Conflict Between Nurses and Clients—and Their Families?

Guttenberg (1983) identifies five common areas of conflict among nurses and their clients and families.

1. **Quality of Care.**

    This is by far the most common area of conflict and the easiest to remedy. Families typically are concerned with how well their loved one is being attended to, how friendly the nurses are, how well the hospital services are provided and coordinated, and how flexible the hospital is with visiting hours and meeting their special needs.

2. **Treatment Decisions.**

    This area of conflict often arises between the family of an elderly adult and the nurse. A physician may order a treatment with which the family does not agree. In this situation it is very important that the nurse *does not* get into defending the doctor's orders or attempting to persuade or establish that she may know what's better for the client. It is important to realize in these situations that it is rarely the treatment issue itself, but more the family's wanting to decide what's right for their loved one. Be sure to clarify the orders and explain to the family that you must carry them out, unless the family wants to discuss or negotiate with the physician themselves over changing the orders.

3. **Family Involvement.**

    For example, in the situation of a young adult diagnosed with cancer, there are issues around the presence of family members during procedures and the extent of their involvement in the overall care. Underlying this is the real issue of the family's need to feel significant and to feel adequate in meeting the young adult's needs.

4. **Quality of Parental Care.**

In this situation, nurses are unhappy with how the parents are participating in their child's care. It is helpful to offer parenting classes, encourage parents to meet other parents, and to model positive parenting techniques.

5. **Staff Inconsistency.**

This is another easily preventable issue. Make sure each shift is consistent with enforcing hospital policies and notifying other shifts of any attempts of manipulation by family members or by clients.

CONFLICT RESOLUTION

What Are the Ways to Resolve Conflict?

Unresolved conflicts waste time and energy and reduce productivity and cooperation among the people with whom you work. In contrast, when conflicts are resolved, they strengthen relationships and improve the performance of everyone involved. The key to successfully managing conflict depends on how you tailor your response to fit each conflict situation, instead of just relying on one particular technique. Each technique represents a different way to achieve the outcome that you want as well as helping the other person achieve at least part of the outcome that they want. How do you know which technique to use? That depends on the following:

◆ How much power do you have in this situation as compared to the other person?

◆ How much do you value your relationship with the person you are in conflict with?

◆ What amount of time is available to resolve the conflict?

An example of a model for conflict resolution can be found in Figure 8–1. This model incorporates several views on conflict resolution. Filley (1975) described three basic strategies for dealing with conflict according to outcome: *win-win, lose-lose,* and *win-lose*. Various authors have identified five responses to resolve conflict. They are as follows: competition, accommodation, avoidance, compromise, and cooperation. Let's look at an example and apply the model.

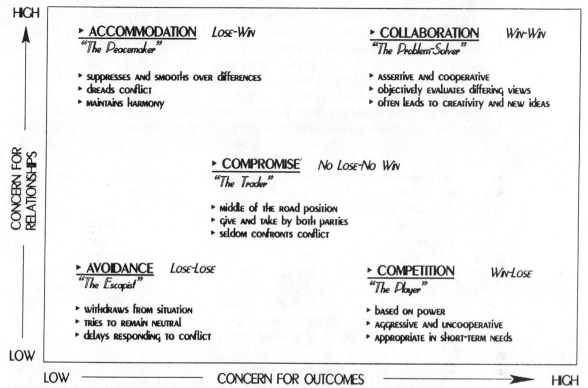

FIGURE 8–1 *Model for conflict resolution.*

(Adapted with permission from Douglas, E., Bushardt, S. (1988): Interpersonal conflict: Strategies and guidelines for resolution. *J AMRA* 56:18, and Sullivan, E., Decker, P. (1988): *Effective Management in Nursing.* Menlo Park, CA, Addison-Wesley.)

....

Suppose the head nurse on your unit has posted the vacations for the month of December. You, as a new graduate, have requested to be off Christmas so that you can be with your family. You notice on the schedule that none of the new graduates on the schedule has received the Christmas holidays off. You feel that this is unfair because you have not had an opportunity to be with your family during the Christmas holidays. How can you resolve this conflict?

....

Competition.   This is an example of the *win-lose situation.* In this situation, force, or the use of power, occurs. It sets up a type of competition between you and your head nurse. Typically, competition is used to resolve conflict when one person has more power in a situation than the other. *In the above situation, the head nurse refuses the new graduate's request for Christmas vacation, explaining to her that the staff with more seniority has priority for vacation at Christmas time.*

Avoidance.   Avoidance is unassertive and uncooperative, and leads to a *lose-lose situation*. In some situations, avoidance is not considered a true form of conflict resolution since the conflict is not resolved nor is either party satisfied. *In the above situation, the new graduate would not have approached the head nurse with the Christmas schedule issue.* Usually both persons involved feel frustrated and angry. There are some situations in which avoiding the issue might be appropriate, such as when tempers are flaring or when strong anger is present. However, it is important to remember that this is only a short-term strategy and that it is most important to get back to the problem after a "cooling off" has occurred.

Accommodation.   *In the above situation, the head nurse would basically put her own concern aside and let the new graduate have her own way, possibly even working in the scheduled slot for the new graduate.* Accommodating is the *lose-win situation*, in which you accommodate the other person at your own expense, but often time end up feeling resentful and angry. Either way, the head nurse loses and the graduate nurse wins in this situation, which may set up conflict among staff and other new graduates. When is accommodating the best response? An example may be when conflict would create serious disruption, such as arguing, or when the person you are in conflict with has the power to resolve the conflict unilaterally? Basically, differences are suppressed or played down while emphasis is placed on agreement in this situation.

Compromise.   Compromising or bargaining is the strategy that recognizes the concern for both the problem and the outcome of the relationship between the two people. It is important to remember that compromise is a moderately assertive and cooperative step in the right direction in which one creates a *modified win-lose situation. In the above situation, the head nurse compromises with the graduate nurse by allowing her to have Christmas Eve off with her family, but not the entire week. The problem lies in the reduced staffing that will occur for a short period of time, which may not be totally satisfactory for either party, but may be offered as a temporary solution until more options become available.*

Collaboration.   Collaboration is the strategy that involves a high level of concern for the problem, the outcome, and the relationship. It deals with confrontation and problem solving. Needs, feelings, and desires of both parties are taken into consideration and re-examined while searching for proper ways to agree upon goals. Collaboration is a *win-win solution*, a commitment to resolve the issues at the base of the conflict. It is fully assertive and cooperative. *In the above situation, you and the head nurse discuss the week of Christmas vacation and the staffing needs and agree that you will work the first three days of that week and the head nurse will work the second half of that week. You also agree to be there the first part of the week to complete the audit on the charts from the previous week for the head nurse. In this situation, both persons are satisfied and there is no compromising what is most important to each person. That is, the head nurse gets her audit completed and the new*

The next group are the maddening ones: the *Clams*. The Clam has an entirely different tactic from the previous three. They just refuse to respond when you need an answer or want conversation. It might be helpful to try to read a Clam's nonverbal communication. Watch out for wrinkled brows, a frown, or a sigh. How to deal with a Clam? Try to get them to open up by using open-ended questions and waiting very quietly for a response. Don't fill in their silence with your conversation. Give yourself enough time to wait with composure. Sometimes a little "clamming" on your own part might be helpful using the technique called "friendly, silent stare" or FSS. The way to set up the FSS is to have a very inquisitive, expectant expression on your face with raised eyebrows, wide eyes, and maybe a slight smile—all nonverbal cues to the Clam that you're waiting for her to speak. When Clams finally open up, be very attentive. Watch your own impulses don't bubble over with happiness that they've finally given you two moments of their time. Avoid the polite ending; in other words, get up and say, "This was important to me. I'm not going to let this issue drop. I'll be back to talk to you tomorrow at 2:00 o'clock." Don't be the nice guy and say, "Thanks for coming in. Have a nice weekend. I'll see you tomorrow." Be very direct and inform the Clam what you're going to do, especially if the desired discussion did not occur.

What Is Anger?

Anger is something that we feel. Usually when we get angry we assume it's because we're upset about what someone has done to us. Often we want to pay them back, or take out our rage on them. Usually when anger occurs, it's hard to see beyond the moment because most people are consumed with thoughts of revenge or the wrongdoing that has occurred to them. Weiss (1991) states, "Anger is often a cover-up emotion . . . that disguises what is really going on inside you." Yet, anger is a signal, and according to Lerner (1985), "one worth listening to." She goes on further to say:

> "Our anger may be a message that we are being hurt, that our rights are being violated, that our needs or wants are not being adequately met, or simply that something is not right. Our anger may tell us that we are not addressing an important emotional issue in our lives, or that too much of our self   our beliefs, values, desires, or ambitions—is being compromised in a relationship. Our anger may be a signal that we are doing more and giving more than we can comfortably do or give. Or our anger may warn us that others are doing too much for us, at the expense of our own competence and growth. Just as physical pain tells us to take our hand off the hot stove, the pain of our anger preserves the very integrity of our self. Our anger can motivate us to say 'no' to the ways in which we are defined by others and 'yes' to the dictates of our inner self."

BOX 8–1

How Do I Resolve Conflict?

Place a 5 beside the sentence you think is most like yourself (the real you), a 4 beside the next, then 3, 2, 1, respectively.

_____ A. When conflict arises, I try to remain neutral.

_____ B. I try to avoid generating conflict; but when it does appear, I try to soothe feelings to keep people together.

_____ C. I try to find fair solutions that accommodate others.

_____ D. I try to cut it off or to win my position.

_____ E. I try to identify reasons for it and seek to resolve the underlying issues.

Reprinted with permission from Blake, R., Mouton, J., Trapper, M. (1981): *Grid Approaches for Managerial Leadership in Nursing*, St. Louis, C.V. Mosby, p. 9.

---

graduate gets to spend half of the Christmas week with her family. What is your particular style for resolving conflict (Box 8–1)?

What Are Some Basic Guidelines for Which Technique to Use?

In some situations, certain techniques and responses work best. You may have to use accommodation or avoidance when you lack the power to change the situation. When you have conflict in a relationship that you value, it might be more helpful to use accommodation, compromise, or collaboration. When there is no immediate, pressing sense of time to solve an issue, then any of the five techniques can be used. However, when you're facing an emergency situation or a rapidly approaching deadline, your best bet is to use competition or accommodation. Just remember these key behaviors in managing conflict:

◆ Deal with issues, not personalities.
◆ Take responsibility for yourself and your participation.
◆ Communicate openly.
◆ Listen actively.
◆ Sort out the issues.
◆ Identify key themes in the discussion.
◆ Weigh the consequences.

Suppose you follow all of these suggestions and you still are confronted with that difficult situation or that difficult person. Read on . . . .

DEALING WITH DIFFICULT PEOPLE

How Do You Deal With Difficult People?

Now that we've discussed what types of conflict management techniques to use, the next issue to look at is techniques to use when handling difficult people. In other words, how do you deal with an abusive doctor or supervisor, or how do you react when someone constantly complains and gripes about something, or how do you deal with the know-it-all who won't even listen to your thoughts on an issue?

I'm sure if you haven't by now, you will, in the near future, run into a *"Sherman tank."* According to Branson (1981), Sherman tanks are the attackers. They come out charging and are often abusive, abrupt, and intimidating. But more importantly, they tend to be just downright overwhelming.

Remember Dr. Smith, who flew into a tirade because you forgot to have a suture removal set at his patient's bedside at 8 AM sharp? My heart was beating so loud I could hear it and was sure everyone else around could hear it too. I was so furious at him for the comments that he made.

One of the important things in understanding Sherman tanks is to realize that they have a strong need to prove to themselves as well as to others that their view of the situation is what's right. They have a very strong sense of what others ought to do or should do, but often lack the caring and the trust that would be helpful in getting something done. They usually achieve what they want, but in doing so, it costs them a lot of disagreements as well as lost friendships and relationships with their co-workers. Sherman tanks are often very confident in themselves and tend to de-value those who they feel are not confident. Unfortunately, they demean others in a way that makes them look very self-important and superior. How do you cope with a Sherman tank? The most important thing is to keep your fear and anger under control and avoid an outright confrontation about who's right and who's wrong. Here are some specific things you should do:

◆ Don't get run over, step aside.
◆ Stand up for yourself. Defend yourself, but without fighting.
◆ Give them a little time to run down and express what they might be ranting about.

◆ Never worry about being rude; get your word in any which way you c
◆ If possible, try to get them to sit down. Be sure to maintain eye con with them while you are stating your opinions and perceptions very for fully.
◆ Don't argue with them or try to cut them down.
◆ When they finally hear you, be ready to be friendly.

Next to the Sherman tanks are the *Snipers*. The Snipers are the pot-sho artists. They are not as openly aggressive as the Sherman tanks, their weapons are their innuendoes and their digs—and their nonplayful teasing, which is definitely aimed to hurt you. Snipers tend to choose a hidden rather than a frontal attack. They prefer to undercut you and make you look ridiculous. So, when you're dealing with a Sniper remember to expose the attack, that is, "smoke them out." Ask them very calmly:

"That sounded like a put-down. Did you really mean it that way?"
or you might say:
"Do I understand that you don't like what I'm saying? It sounds as if you are making fun of me. Are you?"

When a Sniper is giving you criticism, be sure to get group confirmation or denial. Ask questions like, "Does anyone else see the issue this way?", or "It seems as though we have a difference of opinion," or "Exactly what is the issue here or what is it that you don't like about what occurred?" One way to prevent sniping, is by setting up regular problem-solving meetings with that person.

Another difficult person to cope with is the *Constant Complainer*. They often feel as though they are powerless and often get attention, though they seldom get action in what they're doing. A complainer points out real problems, but does it from a very nonconstructive stance. Coping with a complainer can be a challenge. First, it's important to listen to the complaints, then acknowledge them and make sure you understand what they said by paraphrasing it or checking out your perception of how they feel. Don't necessarily agree with what they are complaining about; with a complainer, it's important to move into a problem-solving mode by asking very specific, informative questions and encouraging complaints to be submitted in writing. For example, try communicating with the Constant Complainer in the following manner:

"Did I understand you to say that you are having difficulty with your client assignment?" "Would it be helpful if I went to the pharmacy for you, so that you could complete your charting on your preoperative client?"

No matter what, when feelings of frustration or disappointment or power-lessness take over, there is no doubt anger is in the making. Anger seems to begin in situations fraught with threats and anxiety.

Anger has two faces; one is guilt, which is anger aimed toward ourself at what we did or did not do, and the other is resentment, which is anger directed toward others at what they did or did not do. Regardless, the following is true about guilt and resentment: it accumulates over time and leads to a cycle of negative energy that poisons our relationships and stifles our personal growth.

However, there is another side of the coin. If feeling angry signifies a problem, then ventilating anger does not necessarily solve it. Actually ventilating anger may serve to maintain it if change and successful resolution do not occur. Tavris (1984) suggests that we teach two things about dealing with anger. First, how to think about anger, and second, how to reduce the tension. More about this later on.

Lerner (1985) gives some helpful advice as to how to determine your char-acteristic style of managing anger. Table 8–1 has a summary of five different anger styles. Just think about anger from a cardiovascular point of view. Most authorities consider anger as one of the most damaging and dangerous emotions, because your pulse and blood pressure become elevated, sometimes to dan-gerous highs.

What Is the Solution for Dealing With Anger?

▼

Change the image of it!!

▲

Stop.   Appraise the situation. Don't do a thing. You're at a pivot point. You have two ways to go: one is to get angry, the other is to re-appraise the situation. Try to look at a way to reinterpret the annoying comment.

TABLE 8–1   *Characteristic Styles of Managing Anger*

PURSUERS

- ◆ React to anxiety by seeking greater togetherness in a relationship.
- ◆ Place a high value on talking things out and expressing feelings.
- ◆ Feel rejected and take it personally when someone close to them wants more time and space alone or away from the relationship.
- ◆ Tend to pursue harder and then coldly withdraw when an important person seeks distance.
- ◆ May negatively label themselves as "too dependent" or "too demanding" in a relationship.
- ◆ Tend to criticize their partner as someone who can't handle feelings or tolerate closeness.

Table continued on following page

TABLE 8–1   *Characteristic Styles of Managing Anger Continued*

DISTANCERS

- ◆ Seek emotional distance or physical space when stress is high.
- ◆ Consider themselves to be self-reliant and private persons—more "do-it-yourselfers" than help-seekers.
- ◆ Have difficulty showing their needy, vulnerable, and dependent sides.
- ◆ Receive such labels as "emotionally unavailable," "withholding," and "unable to deal with feelings" from significant others.
- ◆ Manage anxiety in personal relationships by intensifying work-related projects.
- ◆ May cut off a relationship entirely when things get intense.
- ◆ Open up most freely when they are not pushed or pursued.

UNDERFUNCTIONERS

- ◆ Tend to have several areas where they just can't get organized.
- ◆ Become less competent under stress, thus inviting others to take over.
- ◆ Tend to develop physical or emotional symptoms when stress is high in either the family or the work situation.
- ◆ May become the focus of family gossip.
- ◆ Earn such labels as the "patient," the "fragile one," "the sick one," the "problem," or the "irresponsible one."
- ◆ Have difficulty showing their strong, competent side to intimate others.

OVERFUNCTIONERS

- ◆ Know what's best not only for themselves but for others as well.
- ◆ Move in quickly to advise, rescue, and take over when stress hits.
- ◆ Have difficulty staying out and allowing others to struggle with their own problems.
- ◆ Avoid worrying about their own personal goals and problems by focusing on others.
- ◆ Have difficulty sharing their own vulnerable, underfunctioning side, especially with those people who are viewed as having problems.
- ◆ May be labeled the person who is "always reliable" or "always together."

BLAMERS

- ◆ Respond to anxiety with emotional intensity and fighting.
- ◆ Have a short fuse.
- ◆ Expend high levels of energy trying to change someone who does not want to change.
- ◆ Engage in repetitive cycles of fighting that relieve tension but perpetuate the old pattern.
- ◆ Hold another person responsible for one's own feelings and actions.
- ◆ See others as the sole obstacle to making changes.

Adapted with permission from Lerner, H. (1985): *Dance of Anger*, New York, Harper & Row.

For example:

> *"Who does that head nurse think he is to treat me like I'm a dummy!",*
> *or "How could someone be so thoughtless to not remember my birthday!"*
> *You can re-interpret these and say to yourself, "Maybe that person's having*
> *a rough day", or "Maybe if they weren't so unhappy, they wouldn't have*
> *considered doing such a thing."*

The important thing here is to empathize with the person's behavior and try to find justifications with what was so annoying to you.

Look.   What image (shoulds, musts, or need tos) about yourself or another is about to be or has been breached? In other words, what has just occurred that has led you to feel angry at yourself or another?

> *After receiving the end of shift report and making rounds on her clients,*
> *a new graduate goes into a client's room to take vital signs. Within moments*
> *the client has a cardiac arrest. Two hours later while completing her charting,*
> *the new graduate states guiltily, "I should have taken those vital signs earlier.*
> *It just needs to be the first thing I do when I get on the unit. I should have*
> *been on top of this. I must do better."*

Notice the beratement and self-criticism in the new graduate's comments. Guilt, like resentment, can be a habit. It demonstrates—too clearly—how we respond to a situation in a negative manner. To help you get in touch with these feelings, try eliminating the words, "must and should," from your vocabulary for just an hour. It's quite a surprising experience to find out how frequently we use these terms.

Change.   How do you change the image? One of the ways of changing the image is to use humor. Humor makes the anger (guilt and resentment) tolerable. Remember that it's difficult to laugh and frown at the same time. (It only takes fifteen facial muscles to laugh, but twice that many to frown.) If reappraising the situation and humor fail as ways to deal with your anger, some sources suggest to ventilate the anger by getting mad, yelling, shouting, telling someone off, breaking things, etc. While this might momentarily make you feel better, in the long run such outbursts make us feel worse.

Why does this method of ventilating anger, that is, letting it all hang out, make us feel worse? First off, think of all the physiological changes that are occurring in your body: ↑ blood pressure, ↑ pulse, ↑ respirations, muscles contract, adrenalin is released (Sound familiar? It's the "fight or flight" adrenal response.) Can this be a healthy approach to our body to maintain it in a constant state of stress and readiness to respond? Another disadvantage of an uninhibited outburst of anger is that it may lead the other person to retaliate against us.

It might be important for us here to recognize the difference between ventilating and acknowledging our anger. A typical expression of anger might be something like the following:

....

"Hey, you turkey, what do you think you're doing? Don't you know how to put that catheter in? Are you stupid or something? Either you figure it out or you get out of here. You hear me?"

....

This example is both insulting and demeaning as well as accusing. It's likely to lead to some type of provoking comment. On the other hand, when we acknowledge our feelings, we make statements such as, *"I feel angry about . . . "*, *"I feel hurt about . . . "*, *"I feel guilty about . . . "*. Using "I" statements is our first step toward taking responsibility for ourselves by owning up to our own feelings instead of blaming someone else.

Ventilating anger simply doesn't work, unless you want to intimidate those around you, coerce others into submission with a hot temper, or better yet, look childish ranting and raving while beating the floor or each other with foam bats or battacas. So, what does work?

◆ First, acknowledge the anger *(Face it)*: "What am I feeling? Anger? Guilt? Rage? Resentment?"

◆ Second, identify the provoking or triggering situation *(Embrace it)*: "What caused this feeling? Who's problem is it?"

◆ Third, determine what changes need to occur *(Erase it)*: "What can I change? Can I accept what I cannot change? Take action and let go of the rest."

Other ways to deal with anger and get out of the vicious cycle of guilt and resentment include the following:

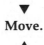

Move.

Get active, try exercise or anything with physical activity, such as walking, aerobics, running. Clean out the garage or a kitchen drawer. If you are sitting, get up. If you are in bed, move your arms around. Just get up and do something!

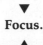

Focus.

Refocus on something positive. Think of your cup as half full, not half empty. Look at the provoking situation: "My head nurse won't give me Christmas off. However, I am not scheduled to work either Christmas Eve or New Year's Eve. So, by working Christmas Day, I'm assured the other days off."

Breathe.

Pay attention to your breathing. Slow it down. Take deep, slow breaths, feeling the air move through your nose and down into your lungs. Check out your body for areas of tenseness, often anger can be felt as a tightness in the chest and abdomen.

Conflict is an inevitable part of our day-to-day experience. How we negotiate and handle conflict and anger may not always be easy. You might be thinking right now, "This looks good on paper. But in real life, it's not that easy to put into practice." If you are feeling this way, take a risk at changing your approach and viewpoint.

▼

The important thing is *learning* about yourself.

▲

How do you deal with conflict? How do you handle difficult people? How do you respond when angry?

SEXUAL HARASSMENT IN THE WORKPLACE

Why bring up the issue of sexual harassment? Because today sexual harassment as a source of conflict has been taken seriously, as evidenced by the widespread visibility and increased recognition of the issue. The potential impact of harassment on nursing students both in the classroom and in the practice area is significant. According to Dowell (1992), nursing administrators and educators must be proactive in writing and implementing policies regarding sexual harassment.

The issue of sexual harassment came to the forefront during the 1991 confirmation hearings of Supreme Court Justice Clarence Thomas (Allen, 1992). Now a once-feared and secretive problem is openly discussed in newspapers and by the media. With the increasing awareness about sexual harassment, we all realized how little we knew about it and what we could do about it. The majority of cases involve women who report being harassed by men. In nursing the stereotype situation of sexual harassment usually involves a nurse (female) and a doctor (male), because of the large number of nurses who are women. However, with the increase in number of men entering the nursing profession, there is the potential for men to experience sexual harassment by women in the workplace.

What Is Sexual Harassment?

According to Friedman (1992, p. 9), "sexual harassment refers to conduct, typically experienced as offensive in nature, in which unwanted sexual advances are made in the context of a relationship of unequal power or authority." He goes on to explain that sexual harassment victims are subjected to sexually oriented verbal comments, unconsented touching, and requests for sexual favors. The typical type problem, also called *quid pro quo harassment*, arises when unwelcome sexual advances have been made and an employee is required to submit to those demands as a condition of employment, or because submission affects employment decisions or employment promotions. Recently, "hostile work environment" as a legal claim has been used to show that "the atmosphere in the work (or other) environment is so uncomfortable or offensive by virtue of sexual advances, sexual requests, or sexual innuendoes that it amounts to a hostile environment," (Friedman, 1992, p. 16). Let's look at a possible example of how this may affect nursing.

> *Tracey, a new graduate working in the surgical area of the hospital, has been receiving compliments by the chief of surgery. Eventually he asked her out and told her that if she would have an affair with him, he would make certain she was promoted to shift supervisor as soon as the position became vacant.*
>
> *Lisa, the evening charge nurse, was quite excited that Tom, a new graduate, was going to work on her unit. Lisa pursued Tom by repeatedly asking him for assistance with patient care and when she called him into her office, she would physically touch him.*

What Can I Do About It?

There are two ways to deal with this type of workplace conflict, informally and through a formal grievance procedure. First, start with the most direct measure. Ask the person to STOP! Tell the harasser in clear terms that the behavior makes you uncomfortable, and that you want it to stop immediately. Also, you might want to put your statement in writing to the person, while keeping a copy for yourself. Tell other people, such as family, friends, personal physician, or minister, what is happening and how you are dealing with it. Friedman (1992) suggests keeping a written journal of harassing events, along with all attempts the victim has used to try and stop the harassment. The need to exercise power and control, rather than sexual desire, is frequently the motive behind the sexual harasser (perpetrator). If sexual harassment is occurring as a result of miscommunication and misinterpretation of actions and is primarily sexually driven, not power driven, then telling the perpetrator to stop will often clear up any misconceptions. However, if the perpetrator is power driven, the harassment will continue as long as he or she views the victim as passive, powerless, and frightened. What may be most difficult for the new graduate is facing the fear that surrounds threats of job insecurity or public embarrassment (Friedman 1992).

If a direct request to the perpetrator to stop does not work, then an informal complaint may be effective, especially if both parties realize a problem exists and want it to be solved. The goal of the informal method is to stop the harassment but not punish the perpetrator. Also, this method assists the person filing the complaint in maintaining some type of harmonious outcome to the relationship. "A formal grievance usually requires filing a written complaint with an official group such as a hearing" (Friedman, 1992, p. 65). This is a legal procedure that is guided and regulated by federal and state laws specific to this type of grievance. Prior to a 1991 amendment to the Civil Rights Act (Title VII), the means of correcting this bad situation—making it right or compensating the victim for difficulty suffered—were quite restricted. What has occurred as a result of this Act is that victims of intentional discrimination may now seek compensatory and punitive damages. Each state has an Equal Employment Opportunity Commission (EEOC), which has as its specific capacity the enforcement of Title VII.

Sexual harassment may be one form of conflict you are faced with in the workplace. Learning to deal with your feelings and being aware of actions to take when this unpleasant situation occurs are important. When resolved in a constructive, positive manner, it allows you an opportunity to feel better about your ability to deal with conflict.

REFERENCES

Allen, A. (1992): Equal opportunity in the workplace . . . sexual harassment. *J Post-Anesth Nurs* 7(2):132.

Bruha, S. (1986): You can conquer conflict. *Nursing 86*(January):81.

Davidhizar, R., Giger, J. (1990): When subordinates go over your head. *JONA* 20(9):29.

Douglass, L. (1984): *The Effective Nurse: Leader and Manager*. St. Louis, C.V. Mosby.

Dowell, M. (1992): Sexual harassment in academia: Legal and administrative challenges. *J Nurs Educ* 31(1):5.

Eubanks, P. (1991): Preventive measures key to sexual harassment policies. *Hospitals* 65(22):35.

Filley, A.C. (1975): *Interpersonal Conflict Resolution*. Glenview, IL: Scott, Foresman.

Friedman, J. (1992): Sexual Harrassment. Dearfield, FL, Health Communications.

Guttenberg, R.M. (1983): How to stay cool in a conflict and turn it into cooperation. *NursingLife*(May/June):25–28.

Isaac, S. (1986): 5 ways to resolve conflict. *Nursing 86*(March):89.

James, J. (1992): Learning the art of verbal self-defense. *Nursing 92*(January):108.

Jones, M.A., Bushardt, S.C., Cadenhead, G. (1990): A paradigm for effective resolution of interpersonal conflict. *Nurs Manag* 21(2):64B.

Lerner, H.G. (1985): *The Dance of Anger.* New York, Harper & Row.

Mallory, G.A. (1985): Turn conflict into cooperation. *Nursing 85*(March):81.

Marriner, A. (1987): How do you spell relief of conflict? Flexibility. *Nursing 87*(March):113.

McDonald, T.S. (1992): When you're feeling defensive. *Nursing 92*(April):122. (Excerpted and adapted from Facing conflicts. *NursingLife.*)

Minard, GF. (1988): Management briefs: Competition vs. cooperation among nurses. *Nurs Manag* 19(3):28.

Roger, J., McWilliams, P. (1991): *You Can't Afford the Luxury of Negative Thought.* Los Angeles, Prelude Press.

Roger, J., McWilliams, P. (1991): *Life 101: Everything We Wish We Had Learned About Life In School-But Didn't.* Los Angeles, Prelude Press.

Rosellini, G., Worden, M. (1985): *Of Course You're Angry.* Minneapolis, Hazelden Foundation.

Rubin, T.I. (1969): *The Angry Book.* New York, Macmillan.

Scafa, W. (1992): Unacceptable advances . . . sexual harassment. *Nursing Times* 88(26):66.

Schutz, C., Decker, P.J., Sullivan, E.J. (1988): *Nursing Management: An Experimental/Skill Building Workbook.* Menlo Park, CA, Addison-Wesley.

Smith, L.E. (1983): Turning negative behavior around. *Nursing 83*(March/April):16.

Sullivan, E.J. (1988): *Effective Management in Nursing.* Menlo Park, CA, Addison-Wesley.

Tavris, C. (1984): Feeling angry? Letting off steam may not help. *NursingLife*(September/October):59.

Todd, S.S. (1989): Coping with conflict. *Nursing 89*(October):101.

Valente, S. (1992): Handling criticism. *Nursing 92*(March):93.

White, T.A. (1985): Nose to nose conflict. *NursingLife*(March/April):49.

Wieland, D. (1985): Working with an angry nurse. *Nursing 85*(July):65.

9

TIME MANAGEMENT

Linda Camin, M.S.N., R.N.

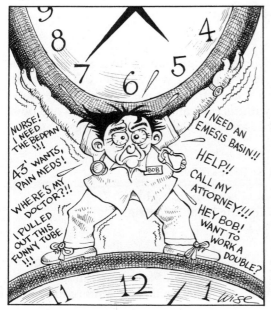

Is time managing you or are you managing time?

Lost time is never found again.
—Benjamin Franklin

After completing this chapter, you should be able to:

◆ Describe your individual time styles.

◆ Increase your organizational skills.

◆ Identify time management strategies for decreasing low payoff, low priority activities

◆ Identify time management strategies for increasing high payoff, high priority activities

S ince you have come this far in becoming a registered nurse (RN), you are already managing time with some degree of success! However, there are so many activities that modern Americans need to accomplish at any one time that deciding "how to get it all done" and "what to do when" is a daily challenge that is sometimes overwhelming. Nursing school really complicates the daily routine. This relentless competition for our attention is aptly described by the term *timelock* (Keyes, 1991).

TIME MANAGEMENT

▼

Time marches on and help is on the way!

▲

Regrettably, there is no way to alter the minutes in an hour and the hours in a day. While we cannot create more actual time, we can alter the *choices* we make in how we use time. The methods and strategies identified by time management experts can help you cope with *timelock* and make choices to use time more effectively. Everyone is busy, but are we doing the right things?

▼

EFFICIENCY VS. EFFECTIVENESS

Efficiency = Doing something right
Effectiveness = Doing the right thing right

▲

This section will introduce you to time-proven principles to guide you in making choices for more effective time management. First, you will learn how to get control of your time, increase your organizational skills, and reduce your time-wasters. Then, you will learn strategies for using your newly acquired hours to achieve your goals. The methods and strategies presented will be applicable in your personal and home life and in your role as a student and, ultimately, a practicing nurse.

Is Balance the Key?

Making time to meet your individual, family, professional, and career needs and goals is vital to overall success. If you neglect your health maintenance needs, completing school or getting to work may be jeopardized. Putting off your school work or household chores to the "last minute" can lead to extreme anxiety and thus stressful behavior, which negatively affects personal health and interpersonal relationships.

Read on and use these principles to meet your time management challenges; they can help you accomplish everything you want to achieve and become everything you want to be.

Do You Know and Can You Follow Your Time Styles?

▼

I am an early bird _____
I am an owl _____

▲

People have different biorhythms that affect their energy level during the day and in different seasons. Do you wake up "raring to go" and enjoy going to bed by mid-evening? Or, do you feel better sleeping until mid-morning and feel more energetic mid-afternoon and evenings? Maybe you prefer to sleep all day and be up all night?

It is not always possible to participate in activities at a time that matches our individual time styles. Obviously, most classes are scheduled during daytime hours and "owls" have to be present and alert. Likewise, "early birds" stay up periodically to participate in late-evening social activities. However, when possible, such as on weekends or days off, you can follow your time style and do those activities that are more difficult (studying for a test) at your times of high energy and do those that are easier (washing dishes) at times of low energy.

Another strategy for maximizing energy and effort is to alternate mental and physical tasks. For example, take a break from studying and vacuum or take a break from charting and ambulate a patient.

▼

Alternating tasks that are mental with tasks that are physical can also help give you an energy spurt to keep going.

▲

When you are working as a nurse, try to be assigned a shift that matches your time style. Studies have shown that when shift rotation is too frequent and does not allow for restoration of biorhythms, more mistakes are made and accidents occur. It may not be possible to get your shift of choice with your first position, but it can be a goal for you as you continue in nursing. If later positions include managerial responsibilities, you will want to consider the time styles of the people you are scheduling. Let's look at the following example:

....

John, who is an early bird, was hired as a new graduate to work the night shift on a medical unit. When an opening for the day shift in renal dialysis became available, John applied for it and was able to transfer to that position.

....

▼

Match your activities to your biorhythms.

▲

What Is Your Dominant Brain Side Times Style?

People also use time in relation to their characteristic brain dominance: left, right, or both.

Left brain dominant people approach time with logic and orderliness. Their thinking structures time by minutes and hours. They tend to schedule their activities in time segments and carry them out in the sequence ordered. Left brain dominant people like to know the rules and "play by the rules." They are usually able to meet their goals. However, if left brain behavior is carried to an extreme, the person is in danger of overwork at the expense of fun, play, and other creative and relaxing activities.

Right brain dominant people resist rules and schedules. They prefer looking at a project as a whole and completing it in their own way and timeframe. These are creative, flexible thinkers. However, their behavior taken to extreme can fail to meet needed completion times, and induce guilt.

Some people are neither left brain nor right brain dominant and thus are more mixed in their behavior. Everyone uses both sides of their brain to some extent and thus has the benefits of their full capacities. They use calendars, lists, and other left brain methods to structure their creativity. Right brain approaches, such as using colored folders and whimsical office supplies, help them "play" into their right brain holistic thinking to solve problems and invent new approaches.

Which are you:

I am left brain dominant
I am right brain dominant
I am left and right brain dominant

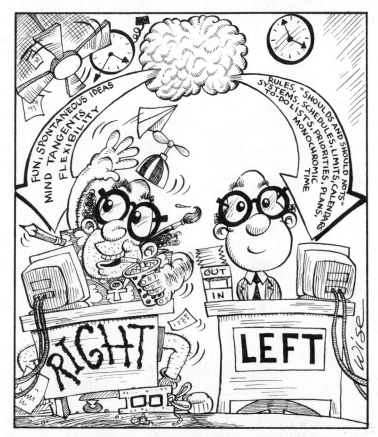

FIGURE 9-1   *Are you right or left brain?*

In addition to assessing your own dominant time style, it is helpful to be aware of the time styles of people you live and work with. Heaping rigid rules on a right brain dominant person will lead to increased resistance and frustration for everyone. Better to assign them clean-up of the kitchen or utility room to be completed by a specific time and if necessary inform them of the consequences of it not being done. It would be appropriate to have some right brain dominant persons on the recruitment and retention committee and some left brain dominant persons on the policy and procedures committee. Knowing your time style can help you maximize your strengths and modify your weaknesses. Individual time styles can be modified but it is wasted energy to fight or work against a person's natural inclination. Now that you are aware of your time style, you can begin to create more time for what you want and need to do by increasing your organizational skills. A little organization goes a long way!

What About Time Managing Your Physical Environment?

▼

A place for everything and everything in its place

▲

Organizing and maintaining your physical environment at home, school, and work can dramatically reduce hours of time and the emotional frustration associated with "looking for stuff."

The Physical Environment

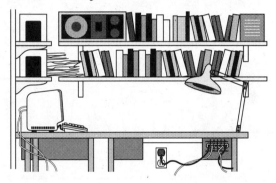

At home, set up a specific work area for such things as school supplies, papers, and books. A separate area, corner, closet, drawer, or cupboard should be set up where you can pay bills, send letters, order take-out food, and take care of other household chores. At school and at work, a locker with extra supplies is also helpful. If none is available, use a compartmentalized carrier of some sort for essential items. At the beginning of your orientation to a new unit, take time for a "scavenger hunt." Tour the area and locate frequently used items.

◆ *Compartmentalize* your areas, carrying bags, even purses. Again, it may not be the time itself spent locating items that is so wasteful, but the accompanying anxiety, fear, or frustration of not finding something or of not having what you need. Men usually carry their keys in a specific pocket; women should keep their keys in a specific pocket of a purse or tote bag. Put papers associated with a class or project in a folder, box or, other designated container.

When practicing nursing, have a pen, pencil, notepaper, scissors, penlight, keys, change, or any other necessary items in a holder that can fit in a uniform pocket and be transferred the next day to another uniform. Such inexpensive serviceable holders can be ordered from nursing journals. Organize supplies for procedures for quick access. An IV start tray or cart with all the needed equipment for insertion of a central line are examples of such time-savers.

◆ *Color-code* files, keys, socks, and whatever you can. Office supply stores are good sources of color-coding items. Color-coding keys with a plastic cover enables you to immediately pick out your car key, house key, or locker key. Drug syringes are color-coded for accurate and rapid identification in a resuscitation situation. One clinical research team copies all their material on purple paper so that all nurses gathering the data can easily identify the correct forms.

◆ *Convenience.* Move and keep items used frequently nearest to where they are used. Keep extra nurse's notes in the area where nurses on the unit chart. Store infrequently used items farther away. A work team needs to agree on where essential items are to be stored in consistently designated places. At home, holiday decorations or out-of-season clothes can be put away in hard-to-reach cabinets or closets.

◆ *Declutter the clutter.* Anything you have not used in a year or more can likely be thrown out or put up for resale. The few items you may wish you had not thrown out can probably be replaced and do not justify the space, moving around, and handling of the other nonused ones. At work, designate one person to clear work areas regularly of clutter.

▼

When in doubt, throw it out.

▲

◆ *Maintenance.* Keep supplies in stock at home and work. Interrupting activities to make a trip for a needed piece of equipment is a definite time waster. If hours are lost looking for or waiting for a wheelchair, more wheelchairs should be purchased. Set up a system with the biomedical department for equipment maintenance. Ensure that when equipment is being serviced a replacement is available immediately. It is also vital to have environmental problems attended to ASAP (as soon as possible). Poor lighting, extreme temperatures, or any other environmental condition in need of repair drains everyone's energy and can be another source of physical and mental frustration. If no one calls maintenance to fix the thermostat in a patient's room, the patient's physical and mental health may be impaired. Likewise, the staff will be interrupted frequently over a twenty-four hour or several day period while everyone lets "the next shift handle it."

How Can I Time Manage the Paper?

The Paper

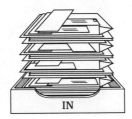

IN

While computers may eventually lead to a "paperless" environment, the paper deluge still is drowning most of us. Handling each piece of paper only one time is a great time-saver. Here are five ways to deal with paper:

- ◆ File it.
- ◆ Forward it.
- ◆ Respond to it—on same sheet if possible.
- ◆ Delegate it.
- ◆ Discard it.

And remember, "when in doubt, throw it out"—especially if you can easily retrieve the information if needed.

For those items that cannot be handled once, use the *A-B-C system*. Sort mail and messages by relative importance. The A pile will require action as soon as possible. The B pile will wait until you can get to it (B items may become A items later, especially if time-dated). The C items can wait until you can get around to doing them. Because of their relative unimportance, most of the C pile items can usually be discarded at some point.

▼

A—Do it now (ASAP).
B—Necessary, but do it later.
C—When I get to it.

▲

In a nursing setting, pace your paperwork by charting throughout the day instead of at the end of the shift. Waiting until the last hour of the shift, when you are likely to be fatigued, reduces accuracy and completeness. Standardized, preprinted change of shift reports, and other kinds of flow charts, also help document objective data effectively and efficiently. There is now "light at the end of the tunnel": bedside and other computers are likely to become the major method of communication in your professional lifetime.

How Can I Time Manage the Phone?

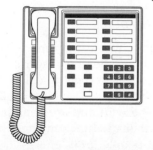

The Phone

Polite comments at the beginning and end of a conversation are necessary to maintain positive interpersonal communications. However, when time limits are necessary, focus the conversation on the business at hand. Some possible phrases include "How can I help you?" or "I called to _____." To end the conversation, summarize the actions to be followed through: "I understand, I am to find out about _____ and get back to you by the end of the week. Thanks for calling."

Having long social conversations to maintain friendships, to touch bases with a relative, to relax yourself, to ventilate, or for a similar social purpose can be combined with routine housekeeping duties. Who hasn't swept the floor, put away dishes, sorted mail, or cleaned out a drawer while chatting with a friend?

▼

The time management principle is don't agonize, organize!

▲

PEOPLE MANAGEMENT

The People

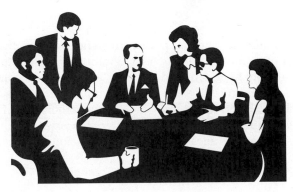

How Can I Effectively Manage People?

Well, this is a big one. You will become increasingly more competent and confident in carrying out the skill aspects of your nursing role and the roles you fulfill in your personal life. Communicating and getting along with other people with various personalities, however, will be an ongoing challenge.

Most people are comfortable to be with and are straightforward and supportive. They *add* to your energy and ability to function effectively and contribute to goal attainment. However, some people *drain* energy from others and/or organizational accomplishment through their whining, overcriticizing, negative thinking, chronic lateness, poor crisis management, overdependency, aggression, and other similar nonproductive behaviors. Occasional exhibitions of such behavior in relation to personal crises that happen to everyone can be dealt with easily. It is the people who have these behaviors as their everyday "modus operandi" (method of operating) who interfere with attainment of individual and organizational goals.

To protect your time and achieve your goals, it may be necessary to limit your time with such individuals. Avoidance is one strategy. Learning to say "no" and assertive communication can help as well. The content and skills in Chapter 7 (Effective Communication) and Chapter 8 (Conflict Management) help you learn to do this.

Even in the best of human relationships, conflict and extreme emotions are inevitable. Lots of time is wasted talking behind people's backs. While this relieves immediate frustration, it does not in itself lead to resolution of the basic problem. It is certainly healthy and wise to ventilate and sort out your feelings with a sympathetic or empathetic person. This will help you feel better and reduce emotions enough to focus on rational approaches for resolving a problem or misunderstanding. It will then be possible to communicate effectively with the person with whom you are having the problem. Remember to work through your feelings and then use your assertive communication skills to communicate directly with the people who are involved.

▼

TIME MANAGEMENT COMMUNICATION SKILLS

Learn to say "NO."
Use assertive communication.
Communicate directly with the person with whom you are having a problem.

▲

What Are Some Survival Strategies for Nurses—and Other People, Too?

▼

Delegation! Delegation! Delegation!

▲

....

Delegation extends from what one can do to what one can control. Moreover, it develops subordinates' initiative, skill, and confidence. A manager needs to devote more time to training and motivating people than to doing the technical work. To accomplish this, activities and tasks should be delegated to the lowest practicable level. (Rowland and Rowland, 1980, p. 55)

....

As healthcare costs continue to escalate, employers of nurses will continue to seek ways of reducing nursing care expenses. It is not cost-effective to pay an RN for activities that a lesser-educated, lesser salaried person can carry out. Nurses are being increasingly required to use their knowledge and manage care that is delivered by other members of the nursing item (i.e., licensed vocational/ practical nurses, nurses' aides, or other assistive personnel).

It is imperative to know the legal aspects of delegation as identified in your state nursing practice act. The act may address specific tasks and activities that RNs may or may not delegate. However, accountability for completion and quality of the task or activity remains with the nurse. Generally, the nurse is responsible for knowing that the condition of the patient, and the skill level of the assistive person, are safe for delegation to occur. Within the limits of legal nursing practice and good nursing judgment, many activities can be delegated.

As an effective and efficient manager of time, you can use delegation skills at home, at work, and in any group activity. When some of your tasks and activities are carried out by others, you will have more time to concentrate on new, other, and higher level activities.

▼

Almost everything can be delegated at one time or another.

▲

Ask yourself: What am I doing? Why am I doing this? Who else can do it now? Who can be trained to do it?

Repetitive, routine tasks are the easiest to delegate or train others to do. While teaching or supervising someone else initially may take more time, the time ultimately gained from not performing the activity yourself in the future far exceeds the initial investment of time. For example, if a person you live with is able to take over the weekly laundry and the laundry has been taking you one hour each week, you will gain four hours a month—forty-eight hours or two days, per year. Perhaps you and another person can take a weekend vacation with the time saved. Similarly, if a nursing assistant makes all the beds for the eight patients you both are caring for, that could gain at least one more hour per day of RN time. This hour could be used for patient teaching or other professional nursing functions. Over a year, considerable RN time would be gained:

▼

**1 hour per day
= 7 hours per week
= 364 hours per year
= 45 days per year**

▲

If there are three nursing assistants working with three RNs, 135 days, or about four and one-half months, of RN time per year on one unit would be gained.

In general, women may have more difficulty than men delegating because of their socialization. Women are socialized into pleasing others as well as anticipating and meeting the needs of others. This results in a "I can do it better myself" belief, which is popularly known as "mama management." Since the majority of the nursing profession remains female, 91.6% female and 8.4% male in 1991 (Davis, 1993), you can understand the magnitude of the problem. In today's society women, men, and nurses have so many responsibilities that sharing and delegating some of them is necessary.

To increase delegation skills, it is sometimes necessary to overcome the "myth of perfection." In teaching or training someone else to do a delegated task, initially they may or may not be able to perform the activity as well as you can; however, it is not important that they do this perfectly or in the way you do it, or even as well as you do. What is important is that they meet the standards required to complete the task adequately. As long as safety is not compromised, it is more effective time management to delegate to others. With experience, most people will improve (and may even surpass you). This is "all to the good" as you move into accomplishing your goals. It is important for the person to whom you are delegating to feel they are not being "dumped on," but are learning new skills for career development and helping the organization improve productivity.

What Do I Need to Know About the Delegation Process in Nursing Practice?

Be sure you know the delegation rules and regulation of your state nursing practice act. You will also need to know the delegation policies and job descriptions of nursing team members in your employing agency.

- ◆ **Assess the patient and the employee.** Begin by assessing the patient to be sure that the patient's condition permits delegation to occur safely. You are responsible for ascertaining that the person to whom you are delegating the task has the knowledge and skill to complete the task safely and competently and in the allotted time period. In new situations, it is better to start with small tasks and gradually increase the complexity and frequency of delegated activities.

- ◆ **Build in authority.** Let the person know who will be responsible and who they can go to if they have questions or need direction.

- ◆ **Set expectations clearly.** Explain what is to be done and, if appropriate, how it is to be done, and by when. Verify that the person understands the instructions.

Here is an example of an RN delegating the taking of vital signs of a patient (Mrs. Parks) to a nurse's aide (NA). The RN knows the delegation rules of her state nursing practice act and the policies in her hospital. She has been taking care of Mrs. Parks all morning. The RN also knows that the NA completed the hospital's NA course three years ago and demonstrated her skills in the learning center last month.

....

RN to NA: "Mrs. Parks in room 109 needs to have her BP checked every 30 minutes. I just checked Mrs. Parks at 12:30 and her blood pressure was 140/90. I will be in a meeting in room 302 for the next hour or so. Do you have time to check Mrs. Parks at 1:00, 1:30, and 2:00?"

NA: "I have a full assignment, but I can do it."

RN: "Thank you. If Mrs. Park's BP changes 20 or more points, please notify the charge nurse. Mrs. Parks may need a change in medication and I have updated the charge nurse. The charge nurse will also be available if you have any questions. When I get back after 2:00, I will check on Mrs. Parks then. Thank you again."

NA: "Fine, see you after your meeting."

Did you notice how the RN clearly identified to the NA what was expected and when it needed to be accomplished? This was an example of appropriate delegation.

A Word About What to Delegate

Again, it is both inefficient and ineffective for a hospital to pay RNs to perform non-nursing functions (e.g., filling water pitchers, running errands) when there is someone present who is able and is being paid less to do it. This is not to say that an RN should never do any of these tasks. Common sense rules that if a nurse is on the night shift with one or two aides or technicians and one is busy and the other on break and a patient is in need of a glass of water then, of course, it will be faster, simpler and more effective for the nurse to fill the pitcher. However, situations such as this one should be the exception, not the rule.

In an employment situation, it is also good sense to first see what the "corporate culture" expects and then "do what the Romans do" to fit in, especially when you are new. When the graduate nurse becomes more of an accepted team member or in a management position, then appropriate delegation will become easier and more accepted.

New graduates also need to be sensitive to when and how to delegate to other nursing team members who—though less educated—may have many more years of experience and/or be senior in age. You can always use your assertive communication skills to try to establish a positive working relationship. For example, "I feel uncomfortable telling you what to do since you have been here so long," or "You have so much experience here—tell me how you like to work with nurses?" The response does not require you meet the other person's preference but at least you have acknowledged their strength and have some clues for proceeding.

Delegating Upward and Across

Delegation is not always a downward process. You can also delegate up the management line or across to peers. If your supervisor has delegated more assignments than you think you can handle, make a list and ask your supervisor which are the highest priority, and which can be given later completion times.

Delegation can also be horizontal as well as vertical. In a group, pieces of a project can be delegated among various members. Even two nurses on a unit can agree to delegate responsibilities for a given period of time. For example, "How about if I cover the call lights for the next thirty minutes while you do your charting, and then we'll switch?"

Real estate agents say the most important thing is "location, location, location." Remember for effective time management—

▼

Delegation! Delegation! Delegation!

▲

We Interrupt This Chapter for a Word About Interruptions

Interruptions are one of the major threats to effective time management. Not only do they take time away from goal-directed activities, but additional time is needed to get refocused and back on track. Of course, some interruptions are inevitable, but they can be minimized. First, begin by recognizing when you are interrupting yourself. Pogo said, "I have met the enemy and he is us." He could paraphrase this to "I have met the interrupter and he is me." Do you start one task and then begin another rather than trying to concentrate on completion? Do you respond to all distractions (television, ringing telephones, chatty friends) at times when task completion is required? In these instances, *you are cooperating with the interruption and allowing yourself to be interrupted.* When possible, in non-emergency situations, use your time management strategies and communication skills to keep you focused on the task at hand. People will accept that you may need to get back to them another time when you have finished what you are doing. Write down when and where you can reach them and then follow through.

Responding to interruptions can also mean you are doing your job. For example, when you are interrupted to answer a patient's call light or answer a physician's telephone call, you are doing your job. These activities are part of your nursing responsibilities. They may not always be of an urgent nature and can be delayed a short time or they may be urgent and necessitate immediate response; either way you will need to deal with them eventually and rather than feeling "interrupted" remind yourself that you are doing—you are accomplishing—your job. There are many aspects of your job that you cannot control, but you can always choose how you respond.

Now, for some uninterrupted time. Relax, refocus, re-energize. Everyone needs some totally uninterrupted time in which to relax, refocus, and re-energize. During clinical experience, or at work or home, spend a few minutes in a quiet place by yourself (nurses' lounge, chapel, empty patient room, bedroom at home) to evaluate what is happening, or what needs to happen next. Take several deep, slow breaths, read, meditate, space-out, relax, and get in touch with yourself. (Parents with small children can take turns watching their children so each adult can have some uninterrupted, private time.) Again, this break from fast-paced activity and relaxation will re-energize you and result in more productive use of time. (If now is a good time to take a break from this chapter, we'll proceed when you get back!)

PROCRASTINATION: THE NEGATIVES AND POSITIVES OF PUTTING THINGS OFF

Everyone procrastinates, especially when a task is unpleasant or overwhelming, or can't be done perfectly. Often more time is spent worrying about or anticipating doing something than it would take to do it! The anticipation itself can also be worse than the actuality—draining energy and accomplishment. Here are some tips for *getting started*.

Have You Considered the Consequences?

Ask yourself what will happen if you do something and what will happen if you don't do it?

▼

If nothing will happen if you don't do something, don't do it!

▲

If there are no negative outcomes if you "don't do something," there is no point in spending time doing it and you can eliminate that activity. (I stopped making my bed and my husband's everyday about fifteen years ago; he has not said a word about it yet and lightning has not struck! I do make the beds when I feel like it or when company comes.) If something will happen if you don't do something then, of course, you need to proceed and get started.

The Earlier, the Better

Most projects take longer than planned and unexpected "glitches" happen: coffee spills all over the notes for the test you started studying for the night before; the person typing a major report due the next day gets called out of town; the person you are preparing for surgery is hard-of-hearing. To compensate for the inevitable delays and avoid crises, *start in advance and plan that your project will take three times as much time as you think.* Schedule times to work on your project and track your progress on your calendar.

"By the Inch, It's a Cinch"

Break a project into small, manageable pieces, and plan to do only the first step. For example, to study for a test, first collect all the related notes and books in one place. Next, review subject areas likely to be tested. If you are having difficulty getting started, plan to work on these steps for five minutes only (anybody can do just about anything for five minutes). Frequently, this will create enough momentum to get you going for longer than the five minutes. When you have to stop, leave yourself a note of what the next steps should be.

Plan Rewards

"Bribing" yourself with a reward can help you get started and keep yourself going. "If I concentrate well for one hour on reading the assigned chapter in *Nursing Today: Transition and Trends,* then I can watch my (favorite) television show guilt-free." Oftentimes, the stress reduction that comes from working on the procrastinated project is reward itself! "If I go to the learning laboratory and review the video on giving injections and practice there, my anxiety will be so reduced that I will feel better—reward enough."

The Myth of Perfection (Mother Was Not Always Right)

Many of us were brought up with the well-intentioned philosophy that "anything worth doing is worth doing well." This usually meant "worth doing perfectly." The fear of not doing something well enough or perfectly also feeds the tendency to proscrastinate.

Certainly everyone needs to make the best effort they can, but not everything needs to be done very well or perfectly. Life-threatening situations, such as those requiring CPR or control of hemorrhage, need to be handled as perfectly as possible. Almost everything else (bedmaking, baths, etc.) can be done to adequate standards without negative consequences.

Consider what the standard needed is—not the standard of perfection possible—and how you can meet it with a minimum—not maximum—amount of time and effort. Remember—

Prioritizing With the A-B-C System

Scan your list and decide which items are A or B or C. The activities that are the most related to your goals are the high payoff ones; they are "A" priorities. Divide the A items into A-1, A-2, and A-3 based on their urgency or time limits. For example, it will be an A-1 priority to get gas for your car if it has an empty tank and you need to get to school or work. It will be an A-1 priority to check a patient's IV drip before it runs out; you need to do this before taking the vital signs of a patient who is in stable condition. Another A-1 activity is reporting to work on time.

The B items also contribute to goal achievement and so are high-payoff, but they are generally less urgent, and so can be delayed for awhile. For example, getting gas for your car when the tank is one-fourth full is a B item. Reading

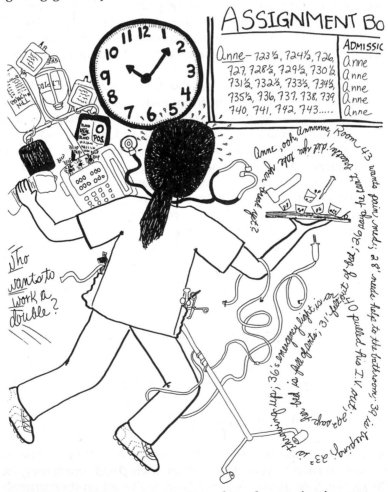

FIGURE 9-2 *Time management and work organization can sometimes be very challenging.*

an article in a nursing journal can be a B item. Eventually, many B items become A items, especially as completion times approach. It is also possible to do some B items in short snatches of time: carry the nursing journal article with you and start reading if you are in a long line or waiting for someone.

The items that do not substantially contribute to goals and are not time-limited are C items. These activities can really wait until you get around to them. Keep a list of things to be done when time permits. On a day when the patient census drops or nursing administration sends you an extra nurse's aide, review your C list. You may have time to watch some new videos in the tape library.

Some C items may not have to be done at all! If you have trouble throwing out mail, announcements of coming events, and so forth put them in a "C" drawer. About once a month, go through the C drawer; many of these will be found to be out-dated and can be thrown out. Of course, some C items become B or A priorities. Many C items will fit the "if nothing will happen if you don't do something, don't do it" category.

The A-B-C system can also help prioritize patient care needs. In some situations, you can put each assigned patient and the related to-do list on a separate index card and put the cards in A-1, A-2 order. As you complete care or a patient's condition changes, you can reorder the cards, which will keep you focused on priorities and eliminate a lot of rewriting. When you are unsure of the priority of patient care needs, consult with your clinical instructor or the nursing supervisor.

Cross out items on your to-do lists, cards, and schedules as you do them. This will give you immediate, positive feedback—an instant reward for your efforts and progress. When the inevitable interruptions occur, scan the to-do list and re-evaluate your priorities in relation to your remaining time.

Train yourself to do the A-1 activity or the hardest task *first*. Attending to the hardest activity first reduces the nagging anxiety that you "should be—" and helps you make progress early to identify, get in control of, and possibly prevent additional problems. This is an example of the classic time management principle, *Pareto's 80/20 rule*.

According to Pareto, an 18th century economist, 20% of the effort produces 80% of the results. For example, salespeople who concentrate 20% of their time on the two of their ten customers who order the most will produce 80% of their commissions. Twenty percent of studying on the hardest course can produce 80% success; attending to the 20% of the sickest patients on the unit will produce 80% of positive outcomes. In your home, 80% of what needs cleaning is in the kitchen and bathroom; spend 20% of your cleaning time on these two rooms and 80% of the cleaning will be done! This does not mean that you don't study for the other courses or clean the rest of the house; it does illustrate that there are proportionally greater results in concentrating at least 20% of your efforts on higher-payoff priorities.

Again, in a nursing situation, it is vital to give the most seriously ill and the most difficult patients high priority and in-depth attention. If there is a patient who is calling the nursing station every ten to fifteen minutes and taking the time of multiple staff members, assigning one nurse to concentrate on that patient's needs will allow the rest of the staff to concentrate on other patient and unit needs.

Scheduling the Priorities

Many goal-directed, prioritized activities need to be scheduled with completion times. This is sometimes called deadlining the to-do list; the term *completion times* seems less stress-producing than *deadlines*. Other than in emergency situations, death is not likely to occur if something is not completed exactly on time. However, it is considerate of people's time to let others affected know about lateness or a change in plans. Careful scheduling can reduce those inevitabilities.

Like others in new situations, student nurses and new graduates are often unclear about or underestimate the amount of time required for a given activity. Seek the advice of clinical instructors and experienced staff nurses on prioritizing, organizing, and scheduling.

All kinds of calendars are available to schedule the to-do activities, first by the month, then by the week, and then by the day (Tables 9–1 and 9–2). Overscheduling, (i.e., scheduling all your A activities in one day or scheduling more tasks than any human being can do in one day) inevitably leads to frustration. Schedule only what can realistically be accomplished and leave extra time before and after every major activity; tasks, meetings, and travel times can take longer than anticipated, and transition time is also needed. As mentioned earlier, alternating physical and mental tasks can be energy-producing. Remember to leave *white space* (nothing) in your schedule so that you will have time for yourself and family.

It will not always be possible to follow your schedule exactly. However, when you do get "derailed," having a plan will help you get back on track with a minimum of time and effort. Knowing your goals and priorities promotes flexible rescheduling, resulting in more effective time management and successful accomplishment.

TABLE 9–1　*Weekly Personal Calendar*

MONDAY	TUESDAY	WEDNESDAY	THURSDAY	FRIDAY
Cleaners 9AM workout	Pick up health insurance forms 3:30PM Carpool	4PM Workout	4–7:00PM Professional organization meeting	9AM Workout

TABLE 9–2 *Daily Nursing To-Do List*

(A) Immediate activities			
A-1		Check IV	Mr. D., Room 20
A-2		Assess chest tube	Mrs. B, Room 15
A-3		Suction ET tube	Ms. P, Room 12

(A) Scheduled items			
A-4	9:00AM	Dressing change	Ms. P, Room 10
A-5	10:00AM	Medications	Ms. B, Ms. P, Ms. J
A-6	12:00PM	CT Scan	Ms. W, Room 25
A-7	2:00PM	Medications	Mr. D, Ms. P
A-8	3:00PM	Change of shift report	

(B) To be done when time allows		
B-1	Diabetic teaching	Mr. X
B-2	Social Service Consultation	Mr. X

(C) If time available	
C	See new videos in tape library
C	Reorganize reference materials on unit

Keeping It Going

Continuously review your lists, schedules, and outcomes and give yourself "a gold star," "a pat on the back," or other positive reinforcement for achieving your goals. As you evaluate and revise accordingly, ask yourself, "Did I have a plan with priorities in writing?" "Was I doing high-payoff activities that pertain to my goals?" "Was I doing the right job at the right time?" "Could it have been done later, or delegated?" "Was the result of a given effort worth the time it took?" "How did I deal with interruptions and other time-wasters?" "To what extent did I reach my goals?" "What is the best use of my time right now?"

No one is perfect. Omissions and errors will occur and are good learning experiences. Don't waste time regretting failure or feeling guilty about what you don't do; consider these learning experiences of "what not to do" and opportunities for learning "what to do." Remind yourself that there is always time for important things, and that if it's important enough, you will do it.

Cross your arms in front of your chest. One arm will be on top of the other. Next, put the bottom arm on top. Awkward, isn't it? Practicing new ways of doing things is awkward at the beginning and takes time. It is estimated that it takes three weeks to integrate a new way of doing something and have it become a habit. It doesn't matter if you don't follow *all* these principles or don't follow them *all the time.* (As one nursing student said, "These time management strategies sound interesting, and some day if I ever get a minute, I'm going to see if they really work!") Using even a few of them will be helpful. Pick at least one new strategy and try it for a month. If you forget, be patient with yourself and try again. Eventually, those that are helpful will become routine, and automatic—providing you with even more time! And then you may want to try some others. One more time, here they are:

- ◆ Efficiency vs. effectiveness.
- ◆ Efficiency = doing something right.
- ◆ Effectiveness = doing the right thing right.
- ◆ Balance = make time for you, for family, and for career.
- ◆ Follow your time styles.
- ◆ Don't agonize—organize!
- ◆ Make a place for everything and put everything in its place.
- ◆ Compartmentalize, color-code, declutter the clutter.
- ◆ Time manage the paper, the phone and the people.
- ◆ Use time management communications skills.
- ◆ Learn to say NO.
- ◆ Use assertive communication.
- ◆ Communicate directly with the person with whom you have a problem.
- ◆ Delegation! Delegation! Delegation!.
- ◆ Reduce interruptions.
- ◆ Practice the 3 R's: relax, refocus and re-energize.
- ◆ If nothing will happen if you don't do something, don't do it!
- ◆ Reduce procrastination with "By the Inch, It's a Cinch."
- ◆ Fight the "myth of perfection."
- ◆ Set goals.
- ◆ Prioritize with the A-B-C system.
- ◆ Use Pareto's 80/20 rule.
- ◆ Schedule your to-do list by the month, week, and day.
- ◆ Evaluate and revise.

Keep it going! It's time to begin now!

　　Note: The author used all of the above time management strategies to write this chapter and completed it only moderately late.

ACKNOWLEDGMENTS

The author wishes to acknowledge Donna Doerr, MSN, RN, and Jennifer Gray, MSN, RN (PhD candidate), for their input on clinical applications of time management, and Virginia Busocker for her clerical assistance and support in completing the manuscript for this chapter.

REFERENCES

Brynes, M.A. (1982): Non-nursing functions: The nurses state their case. *Am J Nurs* 1089.

Covey, S. (1990): *The Seven Habits of Highly Effective People*. New York, Simon & Schuster.

Davis, K. (1982): Non-nursing functions: Our readers respond. *Am J Nurs* 1857.

Davis, R. (1992–93): Mr. RN. *Graduating Nurse* Winter: 40.

Keyes, R. (1991) *Timelock: How Life Got So Hectic and What You Can Do About It*. New York, Harper Collin.

Kramer, M. (1974) *Reality Shock*. St. Louis, C.V. Mosby.

Lakein, A. (1974): *How to Get Control of Your Time and Your Life*. New York, Signet Books.

MacKenzie, A. (1989): *Time for Success: A Goal Getter's Strategy*. New York, McGraw-Hill.

MacKenzie, A., Waldo, K.C. (1981): *About Time! A Woman's Guide to Time Management*. New York, McGraw-Hill.

McGee-Cooper, A. (1985): *Time Management for Unmanageable People*. Dallas, McGee-Cooper and Associates.

McGee-Cooper, A. (1990): *You Don't Have to Go Home From Work Exhausted*. Dallas, Bowen and Rogers.

Moskowitz, R. (1981): *How to Organize Your Work and Your Life*. New York, Doubleday.

Rowland, H., Rowland, B. (1980): *Delegation and Time Management*. p. 47. In Nursing Administration Handbook, Rockville, MD, Aspen Systems.

Smith, M. (1975): *When I Say No, I Feel Guilty*. New York, Bantam Books.

Treuille, B.B., Stautberg, S.S. (1988): *Managing It All: Time-Saving Ideas for Career, Family, Relationships and Self*. New York, Master Media.

Winston, S. (1983): *The Organized Executive*. New York, Norton/Warner Books.

Yager, J. (1989): *Making Your Office Work for You: How to Create a Sense of Comfort, Efficiency and Ease in Your Work Space*. New York, Doubleday.

UNIT IV

ECONOMIC AND POLITICAL ASPECTS OF THE HEALTHCARE DELIVERY SYSTEM

10

Contemporary Healthcare Delivery: Trends and Economics

Joan Jones, M.S., R.N./Susan Houston, Ph.D., R.N.

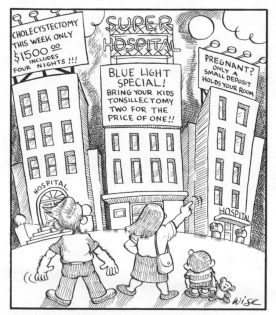

Healthcare consumers are going to be shopping around in order to get the most for their healthcare dollar.

"By identifying the forces pushing the future, rather than those that have contained the past, you possess the power to engage with your reality."
—Megatrends 2000, John Naisbitt and Patricia Aburdene

After completing this chapter, you should be able to:

◆ Discuss how current trends will affect your future nursing practice.

◆ Describe two nursing practice activities that have been influenced by computers.

◆ Discuss the impact of quality improvement activities on nursing practice.

◆ Identify two problems on a nursing unit in which quality improvement efforts would improve patient outcomes.

◆ Identify the purpose of DRGs and Alternate Delivery of Nursing Care Systems.

Dorothy was a little girl from Kansas who experienced another world and another time. That world was influenced and molded by the great Wizard. But Oz wasn't always there nor would he perpetually remain to control the culture of the land. The same is true for our society. Individuals, trends, fads, and demands all influence the path and direction of our world. Our awareness of these demands and our response to them allows us to direct our future. Remember, you do have a choice in creating the future.

The American healthcare system is one of the largest industries in the nation. Changes in the healthcare system are caused by consumer demands, technological advances, and governmental scrutiny. Nursing, as a large subsystem of the healthcare industry, will face the impact of the same dynamic forces on its theoretical viewpoint, its practice models, and its services provided to clients.

Today, the nursing profession is relying on foresight, experience, and nursing visionaries to pave a path toward nursing success. Your contributions can help make nursing an ever more valued resource in the 21st century.

This chapter discusses the predicted trends that will influence the practice of nursing in the future. It also presents activities such as quality improvement, development of new practice models, and computerization that will have a major impact on nursing. Finally, it reviews key economic issues and healthcare system demands so that you will have a clear idea of how cultural changes and external demands will likely influence your practice.

TRENDS AFFECTING HEALTHCARE

> *Imagine activating your voice collar to record your nursing activities. (Beam me up Scottie!!) Picture yourself assuming a yoga position to teach meditation techniques to a cardiovascular patient.*

The future holds many new social, political, and technological changes that will affect nursing directly and help shape this already powerful profession. The optimistic 1990s will mark a major turning point, bringing us into the new territory of the 21st century. The "greying of America," technological advances, "globalization," and social evolution will dramatically change nursing roles and nursing delivery systems.

How Can Nursing Respond to These Trends?

First, we must understand the impact these trends will have on nursing, and then *create* a vision of where we want to be in the future.

▼

"To take advantage of the coming changes, we have to be aware of them." (Galinas, 1990, p. 18)

▲

Creating this vision will allow us to develop educational and service strategies to guide nursing into the twenty-first century. Your contribution to creating this vision is crucial to the future and to the consumers of healthcare. There are ten major trends in nursing. These trends are affecting nursing practice now and will continue to have a major impact into the next millennium.

1. Nursing will assume an undisputed dominant role in the healthcare delivery system, resulting in positions of high esteem with better salaries, incentives, responsibilities, and authority.

2. Care of the geriatric population will become a prominent, respected nursing specialty.

3. Nurses will play a major leadership role in determining and implementing healthcare policies.

4. Nurses will provide the expertise to integrate the multiple facets of healthcare—pharmacology, nutrition, preventive medicine, rehabilitation, etc.—in order to provide holistic care for an individual client.

5. Technological advances will assist the nurse in providing high-quality care that is cost effective.

6. Specific outcome criteria will be important in determining the quality of care and will become healthcare facilities' overriding concern in the future.

7. Case managed care will replace the traditional sick care approach, as prevention will be the key to reducing healthcare costs.

8. Increased numbers of women and nurses will be making policy and governmental decisions affecting healthcare.

9. Education will become more user friendly as the trend moves to a service economy in which knowledge is utilized.

10. Nursing will begin sharing healthcare beliefs, cultural practices, resources, and the expanding body of nursing knowledge as globalization occurs.

Watching a war on TV may sound farfetched, but as a result of the advances in telecommunications, we all actually witnessed parts of Desert Storm. The world is rapidly moving to a worldwide information network that includes laptop computers, fax machines, and cellular phones. Eventually, each person will have their own personalized health status microchip that will match individual needs to healthcare service centers around the world. Naisbitt and Aburdene (1990) predict that the quality of life for rural areas will improve because of electronic and computer innovations. In this new world of information power, nurses will be recognized and rewarded for making use of their intelligence and creativity. Nurses will be required to sort and process information at lightning speed, which will increase the many demands placed upon us, along with the accompanying stress-oriented diseases. Lastly, with the development of nanotechnology, the expanding science of technology that examines or measures information at the molecular level (for example, measuring at one billionth of a gram), nursing will be faced with new ethical concerns. To sum it up:

◆ New nursing care delivery systems must be developed to incorporate the demands of advanced technology.

◆ A shift must be made toward lower-tech, higher-touch therapeutic interventions to offset the technological boom.

◆ Therapies must be developed that combine conventional medical treatments with alternative care approaches (biofeedback, relaxation) in order to deal with stress (Curtin, 1990).

What Is Globalization and How Does It Affect Nursing?

With the trend toward globalization of the world, we will see a universal sharing of attitudes, products, and stocks. Third-world countries will experience a developmental growth and make an even greater contribution to the global market. A religious and cultural resurrection will occur due to the blending of many cultural lifestyles (Miraldo, 1991). We will begin to service the world as one global economy.

◆ Nurses will need to learn about the healthcare beliefs and practices of other cultures.

◆ International nursing forums must meet the need for sharing of nursing practices.

◆ Nursing and healthcare products, publications, methods, and the expanding body of nursing knowledge will find new possibilities in a global economy.

SOCIAL CHANGES AND NURSING

How Do Social Changes Impact Nursing?

Socially, the entire world is evolving. With the demise of socialism and communism, there is a rebirth of progress and growth. People are desiring control over their lives, especially in the area of healthcare (Hadden, 1989). This desire to create and grow will encourage a competitive market throughout the world. According to Coile, "three driving forces—aging, technology, and costs—will reshape health in the future." (1991, p. 10)

Era of the Consumer.   Consumers will make their own choices regarding healthcare—where they will obtain healthcare as well as what type of setting. Consumer choice may initiate voluntary accreditation by institutions in order to ensure quality health services. More unconventional healing alternatives will be available, such as getting in touch with one's own healing powers to mobilize the immune response. The practice of yoga for relaxation, utilization of acupuncture, homeopathy, and chromotherapy are examples of this new wave of increased acceptance of healing therapies. The consumer is a better-informed individual who is taking a more active role in their healthcare.

Medicine and the Public Eye.   The power that medicine now holds in society will be questioned. Medicine will no longer hold the position of high esteem in the public eye. The consumer is tired of paying the high price of medical care and now questions physicians' fees. The public will demand more preventive care rather than focusing on treatment of the illness after it is diagnosed. The "superdoc" fantasy that the physician knows all there is to know and can solve any healthcare problem is a false one that continues to restrict healthcare reforms (Fagin, 1992).

Quality of Care.   Specific outcome criteria will be important as the public judges the value of healthcare. Healthcare will be viewed as a purchase, and the public will make sure they are getting their money's worth. Nurses will be in a position as providers of healthcare to offer the best services for the best price. Into the next century, we will be continuing development of mechanisms to measure the quality of the product. The bottom line in healthcare will be a focus on the value of the product. Quality measures will direct our activities at work and will require us to constantly maintain a level of excellence.

National Health Plan.   The expected introduction of a national health plan in America will reinforce and maintain a focus on the elderly and young populations. Efforts to control costs will further encourage the trend toward shorter hospital stays and an increasing multitude of outpatient options. At the same time, self-care and holistic services will be a growing option for much of the population. Nurses will be in a position to be the major players in the restructuring of this environment.

Aging Population.   Another social influence on healthcare is the increase in the number of people over age 65. Two-thirds of the residents of nursing homes are over the age of 85 (Coile, 1991). As a result of health promotion and disease prevention, people are living longer. The majority of the older generation, those over age 65, have multiple-system problems as well as chronic illnesses. For this group, the cost of healthcare will increase proportionately. As a result, geriatric nursing care along with home healthcare will be areas experiencing significant growth. Provision must be made for the needs of the elderly population. Currently, there is underfunding of healthcare services for the elderly.

New Wave of Technology.   Computers, biosensors, implants, genetics, imaging devices are examples of the emerging technology of the twenty-first century. Medical artificial intelligence, such as computer-assisted surgery, interpretations of electrocardiographic and fetal monitoring, clinical diagnosis, and genetic counseling will have a major impact on our future.

Work Psychology Changes.   Organizations have revolutionized their view of workers from a dependent perspective to an independent perspective. Research and the development of a body of knowledge related to work psychology has now established the concept of leadership as a facilitating role—assisting in moving work groups along the maturity continuum—rather than controlling and making all decisions. This freedom and responsible interaction among employees and employers has encouraged work productivity, and this will continue into the next century.

We must make continued efforts to validate nursing's unique contribution to healthcare. Women are now considered as a potential and expanding labor source (Schwartz, 1989). Not only as an expanding labor source, but also as leaders in the business world. Can you believe that currently over five million women are leading small- to medium-sized companies that are predicted to be the top companies in the future? Healthcare is listed as third out of ten as a "hot career" for women in *Megatrends for Women* (Aburdene and Naisbitt, 1992). Two population groups, women and the elderly, will continue to influence the work environment and cause a restructuring of work ethics and settings. The corporate world will recognize the need to balance personal, professional, and organizational goals.

COMPUTERS IN NURSING

How Are Computers Going to Impact Nursing?

Computer systems are rapidly evolving in the healthcare industry. You can open any nursing-oriented software buyer's guide and find programs to assist you in admitting and discharge, nursing care planning and documentation, staffing, scheduling and continuing education, and healthcare agency orientation. These programs are designed to facilitate your work productivity by assisting you in managing the flow of information, problem solving, and accurate documentation.

Three distinct types of computers exist:

◆ Mainframe
◆ Minicomputer
◆ Microcomputer

Mainframe computers, the fastest and largest computers available, are composed of many pieces of hardware (equipment). They have extensive memory capacity, are generally rented or leased because of their expense, and are usually located in a central area within a facility. They are used to collect, store, and process vast amounts of information. In healthcare agencies, they are used to organize patient data bases, patient billing, budget reports, personnel files, and nursing management information such as staffing and scheduling and incident reports. Smaller computers such as microcomputers can be linked within the mainframe to access information from many locations throughout a facility.

The *minicomputer* is a miniature version of the mainframe with a smaller memory capacity and a slower processing time. These computers may be found in smaller healthcare agencies or in special, more self-contained departments such as the pharmacy (Saba and McCormick, 1986). There may also be multiple access terminals throughout a facility.

The *microcomputer*, known also as the personal computer (PC), home computer, laptop, or notebook computer, has fewer hardware or equipment pieces than the mainframe, and its hardware components differ. These computers can unleash the staff nurse's or nurse manager's creativity. Even though these computers can process only one job at a time, they allow visualization of the input and output and can access a mainframe computer. Most software or programs that enable you to use the PC are user friendly, meaning they guide the user in a step-by-step process. Access to this type of computer can encourage nurses to develop new charting or staffing ideas, record quality assurance findings, or develop patient education materials.

How Will Nursing Balance Computer Technology and Caring?

Computers in healthcare agencies were initially introduced to assist with financial activities such as patient billing. Today computers are being used to directly facilitate nursing activities and patient hospitalization. The initial impact of computers in nursing came with the advent of technological systems developed to monitor patient health status (vital signs, EKG, etc.). Now, scheduling and staffing activities are often computer generated, as are educational programs designed to assist in the orientation and continuing education of nurses. Computers are purported to save nursing time, which is vitally important in this era of nursing shortage. Some staff feel computers are difficult to use, perhaps because of their unfamiliarity and their reluctance to accept them. Some experts feel that the increased use of computers may lead to decreased client contact, however, others feel that bedside computers actually promote more patient-nurse interaction, as tedious tasks are increasingly handled at the bedside. Computer literacy is becoming more important, as this increased knowledge enables nurses to use computer-generated information more efficiently and to incorporate this information into the patient's plan of care. However, current computer-oriented research studies have numerous biases and only partially support the idea that computers reduce the time spent on tasks and allow for increased time for direct patient contact (Hendrikson and Kovner, 1990).

Computers are here to stay, and future efforts in nursing need to include developing techniques that will encourage nurses to become familiar with computer operations, document reduction in nursing errors, and establish a reduction in time spent charting nursing interactions. With the advent of bedside terminals, research will need to validate the computer's contribution to nursing productivity.

Client privacy and confidentiality of healthcare records may pose an ethical issue. The disclosure of information takes on a new perspective with the increasing use of computers in healthcare. Nurses who are computer literate are in a strategic position to safeguard a client's right to privacy and confidentiality.

HEALTHCARE PROVIDER CREDENTIALING AND QUALITY IMPROVEMENT

What Is the Joint Commission on Accreditation of Healthcare Organizations (JCAHO)?

The mission of the JCAHO is to "enhance the quality of healthcare provided to the public" (JCAHO, 1992). In order to accomplish this mission, the JCAHO conducts systematic and intensive surveys of hospitals and other healthcare institutions to determine if accepted standards of structure, process, and outcome are being met. The question being asked is, "Can this healthcare organization provide quality healthcare to its clients?"

The survey and accreditation process JCAHO employs is an intensive procedure, and the accreditation the JCAHO delivers is important to healthcare agencies. Many third-party payors, including Medicare, will only reimburse hospitals that are accredited by the JCAHO. The most favorable accreditation the JCAHO gives is valid for three years.

The arrival of the JCAHO survey team is a time of excitement and anxiety for healthcare providers. The presence of the survey team provides the hospital or healthcare agency an opportunity to display the programs and systems the institution has in place to deliver quality patient care. Accompanying this positive experience is the worry that the JCAHO may find a deficit in the healthcare program, which may result in failure to receive accreditation. Usually the hospital spends a year preparing for the visit by conducting mock surveys and reviewing and revising current practice. JCAHO maintains a free, direct consultation phone line to assist healthcare providers in clarifying and interpreting existing standards.

What Is Quality Assurance?

When asked, "Is nursing a profession?" most nurses will shake their heads up and down, emphatically responding "Yes" to the question. But inherent to professionalism is a dedication to providing quality service to a consumer (Bernhard, 1981). Nursing efforts to monitor and improve patient care services are often recognized as "quality assurance," "quality improvement," or "quality evaluation." Today these programs, whatever they are titled, are nursing's method of monitoring and improving consumer oriented services, a giant step toward professionalism. Quality assurance is a process of evaluating outcomes of care and ensuring that each patient receives a predetermined high standard of care. This process is illustrated in Fig. 10–1.

Quality assurance is usually developed within an organization program unique to each institution. The program generally encompasses a philosophy of quality assurance, methods for accomplishing the process, time lines and report format. However, the purpose of any quality improvement program must be focused on measuring and improving nursing care to clients.

To the new graduate, the word "quality" can seem unconnected to measurement and void of any tangible context. But to consumers, quality means hospital cleanliness, accurate billing statements, courteous environment, nurse competency, available medical specialists, and low mortality rates. With health-

Setting standards
|
Establishing a criteria of achievement
↓
Determining if criteria have been met
↓
Implementing action plans for improvement, and
↓
Re-evaluating standards

FIGURE 10–1   *Quality assurance.*

Primary Nurse:

Initials _____ Signature _____

Associate Nurse:

Initials _____ Signature _____

Associate Nurse:

Initials _____ Signature _____

ETIOLOGIES: renal failure; acute or chronic decreased cardiac output; MI, CHF, LFF; varicosities of legs; liver disease; tissue insult; inflammatory processes; hormonal disturbance

NSG DX: Fluid Volume Excess

Define: The state in which the individual experiences or is at risk of experiencing vascular, cellular or extra-cellular fluid overload.

Potential: _____ Date _____ Initials _____

Potential: _____ Date _____ Initials _____

DEFINING CHARACTERISTICS	EXPECTED PATIENT OUTCOMES	ASSESSMENT	INTERVENTIONS	DATE	EVALUATION OF OUTCOMES*
Edema	Patient will regain fluid balance	Observe electrolyte, albumin, BUN, creatinine, hemoglobin, and hematocrit values	Measure vital signs: _____		
Effusion (pleural, pericardial)	Complications of fluid excess will be avoided	Assess skin turgor and inspect for redness	Daily weight (same scales): _____		
Generalized massive edema	Blood pressure, urine, and serum chemistry within normal limits	Identify contributing factors	Measure I & O: _____		
Weight gain		Assess patient/family knowledge base	Administer drugs as ordered (diuretics, albumin)		
Shortness of breath	Retractable skin turgor		Reposition frequently		
Orthopnea	Clear mentation		Measure abdomen girth: _____		
Intake greater than output	Absence of edema		Evaluate therapeutic, adverse and toxic effects of drugs given		
Third heart sound	Patient and family can explain:		Assist with dialysis		
Pulmonary congestion on x-rays	—reasons for fluid volume excess		Passive range of movement exercises		
Abnormal breath sounds (crackles, rales, rhonchi)	—dietary alterations		Apply elastic stockings as ordered		
Changes in mental status	—medications and treatments for home use		Encourage deep breathing and coughing		
Decreased hemoglobin and hematocrit	—plan for follow-up care		Provide information concerning:		
Changes in blood pressure			—reasons for fluid excess		
Changes in central venous pressure			—reasons for treatment		
Pulmonary artery changes			—dietary alterations		
Jugular vein distention			—purpose for drugs		
Oliguria					

FIGURE 10–2 *Written care plan.*

*Please evaluate patient outcomes and sign each evaluation daily.

(Reprinted with permission of St. Luke's Episcopal Hospital.)

care consuming a larger percentage of the gross national product, healthcare professionals and consumers alike are becoming cost conscious and quality outcome oriented (Miraldo, 1991).

JCAHO has been a leader in demanding evidence of the provision of quality care. The current nursing standards address "the monitoring and evaluation of the quality and appropriateness of the patient care provided by all members of the nursing staff" (JCAHO, 1990). This standard specifically requires nursing staff members to identify quality issues for each unit, methods for monitoring these issues, and methods for evaluating the outcomes. This has special implications for the new graduate in terms of receiving adequate orientation to an agency's quality improvement program and expectations of the nurse concerning his or her participation in quality improvement methods. Today, most of the quality improvement activities are unit-based and require intense staff nurse involvement. This is as it should be, since the nurse on the unit is the one who can best detect and quantify patient needs and outcomes.

Quality improvement approaches offer three perspectives from which to evaluate nursing care provided: structure, process, and outcome. Healthcare institutions' quality improvement methods usually contain a combination of all three perspectives in order to provide comprehensive quality care. The structural perspective encompasses evaluating the physical environment, organizational structure, and licensure of healthcare providers. The process perspective examines what is actually being done for the patient. Standards of care as developed by the American Nurses Association, standardized plans of care, or written care plans represent what the nurse should be doing in collaboration with the patient and colleagues (Fig. 10–2). These plans of care are necessary to ensure that each patient receives at least a minimum standard of the nursing product. The outcome perspective highlights changes in the patient's health status. This perspective has gained momentum over the past few years, and quality improvement efforts are now being concentrated on documenting patient outcomes. Evidence of patient improvement, satisfaction, knowledge of health deviation, and compliance is a major focus of quality improvement methods. This perspective is purported to be difficult for nurses to measure since many patient outcomes are influenced by numerous healthcare professionals. However, creative nurses are constantly developing methods for examining the outcomes of their interventions.

What Are Quality Improvement Methods?

Quality improvement methods differ from institution to institution in terms of what is examined and how it is examined. However, the methods are similar for determining quality nursing care efforts. Quality improvement manuals include a philosophy and objectives of the institution's program. Specific methods for reporting quality measurement results and feedback are also outlined in the manual. The results of quality assurance and method of feedback is dependent on the organizational framework and management philosophy (Fig. 10–3). Indicators of care or problems associated with nursing care can then be identified, most often by the practicing nurse. Methods of determining the severity of the problem or indicators are devised. These methods include chart audits, questionnaires, surveys and reviews for evaluating outcomes of care (Fig. 10–4). To ensure accuracy of measurement, efforts need to be directed at determining the reliability and validity of the measurement tools.

A threshold, or cutoff point, is determined for each indicator.

For example, if a unit or agency is measuring skin integrity, the threshold may be set at 3%, indicating that no more than 3% of the patient population at any given time will show evidence of skin breakdown; if patient knowledge of discharge medications is being examined, a high threshold, such as 96%, would be set to indicate that at any time 96% of the patient population will be knowledgeable concerning their medications prescribed on discharge.

In the past, auditing of these indicators was done randomly, but now, continuous evaluation is being advocated so that prompt action can be taken to identify the problem early and make plans to correct it. Once measurement has occurred and deficits have been identified, action plans are written and implemented to eliminate the problem. The creative genius of practicing nurses is once again called upon to develop methods for eliminating the problems and aligning the indicator measure to the preset thresholds.

What Are Diagnosis Related Groups (DRGs)?

Prospective payment is a relatively new form of hospital reimbursement. With this system, the healthcare agency and providers of care know in advance exactly

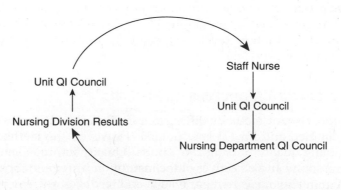

FIGURE 10–3   *Quality improvement (QI) results cycle.*

how much they will receive for the services required to care for a patient with a particular diagnosis. An example of this type of reimbursement might be $1,500, paid for a vaginal delivery, regardless of length of hospital stay or complexity of care. DRGs and prospective reimbursement have turned the delivery of healthcare around 180 degrees. Giving quality care to patients in a timely and cost effective manner has become essential in the present market.

Why do we have DRGs? Several factors forced the government to find a new payment system for Medicare patients. These included:

◆ Spiraling health care costs.

◆ Increasing use of hospital services.

◆ A wide variation in cost of care among hospitals.

DRGs have been criticized for not effectively measuring the "severity of illness" and not adequately measuring the different kinds of nursing resources utilized to care for patients. However, the current trend is demonstrating that clients can be discharged earlier without compromising and actually promoting their healthcare. The DRG system does offer an opportunity for nurses to utilize principles of research to predict nursing resource use by classification of patients. It should be possible to have patient-specific information in a form that will promote a comparison of quality as well as cost (Thompson, 1986).

What Are Health Maintenance Organizations (HMO)?

HMO's are continuing to gain great popularity in the nation and are seen as a component to the solution of rising health care costs. Each member pays a flat fee, therefore, they have an incentive to minimize costs. These organizations provide both inpatient and outpatient care to families or individuals for about the same cost that commercial insurance carriers charge for inpatient care alone. Much of this is accomplished by detailed inpatient utilization review conducted by the HMO. This review has resulted in a reduction in patient length of stay by as much as 45%. It is expected that 70% of all Americans will be enrolled in some type of HMO by the year 1999. (ACHCE, 1984)

What Is on the Horizon with Regards to Patient Models of Care?

A new model of care that is important to consider is the "Planetree Model" or "Humanizing Health Care Experience." This model is currently being implemented in the Planetree unit at the San Jose Medical Center in California. It places personalized health care, not technology, at the forefront of healthcare delivery. Within this model, the patients and family meet with members of their healthcare team and plan care for the patient. Family members actually care for the hospitalized patient—including giving medications, and even cooking some

EVALUATION OF OUTCOMES FOR CARDIOVASCULAR PATIENT   Addressograph

Med Dx: _____

Primary Nurse: _____

Surgical Procedure: _____

Date of Surgery: _____

Expected Status: **Status Criteria:**
WC = Wholly Compensatory   √ = Met   X = Not Assessed at this time
PC = Partly Compensatory   * = Not Met (note significant findings/daily nurses notes)
SE   = Supportive/Educative   − = Unchanged (from previous entry)   Date Admitted _____
                                NA = Not Applicable   Date Discharged _____

EXPECTED OUTCOME	Expected/ Actual Status at DSCHG		HOSPITAL STAY													HOME HEALTH	
Unit Date/Time	Date Initial	Date Initial															
1. Optimal hemodynamic status will be maintained.																	
2. Optimal gas exchange will be maintained.																	
3. Hematologic hemostasis will be achieved.																	
4. Pain will be minimized or alleviated.																	
5. Baseline cardiac rhythm will be maintained.																	
6. Fluid and electrolyte balance will be demonstrated.																	
7. Infection will be minimized or absent.																	
8. Adequate peripheral circulation will be maintained.																	
9. Normal bowel function will be demonstrated.																	
10. Skin integrity is maintained.																	
Signature																	

*For standardized nursing interventions, please refer to patient care standards.

FIGURE 10–4   *Quality Assurance—Evaluation of Outcomes.*

EVALUATION OF OUTCOMES FOR CARDIOVASCULAR PATIENT

Med Dx: _____

Primary Nurse: _____

Addressograph

Expected Status:
WC = Wholly Compensatory
PC = Partly Compensatory
SE = Supportive/Educative

Status Criteria:
√ = Met   X = Not Assessed at this time
* = Not Met (note significant findings/daily nurses notes)
− = Unchanged (from previous entry)
NA = Not Applicable

EXPECTED OUTCOME	Expected/ Actual Status at DSCHG		HOSPITAL STAY														HOME HEALTH
Unit Date/Time	Date Initial	Date Initial															
11. Optimal neurologic status will be maintained.																	
12. Adequate nutritional intake will be achieved.																	
13. Anxiety and fear will be minimized.																	
14. Increased tolerance to activity will be evidenced.																	
15. Optimal involvement in self-care activities will be evidenced.																	
16. Patient's significant others communicate an understanding of disease status and treatment.																	
17. Patient/significant others verbalize understanding of diet, activity, medications.																	
18. Patient/significant others verbalize understanding of discharge instructions.																	
19. Patient/family verbalizes knowledge of available resources during hospitalization and following discharge.																	
Signature																	

*For standardized nursing interventions, please refer to patient care standards.

(Reprinted with permission of St. Luke's Episcopal Hospital.)

FIGURE 10–4   Quality Assurance—Evaluation of Outcomes. Continued

meals for the patient. Patients are also able to read and write on their medical records. There are no barriers to separate the patient from the healthcare team. Instead, patients and families are active participants in the healthcare plan. Some of the benefits of the Planetree Model are:

1. It provides top quality care and helps the hospital to remain on the "cutting edge" of the health care delivery system. Another benefit is that adopting the model allows the hospital to differentiate itself and better market itself in the community.

2. University of Washington at Seattle found in a recent study that patients and nurses are significantly more satisfied with the care provided in the Planetree unit than in other areas in the hospital. Nurses' overall satisfaction with the program is reported to be one of the unit's largest selling points.

3. New York City's Beth Israel Hospital anticipates that the 38-bed Planetree Model unit it plans to open next year will help recruit some of the very best nurses in the marketplace. Some of you may be interested in becoming one of those nurses involved in establishing a Planetree unit.

Another futuristic model that is being evaluated is the healthcare model proposed by the State of Oregon. There are nine (9) principles that the State of Oregon has established in order to provide healthcare for the residents of Oregon. These principles are based on the tenets of making healthcare accessible to all people in the state, as opposed to only certain people being able to receive the care that they need. Health maintenance is the focus of this model.

In the future, an anticipated 70% of the care given to patients will be in the home. This means that nurses in the hospital will be seeing only the most critically ill patients. When those patients are ready to leave the intensive care units (ICUs) and the intermediate care units (IMCs), instead of going to the general floor unit they may even go to another facility, similar to what are called "nursing homes" in Great Britain. This part of the British model of care has been in place for many years and has been reviewed, not only by the United States, but also by Canada, as an improved approach to providing care to their citizens. Extended healthcare facilities are an alternative health care option that is increasing in prevalence. This type of facility offers nursing care to clients who are not ill enough to necessitate hospitalization in an acute care facility.

Preventive medicine and *preventive care* are going to be the buzzwords of the future. Instead of waiting until someone is ill and needs to be hospitalized or we need to step in with emergency treatment, our emphasis will be on preventing disease and keeping people in a state of wellness. Increased emphasis will be placed on nutrition and exercise. Lifestyles will change. The greying of America is also going to continue to affect healthcare. These senior citizens will probably be different from those we have seen in the past. Many of them are the yuppies of today, the baby boomers, who are already very conscious of their health and interested in legislation related to their healthcare. As this elderly group grows, there will be fewer people to provide the tax money to sustain the kind of programs that we have today. Medicare, for instance, will have to change. Not only will we have DRGs, but we may even have something beyond that. There may be a penalty assessed to individuals who do not practice good health habits. For example, you may have to pay a higher premium for your insurance if you smoke.

Nursing has developed a plan for delivery of care called the Nurses' National Health Care Plan (NHCP). It has been endorsed by the National League for Nursing, the American Nurses Association and other professional nursing organizations in the country. This plan positions nurses as the gatekeepers to healthcare services, uses managed care options to contain costs, and provides preventive and primary healthcare to schools, workplaces and community nursing centers as well as hospitals (Hawkins, 1991). The nurse's role will be important in implementing this healthcare plan. The major components of the plan include:

1. Federally defined standard package of essential healthcare benefits, which would include primary care prevention and easy accessibility to the system for all citizens and residents of the United States.

2. A combination of public and private sources that would finance and provide care.

3. Improved consumer access by delivering primary care services in convenient settings such as shopping malls, schools, the workplace, and the home. Healthcare costs would be controlled through managed care. This would result in a reduction of administrative costs.

The implementation of the plan would be done in incremental steps. The highest priority is to allocate resources for pregnant women, infants, and children. This population is essential to our future. At the present time, our morbidity and mortality rates for mothers and babies rank with many third-world countries. Placing initial focus on these groups would represent a cost effective investment in the future health of the nation. As this plan develops, there will be an opportunity for all nurses to participate in its design and implementation.

▼

The role of the nurse in the future will extend beyond our wildest dreams.

▲

Graduates of nursing schools today stand on the threshold of a whole new world, and it is a very good world. The only limiting barriers will be those we erect ourselves. Just as Dorothy in *The Wizard of Oz* found that the tools she needed to positively control her life were talent and knowledge from within, so must we react proactively to a rapidly changing culture.

Significant economic and social trends are dramatically altering the forms of healthcare delivery in the United States and the roles played by nurses in the delivery of that care. Advances in technology, the globalization of culture and communication, ever-widening computer applications, the aging of the population, and movement toward a national health plan are among major developments.

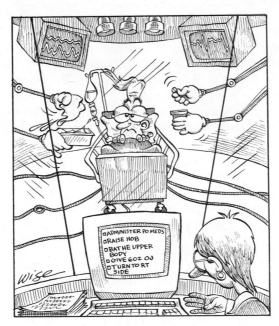

FIGURE 10–5 *Computer technological advances continue to assist the nurse, but it can not replace the humanistic aspect of nursing care.*

© Copyright 1994 W.B. SAUNDERS COMPANY

To cope and to contribute to the future of healthcare, nurses must understand how computers are now being used in healthcare, and they must be able to use computers in a cost effective manner in their nursing practice. They must also understand how the JCAHO evaluates healthcare providers, and they must be familiar with HMOs and the prospective payment system utilizing DRGs.

To participate most fully in the future of healthcare, nurses must also be aware of innovative models of patient care than are being developed, such as the Planetree model, and must be ready to offer ideas that will help create additional models. The NHCP is one plan for delivery of care that has won wide endorsement.

No matter what delivery system is in place in a particular institution, nurses will find that each is vitally involved with ensuring quality and in discovering measurable ways of monitoring that quality. Processes for instituting and maintaining quality differ widely, but what they must have in common is a clear method by which standards are adopted, a reliance on unit-based checks on quality, and an objective means of remedying deficits. For a bright future in the delivery of healthcare, nurses well acquainted with economic and social trends, the latest models of delivery, and the means of ensuring quality care are going to have tremendous impact on the continuing evolution of trends in nursing and overall healthcare.

"The good news: Working together—physicians, nurse, other providers, and consumers of health care—we have all the resources we need here on Earth. Meaningful health care reform, including better primary care, needs common sense, not superhuman rescue fantasies" (Fagin, 1992, p. 543).

REFERENCES

Aburdene, P. and Naisbitt, J. (1992): *Megatrends for Women*. New York, Villard Books.

American College of Health Care Executives (1984): *Health Care in the 1990's: Trends and Strategy*. New York, Arthur Anderson.

American Nurses Association, National League of Nurses, and American Association of Nurse Executives (1991): Nurses National Health Care Plan.

Bernhard, L.A., Walsh, M. (1981): *Leadership: The Key to the Professionalization of Nursing*. New York, McGraw-Hill.

Block, L., Press, C. (1985): Product line development by DRG builds market strength. *Healthcare Finan Manag* December: 50.

Coile, R.C. (1991): Healthcare's future: rising costs and concerns. *Healthcare Trends Transition* April:6.

Curtin, L. (1990): Designing new roles: Nursing in the 90's and beyond. *Nurs Manag* 20(12):7.

Curtin, L., Zurlage, C. (1984): *DRGs: The Reorganization of Health*. Chicago, S-N Publications.

Fagin, C. (1992): The myth of superdoc blocks health care reform. *Nurs Health Care* 13(10):542.

Galinas, L. (1990): Nursing in the 90's, in *Nursing 90 Career Directory*. p. 15.

Glen, J. (1984): Preparing hospital department heads for financial uncertainties ahead. *Hospital Health Services Admin*, 26.

Hadden, R.M. (1981): The final frontier: Nursing in the emerging health care environment. *Nurs Econ* 7(3):155.

Hendrickson, G., Kovner, C.T. (1990): Effects of computers on nursing resource use. *Nurs Econ* 8(1):16.

Joint Commission on Accreditation of Hospitals (1992): Accreditation Manual for Hospitals. Chicago, Joint Commission on Accreditation of Hospitals.

Miraldo, P.S. (1991): The nineties: A decade in search of meaning. *Nurs Health Care* 11(1):11.

Naisbitt, J. and Aburdene, P. (1990): *Megatrends 2000*. New York, William Morrow and Company.

Naisbitt, J. (1984): *Megatrends*. New York, Warner Publisher.

Naisbitt, J., Aburdene, P. (1991): *Megatrends 2000*.

Reinhardt, V. (1984): The health profession's collision course. *Hospitals* August:

Saba, V., McCormick, K. (1986): *Essentials of Computers for Nurses*. New York, J.B. Lippincott.

Schwartz, F.N. (1989): Management, women and the new facts of life. *Harvard Bus Rev* January/February: 65.

Thompson, J., Diers, D. (1986): DRGs and nursing intensity. *Nurs Health Care* 435.

11

Political Action in Nursing

Betty Skaggs, Ph.D., R.N.

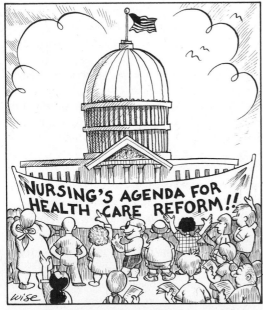

Nurses are playing a major role in the political process for planning the future of health care.

"If you love the law and you love good sausage, don't watch either of them being made."

—Betty Talmadge
The Reader
November, 1977

After completing this chapter, you should be able to:

♦ Define politics and political involvement.

♦ State the rationale for individual nurses' involvement in the political process.

♦ List specific strategies needed to begin to affect the laws that govern the practice of nursing and the healthcare system.

♦ Discuss different types of power and how each is obtained.

♦ Describe the function of a political action committee.

♦ Discuss selected issues affecting nursing:
—Substitution of less-prepared caregivers for RNs.
—Equal pay for work of comparable value.

The quotation above too often reflects nurses' feelings about the legislative process. Politics is associated with wheeling and dealing, smoke-filled rooms, and the exchange of money, favors, and influence. Many believe it is a world that excludes people with ethics and sincerity. Some think only the very rich, the ruthless, or very brave play the game of politics. In the past, nurses seemed to feel that the messy business of politicking should be left to others, while nurses did what they do best and enjoy most—take care of patients.

Today many nurses have come to realize that politics is not a one-dimensional arena, but a complex struggle with strict rules and serious outcomes. In a typical modern political struggle, a rural healthcare center may be pitted for funding against a major interstate highway. Both projects may have merit, but in these times of limited resources not everyone can be victorious. If nurses are to fulfill their mission to "take care of patients," they must engage in the political process.

Today nurses know that if we are to influence the development of public policy, we must be a part of the political process. Nurses must be committed to playing the political game, that is, "the promotion of one's interest group and the use of whatever resources are available to protect and advance that interest" (Kalisch and Kalisch, 1976, p. 80). They must elect the decision-makers, testify before legislative committees, compromise, and get themselves elected to decision-making positions. Nurses know that involvement in the political process is one more tool that we must learn to use if we are to carry out our mission with maximum impact.

According to Joseph Califano, the American healthcare system is "our most rapidly growing, failing U.S. industry" (1978, p. 123). Millions of Americans now receive virtually no healthcare, while countless others receive it only sporadically. Rural and inner-city residents have alarmingly high perinatal morbidity and mortality. Healthcare for rural citizens is virtually nonexistent. Approximately 40 million Americans are without health insurance. Those fortunate enough to have insurance are typically covered only for illness care—rarely health maintenance or promotion. It makes one wonder why they call it "health" insurance!

This assessment, combined with nurses' commitment to the principle that healthcare is a right of all citizens, fuels our desire to become informed consumers and providers of healthcare and to strive to form a collective force to improve the healthcare system.

An example of the force and fury of the nursing collective was the response to the portrait of the nursing profession painted by the TV series, "The Nightingales." Aired by NBC during the 1988 season, the program presented nursing students as vacant females. Offended by the image, the nursing profession rallied. Nurses wrote Aaron Spelling Productions and NBC Entertainment, expressing disgust with the series and promising further action such as a boycott of advertisers who supported the program.

The American Nurses Association (ANA) President Lucille A. Joel offered to provide accurate, positive information about nursing and nursing education. Other nursing organizations orchestrated similar campaigns. In addition, the ANA circulated a list of program sponsors, with the suggestion that nurses let program producers know their feelings about the program.

The result of this collective action is difficult to define precisely, because television networks and producers are reluctant to admit being influenced by what may be perceived as coercive action. The net outcome, however, was that major sponsors such as Sears withdrew their commercial support. This was the blow that probably caused the series to be canceled. Such successes have persuaded nurses that change can be accomplished. And there is an almost limitless number of issues that nurses may confront.

POLITICS AND POWER

What Exactly Is Politics?

Politics, described as "influencing the allocation of scarce resources" (Talbott and Vance, 1981, p. 592), is a vital tool that enables the nurse to "nurse smarter." Involvement in the political process gives the individual nurse a tool that augments his or her power—or clout—to improve care provided to patients. Whether on the unit level, the hospital level, or in the larger community, political skills enable the nurse to identify needed resources, gain access to those resources, and overcome obstacles, thus facilitating the movement of the patient/client to higher levels of health or functioning.

Your hospital is in the process of selecting a new supplier of widgets. You and the other nurses on your unit want to have input into that decision, since widgets are essential to the care of your patients and you have a definite opinion about the type of widget that works best. But the ICU nurses, who are thought to be more important and valuable since the nursing shortage has made them as rare as hen's teeth, have the only nurses' seat on the review committee (and therefore, the director's ear!). You and the nurses on your unit strategize to secure input into this important decision.

Your plan might look like this:

◆ Gather data about widgets—cost, suppliers, possible substitutes, and so on.

◆ Communicate to the head nurse and supervisor your concern with this issue and your plans to get involved in the decision (using appropriate channels of communication).

- State clearly what you want—perhaps request a seat on the committee when the opportunity presents.

- Summarize in writing your request and the rationale, submitting it to the appropriate person(s).

- Establish a coalition with the ICU nurses and/or other concerned individuals.

- Recall that the vice president for purchasing's mother was a patient on your unit and needed widgets in her care and be sure to include this example in your written request.

- Get involved with other hospital issues and contribute in a credible fashion (don't be a single-issue person).

What Other Strategies Would You Suggest?

This vignette illustrates what a politically astute nurse would do in this situation. Even though the example applies to a single hospital, the strategies are comparable to those necessary for getting involved on a community, state, or even federal level. Practicing at the local level will provide good experience for larger issues—you've got to start somewhere. Furthermore, a nurse involved on the local level will be able to hone his or her skills—gaining confidence in the ability to handle similar "exercises" in larger forums.

In our example, the nurse was able to formulate several "political" actions to influence the outcome of the widget decision.

What Are the Skills That Make Up a Nurse's Political Savvy?

Ability to Analyze an Issue (Those Assessment Skills Again!)

The individual who expects to "influence the allocation of scarce resources" must do the homework necessary to be well informed. She or he must know all the facts relevant to the issue—how it looks from all angles and how it fits into the larger picture.

Ability to Present a Possible Resolution in Clear and Concise Terms

The nurse must be prepared to coherently frame and present arguments in support of her or his recommendation. Preparation includes anticipating questions and objections so that a rebuttal will be logical and well developed.

Ability to Participate in a Constructive Way

Too often a person disagrees with a proposal being suggested to a city council (or hospital unit), but only gripes about it. The displeased individual seldom takes the time to study the problem or to understand its connection with other city programs (or of patient care, as a nursing example). Most important, the displeased person seldom suggests an alternate solution.

In short, if an individual's concern is not directed toward solving the problem, she/he will not be seen as a team player, but as a trouble-maker. But constructive responses, perhaps something as simple as posing a single question such as "What solution would you suggest?", may help those involved to think in positive terms and to redirect energy in a more constructive mode. Positive action can produce the kind of creative brainstorming that results in a solution.

Ability to Voice Your Opinion (Understand the System)

When you've done your homework, let the right person know your opinion or solution. For example, communicate your concern and knowledge about the issue to the head nurse and supervisor. Of course, you must make an intelligent and well-informed decision about the person to whom it is best to voice your opinion.

Having a confidant or mentor who knows the environment is one way to acquire this information. Patience and good listening skills are assets that will come in handy! Whatever the technique, studying the dynamics of the institution with all your senses will help you decide on the best person and the most appropriate way to communicate your solution.

Ability to Analyze and Use Power Bases

While discussing issues with colleagues and studying the organization, be alert to the various power brokers. In the widget vignette, the nurse notes the VP for purchasing is an obvious source of power in the hospital. He will certainly concur with, if not make the final decision. But be aware that power does not always follow the lines on the organizational chart. The power of the nurse's aide on the oncology unit who just happens to be the niece of the newly appointed member of the Board of Trustees may escape the notice of some. This person could be used to influence a decision if necessary. Similarly, the fact that the VP for purchasing's mother was on the unit should be filed in your memory for future use.

Facts may be facts, but where you get your information can sometimes make a statement as powerful as the information itself. Most important, having the ability to use many different channels of information will give you the power to choose among them.

What is Power and Where Can I Get Some?

Sanford (1979) describes five laws of power. She recommends that these laws be studied to identify strategies to develop power in nursing. The laws are as follows:

Law 1. Power Invariably Fills any Vacuum.   When a problem or issue arises, the prevailing desire is for peace and order. People are willing to give power to someone interested in restoring order to situations of discomfort.

Therefore, someone will eventually step forward to handle the dilemma. It may be some time before the discomfort or unrest grows to heights sufficient for someone to take the lead. Furthermore, a poorly thought-out solution may be brought forward. Nonetheless, a person exerting power will step forward to offer a solution. In some situations this person may be the previously identified leader, the head nurse, or the chair. More often there is an official power broker influencing the action. Know that there are opportunities to exert influence by stepping forward to fill the vacuum.

Law 2. Power is Invariably Personal. In most instances, programs are attributed to an organization. For example, the program, *Smokefree Class of 2000*, was proposed by the American Cancer Association, the American Lung Association, the American Heart Association, and their state affiliates. If we investigated, we might find that a small group of friends had discussed over a pizza one evening the number of young children smoking. In the course of their conversation, one might have said, "You know, the kids starting school today will graduate in 2000; they will be the "Class of 2000"! And the next person might have said, "Wouldn't it be great if we could convince that group of the dangers. I'm going to propose. . . ."

Initiatives such as this start with a person creating a new approach to a problem. That person exercises power by creating the strategies to carry out such an initiative, thus inspiring people to contribute to the effort.

Law 3. Power is Based on a System of Ideas and Philosophy. Behaviors demonstrated by an individual as he or she exerts power reflect a personal belief system or a philosophy of life. That philosophy or ideal must be one that attracts followers, gains their respect, and rallies them to join the effort. Nurses have the opportunity to ensure that a patient's right to safe nursing care, his or her *right* to health care (versus privilege), access to *preventive* care, and similar values are reflected in policies and procedures.

Law 4. Power is Exercised Through and Depends on Institutions. As single individuals we can easily feel powerless and unable to deal with the complex problems facing a hospital or state. But through a nursing service organization, a state nurses' association, or similar organization we can garner the resources we need to magnify our power. The person-to-person network, the communication vehicle (usually an organization's newsletter or journal), and the organizational structure are established for precisely this function—to support and foster changes in the healthcare system.

Law 5. Power is Invariably Confronted With and Acts in the Presence of a Field of Responsibility. Actions taken speak to the other nurses for whom we act and, most important, the patients for whom we advocate. The individual in the power position is acting on behalf of the group. Power is communicated to observers and is reinforced by positive responses. If the group thinks that its ideals are not being honored, the vacuum will be filled with the next candidate capable of the role and supported by the organization.

Another Way to Look at Power and Where to Get It

French and Raven (1959) described five sources of power. They are (in order of their importance): reward power, coercive power, legitimate power, referent or mentor power, and expert or informational power. The strongest source of power is the ability to *reward*. The best example of using the reward power base is the giving of money. If, for example, one gives a decision-maker financial support for a future political campaign, the recipient will feel obligated to the donor and may from time to time "adjust opinions" to repay these obligations! Today, since caps have been placed on campaign contributions, the misuse of this type of reward has been reduced. An additional source of reward-based political power is the ability to commit voters to a candidate through endorsements. This illustrates the importance of having a large number of members in the organization—in other words, a large voting bloc.

Second in importance is the power to *coerce* or "punish" a decision-maker for going against the wishes of an organization. The best example of this power, the opposite of reward, is the ability to remove the person from office at election time.

Third in importance is *legitimate* power, or the influence that comes with role and position. Influence derives from the status that society assigns individuals as a result of, for instance, their leadership in the church, membership on the school board, or other prominent positions in the community. The dean in your school of nursing had a certain amount of influence just because of who she or he was, right? Our commitment to enhancing nursing's influence explains why we encourage and assist nurses to achieve key decision-making positions—to build our legitimate power base.

The fourth power base is that of *referent* or *mentor* power. This is the power that "rubs off" of influential persons. When representatives of the student body talk with the dean about a problem they are having with a course and receive his or her support, the faculty is more likely to listen sympathetically than if the students were arguing only for themselves. The dean, joining with the students to solve their problem, adds to the students' power. The wish to build this power encourages us to join coalitions, especially those including organizations with greater power than our own.

The last and weakest power base is that of *expert* power. Nurses know about health and nursing care; therefore, we are able to impart knowledge in this area with great confidence and style. Typically, nurses communicate this authority through the letters we write to legislators and through other contacts we make on behalf of nursing and patients.

In summary, power is derived from various sources. Nurses use with greatest frequency and ease the weakest of the power bases, that deriving from their expertise. Although this is an important power base, we must develop and exercise the other types as well. Only then will we realize the full extent of our potential.

What Is Networking?

It's been said that you should never be more than two phone calls away from a resource you need, whether it be a piece of information, a contact in a hospital in another city, or input into a decision you are about to make. The key to successful networking is consciously building and nurturing a pool of associates whose skills and connections augment your own.

As a new graduate, you should begin the important task of networking by selecting one of your instructors from nursing school, an instructor who is able to speak to your performance during nursing school. Ask this person if he or she would be willing to write a letter of reference for your first job. If he or she agrees, nurture this contact from now on. Keep this individual apprised of your whereabouts, your successes, and your plans for the future. He or she will be an important link not only to your school but to your future educational and work undertakings. Again, when you leave a job, find a person to give you a reference and to stay in contact with.

Remember that your network must be nourished. Constant use of your sources without reciprocation will exhaust them and make them unreliable sources of assistance in the future. But if properly cared for, your network will support you for the rest of your career.

BUILDING COALITIONS

A coalition is a group of organizations that share a common interest in a single issue. The groups with whom nurses might form coalitions are as diverse as the topics about which nurses are concerned. For example, nurses are concerned about and lobby for adequate, safe child care, a safe environment, and women's issues. The numerous organizations interested in these diverse issues are potential candidates for a coalition with nursing organizations. It is not unusual for two organizations to be in a coalition on one issue but adversaries on another. Indeed, it's typical in the political arena, where negotiations and compromises are common.

A warning, however: the selection of coalition members should help your organization. Forming coalitions is a strategy to empower oneself. Therefore, solicit organizations enjoying greater power than nursing, not less.

▼

Trade-offs, compromises, negotiations, and other tricks of the trade.

▲

Politics is the art of the possible; not the perfect. Often in the heat of battle we are unwilling to compromise, and therefore sacrifice all.

▼

"To hold out for the ideal often sacrifices an improvement in the real"
(Stevens, p. 210).

▲

POLITICAL SKILLS AND THE GOVERNMENTAL PROCESS

The political skills so far discussed apply to any situation, whether in a family, a hospital unit, or a community. The next part of the chapter will discuss skills that apply specifically to the governmental process.

How Does One Go About Participating in the Election Process?

One key to successful political activity is involvement in the election process. This is the stage where you can get to know the candidates, and they, you. In addition, it is a time when you can make important contacts for that network you are building.

Getting involved in a candidate's campaign is simple. First, study the positions to be filled. Then, with the help of the local nurses' association, the local newspaper, and the Democratic (or Republican) Party for your county or state, select the candidate whose views on healthcare most closely match yours. Next, find the candidate's campaign headquarters. After this, all you have to do is contact the candidate's volunteer coordinator and see when volunteer help is needed. Most campaigns are crying for assistance: folding letters and stuffing envelopes, looking up addresses, and sorting bulk mailings. They will welcome you with great enthusiasm! Be sure to tell the campaign staff that you are a nurse and would be more than willing to improve the candidate's understanding of healthcare issues and to draft the candidate's positions on these issues.

Beware: involvement in campaigns and party organizations can lead to catching the political "bug." Victims of the political bug are overcome by the multitude of opportunities to educate people about the health needs of a county, state, or nation. For example, party platforms are a way to get information about health issues to decision-makers as well as to the electorate. During the past national presidential election, a group of nurses at a state caucus volunteered to write the resolution for the party's position on healthcare. After much work drafting the statement and bringing it before various committees, the group was ecstatic when it passed and became the health statement for their party! See Table 11–1 for an example of a state's healthcare resolution.

TABLE 11–1   *Healthcare Resolution*

Whereas one and a half billion dollars a day is spent on healthcare services that are not comprehensive, nor available to all persons;

Whereas this is a greater percentage of the U.S. Gross National Product (GNP) than any other industrialized country in the world, while those countries do better on key measures of health such as the infant mortality rate and life expectancy;

Whereas according to the Pepper Commission, 31–37 million Americans have no health insurance protection, 20 million are underinsured, and $200 million of the maternal-child health dollars (for services such as care for the pregnant women and infants) were cut earlier in this congressional session from the funding bill;

Whereas every $1 spent on prevention will avoid many more dollars lost in wages, work-time, and more expensive treatment services like emergency or critical care;

Whereas according to Senator Inouye, $1440 per person is spent on curative care, while $0.50 per person is spent on preventive activities;

Whereas every U.S. surgeon general since 1976 has stated that activities promoting health and preventing disease are the most cost-effective approaches to healthcare;

Whereas AIDS has reached epidemic levels, and is rapidly working its way into vulnerable and disadvantaged populations who traditionally have had little access to healthcare;

BE IT RESOLVED,

—that the Texas Democratic Party reaffirms the basic right to healthcare, which in availability must assure quality of care as well as cost-effectiveness,

—that furthermore, the party supports the current efforts of the Congress, particularly the Pepper Commission and the various agencies, to work toward the national goal of Health for All in 2000.

—that furthermore the party affirms the cost-effective, urgently needed preventive approach to healthcare, including guaranteeing that all pregnant women have access to prenatal care, and that every child under 18 has access to healthcare and immunizations,

—and that furthermore efforts be continued to stem the AIDS epidemic and provide healthcare support to HIV+ persons with equitable and affordable access.

(Reprinted with permission from Green SA (1990): Getting involved in a political party. *Texas Nursing* 64(7):13.)

What Is a PAC?

Another way that nurses can influence the elective process is through involvement in an organization's political action committee (PAC). PACs grew out of the Watergate era, when Congress decided that candidates for public office were becoming too dependent on money supplied by special interests—individuals who give large political contributions and thereby exert undue influence over the elected official's decisions.

As a result, Congress limited the amount of money an individual could contribute to a candidate, established strict reporting requirements, and created a mechanism whereby individuals could pool their resources and collectively support a candidate.

The American Nurses Association's National PAC is called ANAPAC. Through this vehicle, nurses across the country organize to collectively endorse and support candidates for national offices. Likewise, state nurses' associations have state-level PACs to influence state elections. There may be local PACs in your area, which endorse candidates in city elections. All PACs must comply with the state and federal election codes and report financial support given to candidates for public office.

Today PACs play an important role in the political process, since they provide a mechanism whereby small contributors like you and I can act as a collective, participating in the electoral process when otherwise we would feel outmaneuvered by the bigger players.

The ANA's Endorsement Handbook stresses three points regarding PACs:

◆ **Political focus.** The only purpose of any PAC is to endorse candidates for public office and then supply them with the political and financial support they need to win an election.

◆ **No legislative activities.** A PAC does not lobby elected officials; that is the job of the state nurses' association and its government-relations arm. A PAC simply provides political support for candidates whose views are generally consistent with those of its contributors.

◆ **Not "Dirty".** A PAC does not "buy" a candidate or a vote; but the very nature of political life suggests that candidates who recognize our ability to affect their electoral prospects will be inclined to listen to our views when considering specific pieces of legislation.

This author wishes to make an additional important point.

◆ **Health concerns only.** Nursing PACs evaluate the candidates on health concerns only. In other words, we might solicit the candidates' ideas about how the state legislature might solve the problem of elder abuse in long-term care facilities. But we as a nursing PAC should not include questions, for instance, about the source of funding for the new state commerce department. The organization speaks for members only on issues covered in our philosophical statements, resolutions, position statements, legislative platforms, or other documents that we as an organization have accepted.

After Getting Them Elected, Then What?

Lobbying is the attempt to influence or sway a public official to take a desired action. Lobbying could also be characterized as the education of the legislator about nursing and its issues. Educating officials, like educating patients, is an important part of the nurse's role.

We can lobby in several different ways. The first and best opportunity to lobby arrives when you first meet the candidate and evaluate him or her as a potential office holder. This is the time to assess the candidate's knowledge of healthcare issues. Take the time to teach as well as learn.

A second opportunity may come when the official needs information to decide how to vote on an issue. Depending on time constraints, the issue, and other considerations, a nurse might decide to lobby the official in person or in writing.

If time permits, the most powerful type of contact is a face-to-face visit. The only way to ensure time with your senator or representative is to make an appointment. Even then you may not be successful.

If an unscheduled visit to the capitol precludes an appointment, the best time to see your senator or representative is early in the day, before the legislative session starts. Contact with a legislative aide or assistant can sometimes be just as effective as time with the official. Busy federal and state officials depend heavily on their staff. Treat staff members with the respect they deserve!

Finally, remember that contact should be made between legislative sessions and during holidays when the official is in his or her home district. The structure and content of the visit should be similar to that of a letter. That is, know your issue, keep it short, identify the issue by its bill number and title, and communicate exactly what action you want the senator or representative to take. Here is a list of specific "do's and don'ts when lobbying." As you try lobbying, add your recommendations to the list.

DO:

◆ Make sure your legislator knows constituents who are affected by the bill; suggest visits to programs in his or her area.

◆ Clearly identify the bill, using title and number, if possible.

◆ Be specific and know about the issue or bill before you write or talk.

◆ Identify yourself (occupation, hometown, member of ANA).

◆ Use your own words; if writing, use your own stationery. No form letters!

◆ Be courteous, brief, and to the point.

◆ Provide pertinent reasons for your stand.

◆ Show your legislator how the issue relates to his or her district.

◆ Respect your legislator's right to form an opinion different from yours.

◆ Present a united front. Keep our internal problems "at home."

◆ Write letters of appreciation to your legislators when appropriate.

◆ Write letters at appropriate times, for example, when a bill is in committee request action that is appropriate for that stage in the legislative process.

◆ Establish an on-going relationship with the public official.

◆ Know issues or problems your legislator is concerned about and express your interest in assisting him or her.

◆ Attend functions sponsored by coalition members. Be seen!

◆ Get involved in your legislator's campaign for reelection—or his or her opponent's, if necessary!

DON'T:

◆ Write a long letter or one on multiple points; deal with a single bill or concern per letter or contact.

◆ Use threats or promises.

◆ Berate your legislator.

◆ Be offended in the event of a cancelled appointment. Things are unpredictable during a legislative session.

◆ Demand a commitment before the legislator has had time to consider the measure.

◆ Pretend to have vast influence in the political area.

◆ Be vague.

◆ Hesitate to admit you don't know all the facts, but indicate you will find out—and do!

If you cannot visit your representative because of time or travel restrictions, a well-written letter will communicate your message. Examine the sample letter in Fig. 11–1. Note that some pointers are listed at the foot of the page. Examples of the proper way to address a public official are presented in Table 11–2.

Although letters are probably the most common method of communicating with elected officials, a phone call is often necessary to relay your opinion before an important vote. Again, the suggested format and content of the phone message is similar to that of a letter or interview. Refer to the list of do's and don'ts when lobbying.

Strategy for types of contact will vary depending on the situation. For

Ima Nurse, RN
123 Main Street
Any Town, USA 12345-6789

The Honorable Y. R. Senator, Jr.
United States Senate
Washington, D.C. 20510

Dear Senator Senator:

I request your support of SB 101 regarding appropriations for nursing education and research. This bill is vital to the country's efforts to improve the number and quality of registered nurses. As you recall, the 1991 Institute of Nursing Study demonstrated the growing demand for Advanced Nurse Practitioners to work with the increasing numbers of people over 65 years of age. This bill will provide funding to increase the number of faculty and student slots in the country's schools of nursing and to support nursing research in gerontological nursing. The expanding numbers of older people in our area of the state are not able to get the healthcare they deserve. I would like to take you to the Senior's Clinic sometime at your convenience. I know that you would be pleased with this service, as are the healthcare providers and the clients.

Will you support this bill? Do you have any questions about it? If so, please contact me.

Thank you for your concern with this issue and your continuing support of healthcare issues.

Sincerely yours,

Ima Nurse, RN

Continued

FIGURE 11–1   *Example of a letter to a public official.*

....

Points to note:

1. Neat, without typos or grammatical errors
2. Correctly addressed
3. Professional letterhead
4. Covering single topic
5. Refers to the bill by number and content
6. States request in first sentence
7. Brief rationale for request
8. Uses RN in inside address and salutation

FIGURE 11–1 *Example of a letter to a public official. Continued*

example, if the bill about which you are concerned is coming up the first time in committee, you may wish to have ten to fifteen people write letters to or call the members of the committee. At this point, the number of contacts with the office is important. The reason is that the legislator's assistant typically answers the phone or opens the mail, notes the subject of the contact, and puts a tally in the "Pro HB 23" or "Con HB 23" column. Therefore, a greater impact will be realized if the contacts pertain to one bill. Bags of form letters, however, have a negative impact on your lobbying efforts. Avoid them at all cost. Similarly, people who call the legislator's office with a script that they don't understand will not further the lobbying efforts of an organization.

On the other hand, if a major, controversial bill is coming up for a final vote in the Senate you will want to activate a state-wide network and bombard the senators with letters, phone calls, and telegrams—as many as possible. The bigger the issue, the bigger the campaign should be.

At several points in a lobbying season, but certainly after contacting him or her for a major vote, a follow-up letter will strengthen your contact with the legislator. In addition to reinforcing the reason for your original contact, thank the official for his or her concern with the issue and work in solving the problem by writing the bill or voting for it (or whatever), and for paying attention to your concern.

In summary, there are some skills to learn for effective political involvement. But most of the skills needed to be politically savvy are ones that will serve you well in everyday professional negotiations.

As you get oriented in your first job and begin to look around at what you

TABLE 11–2 *How to Address Public Officials*

The President

Writing:	The Honorable (Full Name)
	President of the United States
	The White House
	Washington, D.C. 20500
	Dear Mr./Madam President:
Speaking:	"Mr./Madam President"
	President (Last Name)

The Vice President

Writing:	The Honorable (Full Name)
	Vice President of the United States
	Executive Office Building
	Washington, D.C. 20501
	Dear Mr./Madam Vice President:
Speaking:	"Mr./Madam Vice President"
	Vice President (Last Name)

A Senator

Writing:	The Honorable (Full Name)
	United States Senate
	(will have office building and room address)
	Washington, D.C. 20510
	Dear Senator (Full Name):
Speaking:	"Senator (Last Name)"

A Representative

Writing:	The Honorable (Full Name)
	U.S. House of Representatives
	(will have office building and room address)
	Washington, D.C. 20515
	Dear Mr./Ms. (Full Name):
Speaking:	"Representative (Last Name)"
	"Mr./Ms. (Last Name)"

A Member of the Cabinet

Writing:	The Honorable (Full Name)
	Secretary of (Cabinet Agency)
	(will have office building and room address)
	Washington, D.C. 20520
	Dear Mr./Madam Secretary:
Speaking:	"Mr./Madam Secretary" or "Secretary (Last Name)"

The correct closing for a letter to the President is: Very respectfully yours.

The correct closing for all other federal officials noted above is: Sincerely yours.

and your colleagues need to improve, you will agree that political involvement is necessary to reach your goals. This author implores you *not* to wait to be "allowed" to make a difference, *not* to wait to be *invited* to join, and *not* to let someone else do the job. Please step forward! Act like the powerful, informed nurse that you are! Look like the powerful, with-it nurse that you are, and be the powerful, influential nurse that you are. There is much that needs to be done—be a part of the action!

....

Sarah E. Archer (1985) remarked that "If nurses are to fulfill their role as advocates for quality health care, they must realize that caring for and about people is not enough. Nurses must act politically" (Hansten and Washburn 1990, p. 55).

....

CONTROVERSIAL POLITICAL ISSUES AFFECTING NURSING

The Substitution of Less-Prepared Caregivers

Sicker patients, increasing technology, increasing demands for nursing skills, changing opportunities for women, and changing demographics of the population are a sample of the complex factors that are stressing the nursing system. The resulting serious nursing personnel shortage and maldistribution problems threaten the quality and availability of nursing care in most clinical settings in the country.

The solutions, equally complex, range from paying hiring bonuses of thousands of dollars to major recruitment campaigns, such as one designed by the Ad Council: "If caring were enough, anybody could be a nurse."

All agree that these efforts do little for the long-term alleviation of the shortage. One attempt at immediate relief was the program suggested by the American Medical Association (AMA), the Registered Care Technologist (RCT) program. "The AMA characterizes the RCT as a nonleadership, technical role designed to supplement and be additive to nursing at the bedside. The scope of practice would be to continuously monitor and implement physicians' orders at the bedside under constant supervision" (ANA, 1989).

The RCT proposal was not a viable solution to the nursing shortage. Instead nurses agreed that the proposal would further stress existing nursing staff. Furthermore, nurses believed that the RCT would compromise the quality of nursing care and jeopardize the safety of patients.

While nursing has long depended on assistive personnel such as licensed vocational/practical nurses and unlicensed aides, we are committed to the fact that nursing is accountable for the quality of nursing care provided patients.

Nursing is adamantly opposed to the substitution of a less-prepared caregiver, one who is neither trained by, supervised by, nor accountable to the registered nurse.

The Nursing Tri-Council (American Nurses Association, the National League for Nursing, the American Association of Colleges of Nursing, and the American Organization of Nurse Executives), together with most major nursing specialty groups, has therefore professed a commitment to solve the nursing shortage and ensure quality of care by endorsing the ANA's Council on Practice statement on assistive personnel to the registered nurse (Table 11-3):

TABLE 11–3 *American Nurses Association*
Position Statement on Registered Nurse Utilization of Unlicensed Assistive Personnel

Summary: The American Nurses Association (ANA) recognizes that unlicensed assistive personnel provide support services to the RN which are required for the registered nurse to provide nursing care in the health care settings of today.

The current changes in the health care environment have and will continue to alter the scope of nursing practice and its relationship to the activities delegated to unlicensed assistive personnel (UAP). The concern is that in virtually all health care settings, UAP's are inappropriately performing functions which are within the legal practice of nursing. This is a violation of the state nursing practice act and is a threat to public safety. Today, it is the nurse who must have a clear definition of what constitutes the scope of practice with the reconfiguration of practice settings, delivery sites and staff composition. Professional guidelines must be established to support the nurse in working effectively and collaboratively with other health care professionals and administrators in developing appropriate roles, job descriptions and responsibilities for UAP's.

The purpose of this position statement is to delineate ANA's beliefs about the utilization of unlicensed assistive personnel in assisting in the provision of direct and indirect patient care under the direction of a registered nurse.

UNLICENSED ASSISTIVE PERSONNEL

The term unlicensed assistive personnel applies to an unlicensed individual who is trained to function in an assistive role to the licensed nurse in the provision of patient/client activities as delegated by the nurse. The activities can generally be categorized as either direct or indirect care.

Direct patient care activities are delegated by the registered nurse and assist the patient/client in meeting basic human needs. This includes activities related to feeding, drinking, positioning, ambulating, grooming, toileting, dressing and socializing and may involve the collecting, reporting and documentation of data related to these activities.

Indirect patient care activities focus on maintaining the environment and the systems in which nursing care is delivered and only incidently involve direct patient contact. These activities assist in providing a clean, efficient, and safe patient care environment

Table continued on following page

TABLE 11–3 *American Nurses Association* Continued

and typically encompass categories such as housekeeping and transporting, clerical, stocking and maintenance supplies.

UTILIZATION

Monitoring the regulation, education and utilization of unlicensed assistive personnel to the registered nurse has been ongoing since the early 1950s. While the time frames and environmental factors that influence policy may have changed, the underlying principles have remained consistent:

- ◆ IT IS THE NURSING PROFESSION that determines the scope of nursing practice;

- ◆ IT IS THE NURSING PROFESSION that defines and supervises the education, training and utilization for any unlicensed assistant roles involved in providing direct patient care;

- ◆ IT IS THE RN who is responsible and accountable for the provision of nursing practice;

- ◆ IT IS THE RN who supervises and determines the appropriate utilization of any unlicensed assistant involved in providing direct patient care; and

- ◆ IT IS THE PURPOSE of unlicensed assistive personnel to enable the professional nurse to provide nursing care for the patient.

It is the assumption of the ANA that the provision of safe, accessible and affordable nursing care for the public may include the appropriate utilization of unlicensed assistive personnel and that the changes in the health care environment have and will continue to alter the activities delegated to UAPs.

Therefore, it is the responsibility of the nursing profession to establish and the individual nurse to implement the standards for the practice and utilization of unlicensed assistive personnel involved in assisting the nurse in the direct patient care activities. This is accomplished through national standards of practice and the definitions of nursing in state nursing practice acts.

In order to understand the roles and responsibilities between the RN and the UAP the ANA recognizes that the key to understanding is the clarification of professional nursing care delivery and the activities that can be delegated within the domain of nursing. The act of delegation is:

the transfer of responsibility for the performance of an activity from one person to another while retaining accountability for the outcome.

In delegating, it is the RN who uses professional judgement to determine the appropriate activities to delegate. The determination is based on the concept of protection of the public and includes consideration of the needs of the patients, the education and training of the nursing and assistive staff, the extent of supervision required, and the staff workload. Any nursing intervention that requires independent, specialized nursing knowledge, skill or judgement can not be delegated.

Reprinted with permission, American Nurses Association, *Position Statement on Unlicensed Assistive Personnel*, 1992.

TABLE 11–4   *Nursing Salary Comparison to Other Professions*

PROFESSION	AVERAGE BEGINNING	AVERAGE MAXIMUM	SALARY COMPARISON OF REGISTERED NURSE TO OTHER PROFESSIONS' AVERAGE MAXIMUM
Accountants	$24,809	$75,347	154%
Accounting clerks	14,639	24 787	49.3%
Chemists	27,162	88,749	181.4%
Computer programmers	26,103	42,533	115%
Engineers	32,459	95,058	194%
Personnel directors	45,618	101,922	208.3%
Registered nurses	27,225	48,924	
Secretaries	19,844	34,085	69.6%

Source: U.S. Department of Labor, Bureau of Labor Statistics (January, 1992), Occupational Wage Survey: Hospitals. Bulletin 2392, p. 128.

Equal Pay for Work of Comparable Value or Comparable Worth

The concept of comparable worth or pay equity holds that jobs that are equal in value to an organization ought to be equally compensated, whether or not the work content of those jobs is similar. Pay equity relates to the goal of equitable compensation as outlined in the Equal Pay Act of 1963, and "sex-based wage discrimination," a phrase that refers to the basis of the problems defined by Title VII of the Civil Rights Act of 1964.

As long ago as World War II, the War Labor Board suggested that discrimination probably exists whenever jobs traditionally relegated to women pay below the rate of common-labor jobs such as janitor or floor sweeper. One of the first cases was that of the *International Union of Electrical Workers vs. Westinghouse*. The union proved that male-female wage disparity existed and uncovered a policy in a manual that stated women were to be paid less because they were women. Back pay and increased wages were given in an out-of-court settlement in an appellate-level decision.

It was nurses who initiated the action, *Lemons vs. the City and County of Denver*. Nurses employed by the City of Denver claimed under the Civil Rights Act that they were the victims of salary discrimination, since their jobs were of a value equal to various better-paid positions throughout the city's diverse workforce. The court ruled that the city was justified in the use of a market pricing system (a form of pay based on supply and demand) even though it acknowledged the general discrimination against women. The court said that the case (and the comparable-worth concept) had the potential to disrupt the entire economic system of the United States. Because of this judgment and the fact that the nurses were unable to prepare a job evaluation program to substantiate their claim, the judge dismissed the case.

Another important concept in this area is "salary compression." That is, at the beginning of a nurse's career, he or she can expect to enter a beginning staff nurse position earning approximately $26,000. This same nurse can expect to earn a maximum salary of $36,000, or a 38.5% salary progression over a career (Texas Hospital Salary Survey, 1990). A comparison with other professions is shown in Table 11–4.

One explanation offered for the discrepancy is that the salary system for nurses is based on the assumption that most nurses are temporary workers. Therefore salary structures are relatively flat, with essentially no allowances for administrative responsibilities and almost no differential for experience.

Needless to say, much work continues to be done in this important area. Nurses and women in general must continue to strive for equitable compensation based on the inherent value or worth of the work performed, instead of on the basis of historically depressed pay levels or other discriminatory factors. Changes will be achieved as we educate others about inequities, initiate legal remedies in courts and state legislatures, and effect changes in the workplace.

References

American Nurses Association (1989): *Defeating the RCT and Similar Proposals: Workplace Strategies.* Kansas City, MO, American Nurses Association.

Califano, J. (1978): What is wrong with U.S. health care? *Congressional Record* 123 (E4281-E4283).

Flanagan, L. (1990): *Survival Skills in the Workplace: What Every Nurse Should Know.* Kansas City, MO, American Nurses Association.

French, J.R.P., Raven, B. (1959): The bases of social power, in Cartwright, D. (ed): Studies in Social Power. Ann Arbor, University of Michigan, p. 150.

Green, S.A. (1990): Getting involved in a political party. *Texas Nursing.* 64(7):13.

Hansten, R.I., Washburn, M. (1990): *I Light the Lamp.* Vancouver, WA. Applied Therapeutics, Inc.

Jordan, C.J. (1983): The power of political activity, in Stevens, K.R. (ed): *Power and Influence: A Source Book for Nurses.* New York, Wiley, p. 84.

Kalisch, B.J., Kalisch, P.A. (1976): A discourse on the politics of nursing. *J Nurs Admin* 6(2):79.

Mason, D.J., Talbott, S.W. (eds) (1985): *Political Action: Handbook for Nurses.* Menlo Park, CA, Addison-Wesley.

Sanford, N.D. (1979): *Identification and Explanation of Strategies to Develop Power for Nursing.* In *Power: Nursing's Challenge for Change.* Kansas City, MO; American Nurses Association, p. 15.

Schutzenhofer, K.K., Cannon, S.B. (1986): Moving nurses into the political process. *Nurse Educ* 11(2):26.

Stevens, B.J. (1980): Power and politics for the nurse executive. *Nurs Health Care* 1:208.

Stevens, K.R. (ed) (1983): *Power and Influence: A Source Book for Nurses.* New York, J Wiley.

Talbott, S.W., Vance, C. (1981): Involving nursing in a feminist group NOW. *Nursing Outlook* 29:592.

Texas Hospital Association (1990): *Hospital Employees Salary Survey.* Austin, TX, Texas Hospital Association.

12

A Collective Voice in the Workplace

Mary E. Foley, R.N., B.S.N.

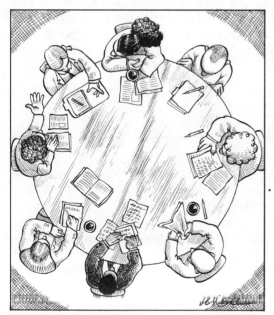

Is there a place for collective bargaining in nursing?

Compromise does not mean cowardice.
—John F. Kennedy

After completing this chapter, you should be able to:

- ◆ Describe the history of collective bargaining in nursing.
- ◆ Compare collective bargaining and other workplace governance structures.
- ◆ Identify the conditions that may cause nurses to seek collective bargaining representation.
- ◆ Identify the steps nurses would take to initiate collective bargaining representation.

You will soon be accepting your first position as a registered nurse (RN). You will not only be adjusting to a new role, but to a new workplace. Even in these times of dramatic change in healthcare, many of you will start your career in a hospital. In fact, recent demographics about nurses show that over two-thirds of nurses in practice are providing care in hospitals.

It is understandable that your major concern may be your personal readiness to practice as an RN. Another legitimate, but often overlooked, concern of new graduates and senior nurses is whether the workplace is prepared to let *you* practice as a professional! As you start your selection process for the first job or the last job of your career, your decision-making process can be made somewhat easier if you employ some of the strategies recommended in materials like *Survival Skills in the Workplace* (Flanagan, 1990).

Hospital structures and governance policies can have a dramatic influence on how much a nurse fulfills her or his obligation to clients and families. Nurses have defined themselves as professionals, and as professionals, must have a voice in and control over the practice of nursing. When that voice and control are *not* supported by the work setting, a conflict will arise.

In some areas of the country, nurses have chosen to gain a voice in and assume control of their practice by using a collective bargaining model. This chapter is intended to give you an idea of why and how that has been accomplished. This chapter will also honestly address some of the controversy that surrounds nursing and unions.

NURSING'S LABOR HISTORY

The first nursing association to represent nurses was the California Nurses Association (CNA). The desire to organize collectively, which came from within nursing, was forced by the wages, benefits, and the conditions of the workplace even before legal protections for employees were legislated. Some believe that when the employers in California saw the alternative—trade unions—they opted for the "lesser of the evils" by cooperating with the CNA proposals of the 1930s and 1940s. Nursing's earliest experiences in the bargaining arena predated the earliest labor law, and occurred in a period when little protection was offered the hospital worker.

Most contracts throughout the nation included no-strike language through the 1960s and 1970s. Table 12–1 highlights the history of labor law in this country.

TABLE 12–1   *A Review of Major Events in the History of the Labor Law*

1935	Passage of the National Labor Relations Act, also known as the Wagner Act: allowed private-sector employees to organize for the purpose of negotiating terms of their wages, hours, and working conditions.
1947	Taft-Hartley Amendments of the National Labor Relations Act: placed specific restraints on unfair labor practices by unions.
1947	Tyding Amendments: Exempted the nonprofit healthcare industry from the National Labor Relations Act.
1974	Repeal of the Tyding Amendments: Extended the National Labor Relations Act to employees of the nonprofit health care industry.
1979	California Court "Sierra Vista" decision: affirmed state nurses' associations, when properly structured, could represent nurses for collective bargaining.
1991	U.S. Supreme Court agreed that the NLRB had ruled properly when it determined registered nurses are entitled to separate and distinct bargaining units.

COLLECTIVE BARGAINING IN NURSING

Is There a Place for Collective Bargaining in Nursing?

Should nurses use collective bargaining if they are professionals? Is nursing a profession or an occupation? These are the kinds of questions nursing has debated, and continues to debate, throughout its history.

A profession can be defined as a vocation that requires a long period of specialized education to prepare one for service to society. Because of their expertise and the value of their service, society grants professionals a measure of autonomy in their work. This autonomy permits professionals to make *independent* judgments and decisions based on a theoretical base that is learned through study and practice.

Conflict arises for nurse-employees because of the pressures as they advocate for their professional role in client care and the healthcare institutions' demand for productivity and cost savings. In addition, nurses are no longer immune to job security issues. For example, as cost containment has become the watchword of the hospital industry, staff "down-sizing" and increased nurse workloads have occurred as the client population's acuity level has risen. In other words, the clients are sicker, and yet are moved more quickly through the acute care setting, by use of such innovations as same-day surgery, same-day admissions, and early discharge. Add periodic shortages of nurses prepared for acute care, long-term care, and home care, and substitution of nurses with unlicensed assistive personnel, and a soon to be reformed health system, and tensions are understandably high.

A study conducted by a Kansas City labor relations consulting firm defined why hospital employees and nurses joined unions, and how union organizers garnered their support. Their conclusion confirms what has been confirmed again and again:

> A myth widely subscribed to by hospital management is that big powerful unions organize professional nurses. In fact, unions do not organize nurses; professional nurses organize themselves. They do this because administrators and nursing supervisors fail to recognize and address nurses' individual and collective needs. (Stickler and Velghe, 1980, p. 14)

In addition, a study from the University of California, Berkeley, found that nurses who engage in collective bargaining believe it is the only solution to a management-employee power struggle. They conclude that nurses decide to unionize because of their "inability to communicate with management and their perception of authoritarian behavior on the part of management" (Parlette et al., 1980, p. 16).

Nursing has used collective action to its benefit, achieving professional goals while protecting and promoting public interest through lobbying efforts in the political arena. Many nurses support collective bargaining in the workplace as a way to control their practice by redistributing power within the healthcare organization. Virginia Cleland (1981) stated, "The power bestowed upon the nursing profession should derive not from the hospital administrator's benevolence, but rather from the public's view of the value of services provided by the practitioner" (p. 17). Ada Jacox (1980) has criticized nursing departments that fail to acknowledge that nurses are professionals. In her view (and the author's) the authority for nursing practice must rest within the profession. She suggests that collective bargaining through the professional organization may be a way for nurses to achieve collective professional responsibility.

If I'm a Nurse, Who Should Speak for Me?

As you choose a job with a union in place, or about to choose a union, what have been the choices for nurses? Meatpackers, Paperhangers, United Food and Commercial Workers and Longshoremen, Teamsters, Local 1199 AFL-CIO, the Service Employees International Union, the Association of Federal, State, County and Municipal Employees (AFSCME), and the American Federation of Teachers (AFT) are among the competitors.

Competition for nurses has become intense, especially as traditional union membership has declined. Some of these unions offer organizations the image of endless resources and lengthy experience in labor relations.

▼

Traditional trade unions, however, are reluctant to become involved in worker control issues—control of practice that many nurses seek when they pursue collective bargaining—and often focus only on wages and benefits.

▲

If nursing goals are to be set by nurses, it is this author's firm conviction that nurses must represent themselves. As Jacox, Cleland, and many other nursing leaders have stated, the professional association has the means and responsibility to represent nurses. The national professional organization for nursing is the American Nurses Association (ANA) with its constituent units, the state and territorial nursing associations. Through its economic security programs, ANA recognizes state nursing associations as the logical bargaining agents for professional nurses. These professional associations are indeed multipurpose; their activities include economic analysis, education, nursing practice, research, collective bargaining, lobbying, and political action.

Legal Precedents for State Nursing Associations

The legal precedent which determined that state nursing associations are indeed qualified under labor law to be labor organizations is the 1979 Sierra Vista decision. This author contends, not only are they proper and legal, but that they are the preferred representative for nurses in this country for purposes of collective bargaining.

▼

The state nurses' association is really the only safe ground, what I could call the neutral turf, on which professional nurses can meet and discuss issues as colleagues, issues that are of a generic and important nature to all nurses, regardless of title.

▲

It is in the nursing associations that staff nurses, educators, advanced practice nurses, and administrators are able to talk as nurses. Issues associated with clinical ladders, staffing, unlicensed assistive personnel, client acuity, the reimbursement climate, and regulatory matters affect all nurses and benefit from our collective thinking and the application of our collective resources.

Nurse Participation in Collective Bargaining

If the ANA and state nursing associations are logical bargaining agents for professional nurses, why are so few nurses joining associations and even fewer pursuing collective bargaining? Most persons join an organization only in response to a particular incentive or when coerced. Otherwise, people will "free ride"—enjoy whatever collective goals are obtained without helping to pay for them (Olson, 1977).

Collective bargaining for nurses usually occurs in states where there is also significant union activity. Fewer than one-half of the state nursing associations engage in collective bargaining. Some state associations have left the arena because of external pressures: challenges by competing unions, excessive resistance by employers, or state policies that make unionization difficult, such as right-to-work laws. (In states with right to work laws, it is illegal to negotiate an agency shop requirement, so membership and dues collection can never be mandatory even if the workers are covered by a collective bargaining agreement.) Philosophical conflicts regarding the benefits and risks of professional association bargaining have also led nurses in some states to abandon the activities.

A recent article discussed the compatibility of unionization and professionalism. The conclusion confirmed that when "substantial" and "unambiguous" support for professional values were included in the bargaining agreements, the two are viewed as compatible (Rabban, 1991). How will collective professional goals be achieved if so many nurses depend on the time and finances of so few? There are over two million professional nurses in the United States, but only about 150,000 nurses are organized by state nursing associations, and 125,000 nurses by other unions. Some, including the author, believe that the ANA's efforts to address workplace concerns will result in larger numbers in the near future, but for now, there are too few nurses involved in collective bargaining and the nursing associations.

Where Does Collective Bargaining Begin?

Electing the Collective Bargaining Agent

Nurses in the private sector are guaranteed legal protection, as stated in the National Labor Relations Act, if you seek a collective bargaining agent. Once a drive for such representation is underway, and 30% of the employed nurses in an institution have signed cards signaling interest in representation, both the employer and the union are prohibited from engaging in antilabor action. Employers are prohibited from firing the organizers, refusing to allow dissemination of union information in the workplace, and ignoring the request for a vote for union representation. After the organizing campaign, a vote is then taken, and 50% plus one of those voting selects, or rejects, the collective bargaining agent.

Your employer may choose to bargain in good faith on matters concerning working conditions by recognizing the bargaining agent before the vote. This usually occurs only if management believes a large majority supports the foundation of a union. In other cases, your employer may appeal requests for representation to the National Labor Relations Board (NLRB). Before and during the appeal, other unions may intervene and try to win a majority of votes.

Arguments are made before the NLRB as to why, by whom, or how the nurses are to be represented. For example, the hospital may raise the question of "unit determination." The original policy interpretation of the labor law simultaneously limited the number of individual bargaining units an employer or industry would have to recognize, yet allowed for distinct groups of employees, like nurses, to have separate representation. Nurses historically had been represented in all-RN bargaining units, and the largest majority of bargaining units throughout the country reflect that pattern.

Milestones in Collective Bargaining

During the late 1980s, the demand for representation by nurses was growing, and yet efforts to organize nurses for collective bargaining were being stymied by the precedent set in what was called the St. Francis II case. That precedent stopped approving all-RN bargaining units. The ANA decided that this NLRB decision had to be challenged. The chief opposition to nursing was the American Hospital Association (AHA). A legal battle then ensued with the ANA and other labor unions against the AHA. The ANA was able to convince the NLRB to hold national hearings on this controversy. The NLRB issued a ruling that reaffirmed the right of nurses to be represented in all-RN bargaining units. That ruling was challenged by the AHA in an Illinois federal court, and an injunction was imposed at that time. The ANA deemed it essential to take this issue to the highest court in the country, so it could be finally settled. Hence, the ANA, with the NLRB, appealed the case to the U.S. Supreme Court. In May 1991, to the satisfaction of nurses throughout the United States, the U.S. Supreme Court confirmed that the NLRB had ruled properly and correctly in determining that nurses in this country have a right to be represented for purposes of collective bargaining in all-RN bargaining units.

Nurses represented by a bargaining agent have the right to drop or change (decertify) that agent by similar campaign of signatures (30%) of the affected members, followed by a vote, again requiring 50% plus one (a simple majority) in a unit-wide election. While the election process may ensure fair representation and an agent's accountability, election campaigns can be destructive and diversionary when initiated for frivolous (of little or no weight or importance, not worthy of serious notice) reasons. An example could be a competing union that promises it can "do better" for the membership if only the nurses will decertify their current union and elect the competitor. Such campaigns have occurred in Washington, Florida, and New York.

CONTRACTS

What Can a Contract Do?

Generally speaking, what can a union contract do in a hospital setting? A study of thirty-six nationwide hospitals, which all had extensive experience with collective bargaining, illustrates the positive effects a union can have:

1. Unions stimulate better hospital management by fostering formal, central, and consistent personnel policies with better lines of communication.
2. Unions "force" improvements in the workplace so that recruitment and retention become easier (Juris and Maxey, 1981).

Wages

Wages are the foundation of a contract. Wages are the remuneration one receives for providing a service and reflect the value put on the work performed.

Nurses' wages have experienced dramatic increases during the 1980s as a direct result of the highly publicized shortage of nurses. Collective bargaining agreements from New York to California have reflected some wage gains which, it is hoped, will place nursing wages and benefits in a competitive position as women and men make choices about their careers.

One of the major objectives of the bargaining environment during the 1980s shifted the focus away from wages paid to the novice nurse to those paid to the experienced nurse. Little or no salary increase was given to experienced and reliable nurses who continue to work for the same employer. Nurses have also experienced "wage compression." This economic concept means that nurses who have been in practice for ten and twelve years were beginning to make less money than new graduates in their first nursing jobs. Morale was deteriorating and, in fact, there were incentives for experienced nurses to leave jobs for a new position elsewhere, just so that the starting wage could reflect an increased salary.

Many studies have documented that, sometimes after five years, a nurse begins to practice with a level of intuition and expertise that is beneficial to the clients and the practice environment (Benner, 1982). As a result, many contracts now include tenure steps that reward nurses who have been in practice for many years in the same institution (longevity). This provision helps ensure the salary growth over what is now a lifetime of employment. Salary increment steps now continue to the tenth, fifteenth, and even the twenty-fifth year in some hospitals.

A 1990 article on the history of nursing's efforts to receive adequate compensation reaffirms the need to continue efforts on behalf of nursing salaries (Brider, 1990). The author correctly states that " . . . from its beginnings, the nursing profession has grappled with its own ambivalence: how to reconcile the ideal of selfless service with the necessity of making a living" (p. 77). The article cited the nurses who recorded both their joy in productive careers and their disappointment with the way their work was valued. Nursing has certainly come a long way from the early 1900's $8 to $12 a month "allowance," and yet the challenge remains to bring nursing into line with comparable careers. Hospital based salaries in 1990-1991 increased an average of 9%. Hospital industry surveys and the Bureau of Labor Statistics both report average hourly wages as $16.41 an hour. In 1989, the hospital salaries were $13.00 on average. The long-term University of Texas study of over sixty South/Central medical centers reveals that despite the increases, nurses are barely keeping ahead of inflation, and the actual adjusted increase is just under 2% for that same period. The problems of wage compression were addressed in relation to the nursing shortage, and it is encouraging to note an improvement in the maximum wages, which are those paid to the more senior staff.

Seniority Rights

Nurses who remain on staff at an institution accrue seniority rights. These rights arise from the idea of rewarding permanent employees for their service, and viewing them as assets. In nursing employment contracts, there are provisions ("seniority language") that give senior nurses the right to accrue more vacation time and to be given preference when requesting time off, new positions, or relief from shift rotation requirements. In the event of a staff layoff, the rule that states "the last hired become the first fired," protects senior nurses. Seniority rules may be applied to the entire hospital nursing staff or be confined to a unit, while transfers and promotions must reward the most senior, *qualified* nurse in the institution.

Resolution of Grievances

Methods to resolve grievances, which are sometimes explicitly spelled out in a contract, are an important element of any agreement. A grievance can arise when provisions in a contract are interpreted differently by management and an employee(s). This often happens when issues relating to job security (a union priority), job performance, and discipline (a management priority) arise. "Grievance mechanisms" are employed in an attempt to resolve the conflict with the parties involved. The employer, the employee, or the union may issue a grievance. Nurses who are covered by contracts should be represented at any meeting or hearing that they believe may lead to disciplinary action being taken against them. Such representation can be provided by a co-worker, the elected nurse representative, or a member of the labor union's staff.

If the "grievance mechanism" does not lead to a resolution of the issue, some contracts allow for referral of the issue to arbitration. A knowledgeable but neutral arbitrator acceptable to both parties (union and hospital) will be asked to hear the facts in the case and issue a finding. In pre-agreed, binding arbitration, the parties must accept the decision of the arbitrator. For example, some hospital contracts require that when management elects to discharge (suspend or terminate) a nurse, the case must be brought to arbitration. When a nurse is suspended, the case is presented to an arbitrator chosen from an established list of arbitrators. Based on the arbitrator's finding, the nurse may be reinstated, perhaps with back pay, remain suspended, or be terminated. If the contract states that the arbitrator's decision is final and binding, there is no further contractual avenue for either party to pursue.

Arbitration

Arbitration has also been used to resolve issues involving the "integrity of the bargaining unit." Arbitrators have been asked to decide if nurses remain eligible for bargaining unit coverage when jobs are changed and new practice models are implemented.

Mediation, arbitration, and fact-finding have all been used to resolve conflicts in union contracts. There is strong support for use of these methods, yet hospital management personnel often resist using them. Nurses have usually fared well when contract enforcement issues have been submitted to an arbiter, and facts, not power or public relations, have determined the outcome.

What Are the Elements of a Sound Contract?

MEMBERSHIP.   The inclusion of union security provisions is an essential element of a sound contract and one of the defined goals of collective bargaining (union integrity). Security provisions include measures such as enforcement of membership requirements (this means collection of dues and access by the union staff to the members). A modification of the closed shop is the "agency shop," in which new employees are required to join the union within a given period of time.

OBJECTION TO AN ASSIGNMENT.   The right and means for a nurse to register objection to a work assignment are considered an essential element in a union contract. Professional duty implies an obligation to complete an assignment despite the nurse's disagreement with it. Nurses cannot abandon their post without risking disciplinary action. Some contracts and national proposals "endorse objection" (support nurses who disagree in writing with an assignment) when the assignment could violate the client protection language of the state nurse practice act. An "assignment-despite-objection" report is submitted to the nursing administrator and the bargaining agent simultaneously, thus officially registering the complaint. Inadequate staff, poorly prepared staff, high client acuity, and excessive use of registry personnel are all problems that motivate nurses covered by union contracts to submit "assignment-despite-objection" reports. Constructive follow-through by management may improve the situation in the future, just as inaction could serve as a basis for a grievance and/or negotiated change in the contract. Ideally, the professional performance or professional practice committee (one that is mandated by contract) at the facility will work with nursing administrators to address nurses' complaints and decide if they reflect a pattern or remain unresolved. When a nurse registers a complaint, she alerts management to a problem. This act can also be constructive in that it can help a nurse vent her frustration and anger, and help her turn a bad experience into a positive effort.

STAFFING.   Staffing requirements are mandated by various agencies. For example, Medicare, state health department licensing requirements, and the Joint Commission on Accreditation of Health Organizations each publish staffing standards. However, standards that outline nurse:client ratios do not address the issue of what qualifications the nurse must have. For example, a standard that requires one nurse per client in the ICU does not mandate that the nursing staff needs to have had certain education and experience to work in the ICU.

Staffing issues were at the root of the historic 1974 Bay Area (California) strike. Management resisted CNA and staff nurse review of staffing and specialty area qualifications. After a twenty-one-day strike, involving forty-two northern California hospitals and clinics, the final agreement included these key provisions:

1. Staffing systems must be clearly spelled out, and the bargaining agent must be made aware, in writing, of any changes.
2. New employees will not be counted as staff during orientation.
3. The hospital will not, except in emergencies, assign an unqualified nurse to the ICU, respiratory care unit, burn unit, postanesthesia recovery room, intensive care nursery, or renal dialysis unit.
4. The hospital will employ full-time specialty unit staff prepared through inservice or other programs, for nurses on staff, and will use a pool of qualified regular and short-hour nurses to fill vacancies.

RETIREMENT.   Most pension or retirement programs for nurses have either been the Social Security system or a hospital pension plan. Individual retirement accounts (IRA), which are transferable from hospital to hospital in case of job change, are relatively rare and should be a topic for negotiations. In fact, the ANA has considered creating a national pension plan to which a nurse could contribute through his or her lifetime of employment, irrespective of geographic location or place of employment. While this plan could be complicated by conflicting state laws governing pension plans, a precedent was set as long ago as 1976, when the California nursing contracts mandated employer contributions to individual retirement accounts for each nurse with immediate vesting (eligibility for access to the fund) and complete "portability" for the participants (that meant the nurse could take her pension to another hospital and continue to add to it, within the state of California).

One of nursing's most attractive benefits has been a nurse's mobility, the opportunity to change jobs at will. A drawback of this mobility, however, is the loss of long-term retirement monies. Pension programs should be looked at not as a reward for continued service, but as a basic protection earned by employees as part of their benefit program. With financial cutbacks in the hospital industry, retirement plans are in danger of being targeted as "givebacks" in negotiations. This means "givebacks" are rights or benefits that can be traded away in lieu of another issue or benefit that may be more pressing at the time. Health insurance coverage persists as a key topic of employee concerns and has been at the root of the majority of labor disputes in all industries in the last few years. It is not inconceivable that nurses may be asked to trade off long-term economic security (pensions) for short-term security (health benefits, wages, etc.).

OTHER BENEFIT ISSUES.   All employees in the United States have been experiencing a dramatic reduction in their health benefit's packages. This trend is reflective of the crisis of the healthcare system and the escalating costs of healthcare. Most of the labor disputes of the last five to six years are the result of efforts to reduce or eliminate health benefit packages for employees or their dependents. Nurses have not been immune to the reduction in health benefits and access to health care benefits will continue to be a major issue for nurses and all employees until substantial reform is accomplished.

Other issues that have affected nurses as employees are family leave policies, availability of daycare services, long-term disability insurance, and access to health insurance for retirees. An issue of special concern to nurses involves the scheduling of work hours. While some men have been joining the nursing profession, nursing remains a 97% female occupation. That reality must be addressed by benefit packages that provide flexibility for women who assume multiple roles in today's society. Women, and nurses in particular, provide care to both children and parents. Nurses are asking nursing contract negotiators to secure sick leave policies that permit use of sick time for family needs, scheduling that is both flexible and allows for part-time employment and work-sharing.

HEALTH HAZARDS.   Nurses are using collective action to protect themselves against the health hazards and unsafe working conditions and to advocate for positive health and safety programs. Right-to-know provisions (knowledge of where and what a substance is and how to use it safely) and job security in the case of reassignment can be written into contracts. Such agreements have been included in contracts in the District of Columbia and Illinois. Nationally, the ANA is urging the Occupational Safety and Health Administration (OSHA) to provide hazardous substance information to health workers. Nursing associations and unions have advocated for inclusion of strict infection control guidelines for healthcare facilities to protect workers from blood-borne pathogens including hepatitis B and human immunodeficiency virus. Nursing has played a major role in designing and advocating stringent ongoing education and training on universal precautions, provision for safe equipment and research and development of safer needle devices, postexposure protocol, employer-provided hepatitis B vaccine. Additional health and safety concerns include the reemergence of tuberculosis, and a high incidence of violence in healthcare settings. Some state nurses' associations have introduced legislation to rectify workers' compensation policies once an exposure has occurred in the workplace. The ANA and other unions have used collective bargaining agreements, aggressive government relations campaigns, and nursing practice networks to educate nurses about workplace risks.

Collective Bargaining and Nursing Practice

How Can Nurses Control Their Own Practice?

Hospital management representatives often ask staff nurses what they mean when they say their goal is to control nursing practice. These managers seem unclear about what it is we consider "appropriate practice issues," and they react negatively to the concept of "control." The essence of the professional nurse contract is control of practice. For example, nurse councils or professional performance committees provide the opportunity for nurses within the institution to meet regularly. These meetings are sanctioned by the contract. The elected staff nurse representatives may, for example, have specific objectives to:

- ◆ Improve the professional practice of nurses and nursing assistants.
- ◆ Recommend ways and means to improve client care.
- ◆ Make recommendations to the hospital management when, for example, a critical nurse staffing shortage exists.
- ◆ Identify and recommend elimination of hazards in the workplace.

The importance and relevance of such professional practice committees was documented by a 1986 review of state nursing association contracts. When 381 agreements were analyzed, 424 references to professional practice committees were identified.

Nurse Practice Committees

Nurse practice committees should have a formal relationship with nursing administration. Regularly scheduled meetings with nursing and hospital administrators can provide a forum for discussion of professional issues in a "safe" atmosphere. Many potential contract conflicts can be avoided by discussion before contract talks begin or grievances arise. Ideally, physicians should be a part of these forums; and joint practice language has been proposed in some contracts.

Current nursing concerns continue to focus on staffing ratios, client acuity, the use of client classification systems, and the training of and appropriate use of nursing assistants.

There are cycles of shortages of RNs and, in some cases, cost containment efforts have led to the reduction of nursing staff. Issues related to the "staff mix" (number of full-time RNs, licensed vocational/practical nurses, aides) has become an important workplace issue. Since a principle of professional nursing practice requires nurses to be involved in making decisions that will affect their working conditions and quality of the care, it is reasonable to expect nurses to use their union contract to assist them in dealing with issues such as "staff mix." When nurses refer to "control of nursing practice," they are not talking about infringing on rights or the responsibilities of managers to ensure financial stability and administrative order. Rather, nurses are referring to the elements that affect professional practice, for which they, as licensed professionals, are responsible.

Concept of Shared Governance

Many facilities are implementing a variety of practice models that they call shared governance. Shared governance is defined as an arrangement of nurses (staff and managers) that attempts to emphasize principles of participatory management in those areas related to both the governance and practice of nursing (Porter-O'Grady and Finnigan, 1984). Also labeled as self-governance, participative decision making, staff by-laws, and decentralized nursing services, these are all structural activities meant to address nurse participation in control of practice. The concept of shared governance has worried unions that represent nurses in collective bargaining. The historical precedents of shared governance in an academic setting mandate caution when applied to healthcare settings. It is necessary to avoid a legal finding that the nurses, who are part of a shared governance model, have become so involved in the governance activities of the facility that they are no longer eligible for representation by a bargaining agent. That is exactly what happened in the Yeshiva faculty precedent (Yeshiva, 1980).

Some shared governance models make no effort to hide the fact that their expressed purpose is to involve nurses in decision making and yet retain the unilateral decision-making authority by managers. That certainly would violate the principles of professional participation in decision making and would be a major disadvantage to nurses employed by institutions if shared governance models are adopted in lieu of collective bargaining agreements. In an environment where collective bargaining already exists, it is also probably unnecessary to adopt a totally new model to achieve shared governance if, in fact, the professional practice committee is involved, as it should be, in providing staff nurse input into decisions that affect the professional practice of nursing. To preserve bargaining rights, the model must be compatible with collective bargaining rights and must clearly define the demarcation between professional and management issues.

Clinical or Career Ladder

The clinical ladder (Huey, 1982; Wieczorek, 1982, 1983), or career ladder, has a place in collective bargaining agreements. The clinical ladder has been designed to permit recognition of the long-term career nurse who wishes to remain clinically oriented. The notion and the tools to reward the clinical nurse with pay, and status, along a specific tract or "ladder" is the result of the great contributions of a nurse researcher, Dr. Patricia Benner. Her descriptions of changes in the growth and development of nursing knowledge and practice have led to the development of a ladder that can identify and reward the nurse along the steps from "novice" to "expert" (Benner, 1984). Reports issued by the National Commission on Nursing (1983), the Institute of Medicine (1983), and the Department of Health & Human Services Secretary's Commission on Nursing report (1988) all cited the career ladder as an effective tool for use in the retention of career-minded nurses.

Negotiations

The principles of successful negotiations are difficult to articulate. Nurse negotiators are elected by their peers, and must represent a diverse population (a multitude of specialty areas, educational backgrounds, and practice needs). Nurses have little or no introduction to labor practices or procedures in nursing education programs so they must learn on the job. Foreign nurses are at a greater disadvantage because they are unfamiliar with cultural factors that affect negotiations, such as power, politics, economics, and competition.

Negotiations are held before a contract is agreed to and again just prior to the time it expires. Nurses in the bargaining unit will elect a negotiating team to represent them. These nurses may be assisted by labor union staff, skilled negotiators, economists, and/or legal staff.

Professional goals and practice needs should be discussed in negotiations, but personnel directors, hospital administrators, and hospital lawyers often seem to have difficulty relating to discussions of nursing practice concerns. Nursing directors usually remain in the wings, only joining the discussion when invited by the hospital administrators. Resolution of disagreements about professional issues necessitates a long and thoughtful process. Complex issues, like recruitment, retention, staffing and health and safety, can be better addressed in a more deliberate and collegial setting.

What nurses may want, and what nurses can achieve during negotiations may be worlds apart. While a survey of the nurses may produce a "wish list," it must be pared down to only those issues that are of greatest importance to the whole and have the most chance of surviving the give and take of collective bargaining. If nurses are not helped to understand the negotiation process, they could begin to feel that their individual needs are not being attended to.

Strikes and Other Labor Disputes

Just what can nurses do in the face of a standoff during contract negotiations? Nurses' options are quite different from those of just fifteen years ago, when nurses felt a greater sense of powerlessness. At that time, despite nurses' threats of sickouts, walkouts, picketing, or mass resignations, the employer maintained an effective power base. Threats of group action attracted public attention, but nurses' threats had little effect on employers because nurses represented through the ANA had a no-strike policy. As negotiations became more difficult, it was apparent that nurses were in a weaker bargaining position, due to the no-strike policy. The ANA responded to the state nursing associations and, in 1968, reversed its eighteen-year-old, no-strike policy.

Strikes are the ultimate last resort and are used only after every other recourse fails. Nurses who strike take their appeals to the "street," hoping for positive public response. Many nurses are uncomfortable with the idea of "abandoning" their clients. This runs counter to the service ideal. It is important for nurses who contemplate striking to discuss plans for client care with nurses who have previously conducted strikes so that they will be assured that plans to care for clients are adequate.

When an impasse is reached in hospital negotiations, national labor law requires nurses to issue a ten-day notice of their intent to strike. In the public's interest, every effort must be made to prevent a strike. Mediation is mandated by the NLRB, and a board of inquiry to examine the issue may be created prior to a work stoppage. The hospitals are supposed to use this time to reduce the client census and to slow or halt elective admissions. In the meantime, the nurses' strike committee will develop schedules for coverage of emergency rooms, operating rooms, and intensive care areas. This coverage is to be used only in the case of real emergencies. Planning client care coverage should reassure nurses troubled by the strike scenario. Nurses who agree to work in emergencies or at other facilities during a strike often donate their wages to funds set up for striking nurses.

Employer Strategies

During the 1980s, a growing antiunion sentiment in this country provided ample opportunity for hospital management to regain their right to "rule the roost." The disdain for nurses' unions seems to stem from a general dislike of having nonmanagement personnel observe or judge how hospital managers do their job. Indeed, the principles of productivity and efficiency, advocated by hospital managers, can clash with the practice of professional nursing care. One definition of collective bargaining defines it as a struggle for power in which the opposing parties, the employer and the collective bargaining agent, rival and manipulate each other in an effort to improve and advance their respective positions. In the healthcare setting, the broadly defined bargaining objectives include:

1. To protect the economic position and personal welfare of the worker.
2. To protect the union's integrity as an ongoing institution.
3. To recognize the outer limits imposed on collective bargaining outcomes by the economic conditions of the industry and the employer and by the climate of opinion (Stern, 1982, p. 11).

The National Labor Relations Act governs labor practices and prohibits certain unfair practices once an organizing campaign has been initiated. An employer cannot engage in interference, domination, discrimination, or refusal to bargain, and cannot unjustly discipline an employee simply for his union activities.

Before 1983, Medicare allowed hospitals to include antiunion expenses in their bills. Hospitals, like private industry, have hired expensive, antiunion "industrial relations" firms to coach management in techniques to quickly detect prounion sentiment. However, this practice demonstrates the fine line between legal and illegal activities. One wonders why that same money could not be used to compensate nurses, to improve client care and nurses' working conditions, or to introduce positive approaches to conflict resolution.

Business and labor are both in search for more positive ways in which to work together. National grants have been sponsored by the Department of Labor and the Federal Mediation and Conciliation Service to undertake alternatives to traditional bargaining. At least two midwestern nursing organizations utilized "win-win" bargaining techniques and found them to be constructive methods of negotiation.

FUTURE TRENDS

What Lies Ahead?

It is a well-known fact that the nursing community was struck in the late 1980s with a deeply entrenched, widespread, and possibly permanent imbalance between the demand for nurses and the ability of nursing education to supply adequately prepared registered nurses to meet future public needs. For about two years, it was common to pick up publications or turn on a national talk show, whether it be radio or television, and find coverage of the shortage of nurses. The attention was well deserved, since the public should be concerned about an inadequate supply of nurses. That attention helped nursing advocates for better wages and working conditions, and led to large increases in applicants to schools of nursing.

Data on the status of the nursing shortage confirms a serious problem with vacancy rates in the 1980s. Generally, a vacancy rate higher than 10% is considered serious. For the period of 1986-1989, the rates were consistently above 10% for hospitals, and in 1989 was 12.7% (McKibbin, 1990). The same source, AHA, reported a 1990 vacancy rate of 10.96% (ANA staff, personal communication, 1991). In some cases, the vacancy rate may be lower if positions for registered nurses have been eliminated or changed to another personnel category. It may be no surprise to learn that vacancy rates for other health facilities, nursing homes specifically, are even higher, at 18.9%. Home care agencies and HMO settings all reported vacancies over 10% in 1989. Efforts to improve the wage and benefit package, with specific attention on the tenure steps and career earning patterns, have begun to address the competitive wage environment which women and men find themselves in as they make early or mid-career decisions. The question of job satisfaction, however, must not be overlooked. In survey after survey, the number one reason why nurses are unhappy with their nursing practice environment is their dissatisfaction with the care that they are able to give in the current environment. Nurses throughout the country have felt firsthand the effects of cost containment of the mid-1980s. Those effects have been detrimental to the quality of care that the professional nurses are charged to provide. There were wholesale reductions of staff in response to prospective payment systems and cost containment in the 1980s. Healthcare facilities reduced transport, clerical, and other non-nursing ancillary personnel. Nurses were expected to assume not only the increasingly demanding duties of a professional nurse, in an era of what we call the quicker and sicker client load (higher acuities and shorter inclient stays), but they were also expected to pick up the non-nursing duties. In some studies, it has been documented that up to 50% of a nurse's time is spent performing non-nursing duties (ANA News, 1989). Improper utilization of an already scarce resource is a tragedy.

Some of the short-sighted solutions to the long-term problem of adequate nurse supplies served to unify nursing during the 1980s. For example, the American Medical Association (AMA) proposed the training of an alternative healthcare provider who would work beside, but not with, nurses, particularly in the acute care facilities. The "registered care technician" (RCT) proposal was designed to provide client care services the doctors believed were missing. While there is little disagreement that nurses and physicians need to provide care to the public, this goal should be achieved through a collaborative and cooperative problem-solving approach. The ANA viewed the AMA proposal as anything but collaborative and cooperative. Response by nurses and their unions helped to minimize the success of the AMA's RCT campaign. A key question relates to how nurses can create categories of personnel who will assist the nurse, and still retain control of nursing practice.

Encroachment is a term that encompasses the multitude of providers who threaten the integrity of nurses' practice. Concerns about encroachment arise from proposals that would allow a provider of respiratory or pharmacy services to expand their practice into the sphere of nursing care. At the other end of the spectrum, unlicensed assistive personnel must be assigned or delegated nursing duties that do not exceed their knowledge and training. It is necessary for the bargaining agent to have a well-grounded and thorough operating knowledge of nursing, its definition, scope of practice, and standards. I believe that only a state nurses' association, in collaboration with the ANA, can simultaneously promote nursing practice and perform superior workplace advocacy.

What lies ahead for collective bargaining and all forms of collective action for nurses must be viewed within a context of the larger changes occurring in the healthcare system and in the financing mechanisms. As this chapter is being prepared, there is a heightened awareness by both the politicians and the public that there is something grievously wrong with not just how we pay for our healthcare, but what we are receiving at that high cost. This issue of health access is one that will probably be with us for the rest of our professional lives. As nurses advocate for improved access to health services, those services will, by necessity, be delivered in environments and by providers that have not traditionally been a part of our so-called medical care system. Just as cost containment of the 1980s brought emphasis on home care, early discharge, and alternatives to institutional care, remedies to improve access will include school-based care, workplace-based care, and community care.

In my best crystal ball/tea leaves mode, I am challenged to predict what healthcare will look like after the reform agendas of the 1990s are complete. As this chapter is prepared, the newly elected Clinton Administration is preparing a healthcare reform proposal. Implications for nursing include:

◆ Guaranteed access to care by all residents of the United States.

◆ An emphasis on primary, preventive care delivered in a continuum of care.

◆ Enhanced utilization of nurses in advanced practice (nurse practitioners, certified nurse midwives, and clinical specialists).

◆ Expanded community based care.

◆ Utilization of acute care facilities for briefer, more intense care.

◆ Cost containment efforts to deliver quality care at the lowest cost and more efficiently.

◆ Healthcare institution mergers, closure, and integration of services and product lines to meet varying community needs.

◆ An increasing reliance on the skills and voice of nurses to ensure quality care.

The workplace advocacy goals for nursing during this transition will be focused on quality of care issues and assisting nurses as they expand their skills into community settings.

Nurses who are not organized for collective bargaining purposes should examine their work setting. If collective bargaining could improve the lines of communication and management authority, benefit packages, or practice controls, explore the possibility of an organizing campaign. Organizing and retaining nurse interest is a serious and strenuous undertaking. The benefits and protections that accrue when nurses act collectively strengthen nursing, and help nurses everywhere to improve client care.

The multipurpose functions of the professional nursing association will preserve the future of nursing. This chapter cannot stand alone, nor can the nurses in the workplace stand alone if they are to offset the forces that negate contributions of nurses. Political action and lobbying, research, and education are necessary to further the cause of nursing and to meet the public's healthcare needs. While nursing works to change the health system and improve citizens' access to care, nurses will continue to depend on collective action and a collective voice to advocate for optimal working conditions and standards of practice. Welcome to nursing! Join us in our efforts to unify our skills, knowledge, and our voices as we celebrate our past and create our future.

REFERENCES

American Nurses Association activities. (1946): *Am J Nurs* 46:728.

American Nurses Association news. (1989): *Am J Nurs* 9:1223, 1231.

Becker, E., Sloan, F. (1982): Union activity in hospitals: Past, present, and future. *Health Care Finan Rev* 3:1.

Benner, P. (1982): From novice to expert. *Am J Nurs* 82:402.

Brider, P. (1990): The struggle for just compensation. *Am J Nurs* 10:77.

Cleland, V. (1981): Taft-Hartley amended: Implications for nursing—the professional model. *J Nurs Admin* 11:17.

Flanagan, L. (1984): *Collective Bargaining and the Nursing Profession.* Kansas City, MO, American Nurses Association.

Flanagan, L. (1990): Survival Skills in the Workplace: What Every Nurse Should Know. Kansas City, MO, American Nurses Association.

Huey, F. (1982): Looking at ladders. *Am J Nurs* 82:1520.

Institute of Medicine, Health Care Services, Nursing and Nursing Education Committee (1983): *Nursing and Nursing Education: Public Policies and Private Actions.* Washington, DC, National Academy Press, p. 27.

Jacox, A. (1980): Collective action: The basis for professionalism. *Supervisor Nurse* 11:22.

Juris, H., Maxey, C. (1981): The impact of hospital unionism. *Modern Healthcare* 11:36.

McKibbin, R. (1990): *The Nursing Shortage and the 1990s: Realities and Remedies.* Kansas City, MO, American Nurses Association, p. 4.

News and background information. (1984): *Labor Relations Report* 116:11.

Nurse membership in unions. (1937): *Am J Nurs* 37:766.

Olson, M. (1977): *The Logic of Collective; Action*. Connecticut, Harvard University Press.

Parlette, G.N., O'Reilly, C.A., Bloom, J.R. (1980). The nurse and the union. *Hosp Forum* 23:14.

Porter-O'Grady, T., Finnigan, S. (1984). *Shared Governance for Nursing: A Creative Approach to Professional Accountability*. Gaithersburg, MD, Aspen Systems.

Rabban, D. (1991): Is unionization compatible with professionalism? *Industrial and Labor Relations Review*, 45(1), 97-110.

Secretary's Commission on Nursing. (December 1988): Final Report. Washington, D.C., Health and Human Services, Office of the Secretary.

Shramm, C. (1982): Economic perspectives on the nursing shortage. In L. Aiken (ed); *Nursing in the 1980s: Crises, Opportunities, Challenges*. Philadelphia, J.B. Lippincott.

Stern, E. (1982): Collective bargaining: A means of conflict resolution. *Nurs Admin Quart* 6:9.

Stickler, K.B., Velghe, J.C. (1980): Why nurses join unions. *Hosp Forum* 23:14.

Wieczorek, R.R., et al. (1982): A clinical career pathway, Part 1. *Nurs Health Care* 3:533.

Wieczorek, R.R., et al. (1982): A clinical career pathway, Part 2. *Nurs Health Care* 4:318.

Yeshiva, supra, 103 LRRM at 2553 (1980).

Ethical and Legal Issues in Nursing

13

Ethical Issues

Alice Pappas, Ph.D., R.N.

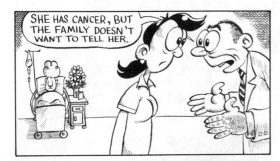

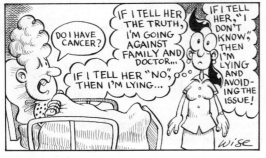

Ethical dilemmas are not easy situations.

People of Orphalese, you can muffle the drum, and you can loosen the strings of the lyre, but who shall command the skylark not to sing?
—Kahlil Gibran, *The Prophet*

After completing this chapter, you should be able to:

◆ Define terminology commonly used in discussions about ethical issues.

◆ Analyze personal values that influence approaches to ethical issues and decision-making.

◆ Discuss the moral implications of the ANA and ICN codes of ethics.

◆ Discuss the role of the nurse in ethical healthcare issues

C oncern with ethical issues in healthcare has increased dramatically in the last two decades. This interest has soared for a variety of reasons, including advances in medical technology; social and legal changes involving abortion; euthanasia, patient rights, and reproductive technology; and a growing concern with the allocation of scarce resources. Nurses have begun to speak out on these issues and have focused attention on the responsibilities and possible conflicts that nurses experience as a result of their unique relationship with patients and their families.

UNDERSTANDING ETHICS

Let's begin with a definition of commonly used terms (Table 13–1).

What Are Your Values?

Clarification of your values is suggested as a strategy to develop greater insight into *yourself* and *what you hold dear*. Values clarification involves a three-step process: choosing, prizing, and acting upon your value choices (Steele, 1983). Opportunities to make choices and improve your decision-making are included

TABLE 13–1 *Definition of Terms*

Ethics—rules or principles that determine which human actions are right or wrong.

Bioethics—ethics concerning life.

Bioethical issues—subjects that raise concerns of right and wrong in matters involving human life. i.e.: Euthanasia, Abortion.

Ethical dilemma—[1]a situation involving competing rules or principles that appears to have no satisfactory solution. [2]A choice between 2 or more equally undesirable alternatives.

Moral reasoning—a process of considering and selecting approaches to resolve ethical issues.

Moral or ethical principles—fundamental values or assumptions about the way individuals should be treated and cared for. These include **autonomy, beneficence, nonmaleficence, justice, fidelity,** and **veracity.**

Values—beliefs which are considered very important and frequently influence an individual's behavior.

Moral uncertainty—a situation which exists when the individual is unsure which moral principle or values apply in a given situation.

in the following pages. You will, it is hoped, gain more understanding about your values as well as the underlying motives that influence them. It is not intended as a "right" or "wrong" activity, rather, a discovery about the "what" and "whys" about your actions. Don't be surprised if your peers or family hold different views on some topics. And, remember: the values that are "correct" or "right" for you may not always be the "right" values for others. Your values may also change over time as you face different life experiences.

In Boxes 13–1 and 13–2 write down your responses and consider the possible reasons(s) for your choices. Doing the exercise in Box 13–1, Listing Values, is suggested as a means of *clarifying your values*. Discuss your answers with peers and decide how comfortable you are in defending your values, especially if they differ from the values of your peers. Box 13–2 involves reproductive issues and has been included here because of the proliferation of reproductive technology and the continuing moral and political debate regarding abortion.

MORAL/ETHICAL PRINCIPLES

What Is the Best Decision? And How Will I Know?

Despite different ideas regarding which moral or ethical principle is most important, ethicists agree that there are *common principles or rules* that should be taken into consideration when an ethical situation is being examined. As you read through each principle consider instances when you have acted on the principles, or perhaps felt some conflict when you tried to determine what was the best action to take.

Autonomy—A Patient's Right to Self-Determination Without Outside Control

For example, autonomy implies the freedom to make choices and decisions about one's care without interference, even if those decisions are not in agreement with those of the healthcare team. This principle assumes rational thinking on the part of the individual and may be challenged when the rights of others are infringed upon by the individual.

> **Point to Ponder:** What if patients want to do something that will cause them harm?

Beneficence—Duty to Actively Do Good for Patients

For example, deciding what nursing care should be provided for patients who are dying when some of that care may cause pain. In the course of doing good for patients, harm sometimes occurs.

BOX 13–1

Listing Values

List ten values that guide your daily interactions.

1. _____
2. _____
3. _____
4. _____
5. _____
6. _____
7. _____
8. _____
9. _____
10. _____

Choose a partner (if available).

1. Discuss with a partner each of the values you listed and how they guide your interactions.
2. Compare your list of values with your partner's and discuss similarities and differences in the two lists.
3. Prioritize your list and discuss why you feel some are more important than others.

Reprinted with permission from Steele, S., Harmon, V. (1983): Values Clarification in Nursing. 2nd ed. East Norwalk, CT, Appleton-Century-Crofts, p. 90.

Point to Ponder: Who decides what is good? Patient, family, nurse, physician?

Nonmaleficence—Duty to Prevent or Avoid Doing Harm Whether Intentional or Unintentional

For example, accepting an assignment to "float" an area you are unfamiliar with, including the responsibility to give medications you are unfamiliar with.

BOX 13–2

Reproductive Exercise

Identify your degree of agreement or disagreement with the statements by placing the number that most closely indicates your value next to each statement.

1 = Strongly Disagree
2 = Disagree
3 = Ambivalent
4 = Agree
5 = Strongly Agree

_____ 1. Contraception is a responsibility of all women.

_____ 2. Some types of contraception are more valuable than other types.

_____ 3. Abortion as a form of contraception is completely unacceptable.

_____ 4. Abortion decisions are the responsibility of the pregnant woman and her physician.

_____ 5. The birth of a "test tube baby" is a valuable medical advance.

_____ 6. Genetic screening should be done frequently.

_____ 7. Genetic counseling should provide information so that clients can make informed choices about future reproductive decisions.

_____ 8. Amniocentesis should be required as part of prenatal care.

_____ 9. Genetic engineering should be advanced and promoted by federal funding.

_____ 10. Artificial insemination should be available to anyone who seeks it.

_____ 11. Sperm used in artificial insemination should come from all strata of society like blood transfusions do.

_____ 12. Fetal surgery should be done even when it places another fetus at risk (i.e., a twin).

_____ 13. Surrogate mothers play an important role in the future of families.

_____ 14. Fetuses who survive experimentation should be raised by society.

_____ 15. Women should be encouraged to participate in fetal research by carrying fetuses to desired dates and then giving the fetus to the scientist for research.

Continued.

BOX 13–2
_____

Reproductive Exercise Continued
_____

____ **16.** Contraception is reserved for women of legal ages.

____ **17.** Adolescents should require a parent's signature for abortion.

____ **18.** Information about genetically transmitted diseases should be provided to all pregnant women.

____ **19.** Women at high risk for genetically transmitted diseases should be encouraged to have amniocentesis.

____ **20.** Infants born with severe defects should be allowed to die through a natural course.

Point to Ponder: When a unit is short-staffed, is it acceptable to refuse to float there?

Fidelity—The Duty to be Faithful to Commitments

It involves keeping promises and information confidential as well as maintaining privacy. For example, maintaining patient confidentiality regarding a positive human immunodeficiency virus test.

Point to Ponder: To whom do we owe our fidelity? Patient, family, physician, institution, profession?

Justice—The Duty to Treat All Patients Fairly, Without Regard to Age, Socioeconomic Status, or Other Variables

This principle involves the allocation of "scarce healthcare resources." For example, on what basis should scarce ICU beds be allocated?

Point to Ponder: What is fair and who decides?

Veracity—The Duty to Tell the Truth

For example, a patient who suspects that his diagnosis is cancer asks you, "Nurse, do I have cancer?"

Point to Ponder: Is lying to a patient ever justified?

Each of the aforementioned principles sounds so right, yet the "point to ponder" questions indicate that putting them into practice is sometimes easier said than done. Reality does not always offer textbook situations that allow flawless application of the principles. You will encounter clinical situations that challenge the way in which you apply the principle, or cause two or more principles to be in conflict, creating moral uncertainty or an ethical dilemma.

Which Principle or Rule Is Most Important?

Current thinking on the part of ethicists favors autonomy and nonmaleficence as preeminent because they emphasize respect for person and avoidance of harm. However, there is no universal agreement. Traditional and contemporary models of ethical reasoning offer world views from which these principles can be derived, interpreted, and comparatively emphasized. However, they are not without their critics, including nurses. In recent years, nursing ethicists have advanced a new approach to ethical issues emphasizing an "ethic of caring" as the moral foundation of nursing. The nursing profession is being encouraged to consider all ethical issues from the central issue of caring. Because caring implies concern for preserving humanity and dignity, and promoting well-being, awareness of rules and principles is important, but not enough. In fact, reliance on rules and principles alone may not adequately address the ethical issues that nurses confront, such as suffering or powerlessness. Research regarding the application of caring to ethical issues is underway, but a practical model for applying this "ethic of caring" to clinical situations does not yet exist.

So How Do I Make an Ethical Decision?

At the present time, there are a number of approaches to ethical decision-making. The following is a brief overview of the three most commonly applied models. An overview of each is presented, emphasizing their origin, usefulness, and possible drawbacks. The first two types are considered normative because they have clearly defined parameters or norms to influence decision-making. The third type is a combination of the previous models.

Deontological

Derived from Judeo-Christian origins, this normative approach is duty focused and centered on rules from which all action is derived. The rules represent beliefs about intrinsic good that are moral absolutes revealed by God. All persons are worthy of respect and thus should be treated the same.

▼

All life is worthy of respect.

▲

As a result of the rules and duties that the deontological approach outlines, the individual has clear direction about how to act in all situations. Right or wrong is based on one's duty or obligation to act, not on the consequences of one's actions. Abortion and euthanasia are not acceptable actions because they violate the duty to respect life. Lying is never acceptable because it violates the duty to tell the truth.

Teleological

Derived from humanistic origins, this approach is outcome focused and emphasis is placed on results. Good is defined in utilitarian terms: that which is useful is good. Human reason is the basis for authority in all situations, not absolutes from God. Morality is established by majority rule and results of actions determine the rules. Because results become the intrinsic good, the individual's actions are always based on the probable outcome.

▼

That which causes a good outcome is a good action.

▲

Simplistically, this view is sometimes interpreted as "the end justifies the means." Abortion may be acceptable because it results in fewer unwanted babies. Euthanasia is an acceptable choice by some patients because it results in decreased suffering.

Situational

Derived from humanistic as well as Judeo-Christian influences and most commonly credited to Joseph Fletcher, an Episcopalian theologian, this view holds that there are no prescribed rules, norms, or majority focused results that must be followed. Each "situation" creates its own set of rules and principles that should be considered in that particular set of circumstances. Emphasizing the uniqueness of the situation, and respect for the person in that situation, Fletcher appeals to love as the only norm.

▼

Decisions made in one situation cannot be generalized to another situation.

▲

Abortion is the best choice for an unmarried 16-year-old because it gives her the opportunity to finish school and mature, but may not be the best answer for all girls in such a situation. "Pulling the plug" on a terminally ill patient who does not want any more extraordinary care is an act of love.

In Table 13–2 there is a brief comparison of the relative advantages and disadvantages of each approach. Remember that there is no perfect world view. If there were, debate would stop and the need for continued ethical deliberation would cease. The ethical models presented here are not intended to be all-inclusive or exhaustive in depth. Rather, they should whet your appetite for further content. Many journals and texts are devoted to the topic, and you are encouraged to see how ethicists apply these and other models to issues that affect your area of practice.

How Do I Determine Who "Owns the Problem"?

The decision to choose a particular model of ethical reasoning is personal and based on your own values. Familiarize yourself with various models in order to decrease your own moral uncertainty and gain some understanding of the values of others. The following guidelines are suggested as a means of analyzing ethical issues that will confront you in nursing practice. You may not be a pivotal decision-maker in all situations, but these guidelines can assist you.

TABLE 13–2 *Three Approaches to Ethical Decision Making Comparison of Advantages and Disadvantages*

ETHICAL APPROACH	ADVANTAGES	DISADVANTAGES
Deontological	Clear direction for action. All individuals are treated the same.	Perceived as rigid. Does not consider possible negative consequences of actions.
Teleological	Interest of the majority protected. Results are evaluated for their good and actions may be modified.	Rights of individual may be overlooked/denied. What is a good result? Who determines good? Morality may be arbitrary.
Situational	This approach mirrors the way most individuals actually approach day-to-day decision-making. Merits of each situation are considered. Individual has more control/autonomy to make decision in his/her own best interest.	What is good? Who decides? Possible morality is arbitrary. Lack of rules of generalizability limits criticism of possible abuse.

▼

Who owns the problem?

▲

First, Determine the Facts of the Situation and make sure you have collected enough data to give yourself an accurate picture of the issue at hand. When the facts of a situation become known, you may or may not be dealing with an ethical issue.

....

As an ICU nurse, you believe that the wishes of patients regarding extraordinary care are being disregarded. In other words, resuscitation is performed despite expressed patient wishes to the contrary.

....

You need to:

1. Determine whether discussion about extraordinary care is taking place between patients, families, and attending physicians.
2. Clarify the institution's policy regarding cardiopulmonary resuscitation (CPR) and do not resuscitate (DNR) orders.
3. Determine what input families have had into the decisions (i.e., whether the families are aware of the patient's wishes).
4. Explore the use of living will documentation at your institution, and determine if patients are familiar with the use and possible limitations of living wills.
5. Share your concerns with the attending physicians to obtain their view of the situation.
6. Discuss the situation with your clinical manager to clarify any misconceptions regarding policy and actual practice.

Second, Identify the Ethical Issues of the Situation. In the ICU scenario, if competent patients have expressed their wishes about resuscitation, this should be reflected in the chart. If a living will has been executed and is recognized as valid within your state, its presence in the chart lends considerable weight to the decision. The patient should be encouraged to discuss his decision with family to decrease the chances for disagreement if the patient can no longer "speak" for himself. If immediate family members disagree with the living will, the physician may be reluctant to honor the will, at least in part, because of concern regarding possible liability. If the living will was executed without prior or subsequent discussion with the attending physician, there may be reluctance to honor the will because the physician was not informed of the patient's decision. The physician may feel that the patient did not make an informed decision. A durable power of attorney for healthcare (DPAHC), however, combined with a living will and completed prior to the patient's present state of incapacitation, would stand as clear and convincing evidence of the patient's wishes, preventing such a problem. The above example illustrates the existence of some values and principles in possible conflict.

....

Patient: Values autonomy, including right to decide when intervention should stop.

Family: May value life at all cost and be unwilling to "let go" of the patient when a chance exists to prolong life.

Physician: May feel that the patient has a fair chance to survive and that the living will was executed without being "fully informed." The duty to care/cure may outweigh the physician's belief in the exercise of patient autonomy and fidelity.

Nurse: Values patient autonomy and the need to remain faithful to the patient. Concern for the needs of the family may cause some conflict, as well as respect for the physician-patient relationship.

Institution: Examination of institutional policy may reveal conflict between stated policy (honoring living wills) vs. actual practice (code all patients unless written physician orders indicate otherwise).

....

In this situation, the ethical components of this second step involve autonomy and fidelity vs. beneficence.

Third, Consider Possible Courses of Action and Their Related Outcomes.   Having collected data and attempted discussion on the issue with all involved parties, you are faced with some options:

1. Advocate for the patient(s) with physicians and families by facilitating communication.

2. Encourage patient(s) and families to share feelings with each other regarding desires for care.

3. Encourage families, patients, and attending physicians to discuss the situation more openly. If the advocacy role does not bring about some change in behavior, consider the possible input and assistance of an *interdisciplinary ethics committee* (IEC). In the last decade, such committees have evolved in response to the growing number of ethical issues faced in clinical practice. At present, over 60% of hospitals have such a committee, and it may become an integral aspect of every institution if Medicare reimbursement is linked to their presence. The IEC is typically composed of physicians, clergy, social workers, lawyer(s), and increasingly, nurses. Any health team

member can access the committee with the assurance of receiving at least a helpful, listening ear. If necessary, the committee will convene to review a clinical case and will offer an unbiased opinion of the situation. They may be helpful in clarifying issues or in offering moral support, or be persuasive in suggesting that involved parties (family, physician, patients, nurse) consider a suggested course of action. The authority of an IEC is usually limited, as the majorty of IECs are developed with the understanding that the advice and opinions offered are not binding to the individual. However, it can serve as a potent form of moral authority and influence if utilized.

Taking the initiative to express your values and principles is not necessarily easy. As a new graduate, it may seem safer to "swallow hard," remain quiet, and invest your energies into other aspects of your role. You may risk ridicule, criticism, and disagreement when you speak out on an ethical issue, especially if your view is different, or unpopular. However, you risk something far more important if you do not. Silence diminishes your own autonomy as a person and as a professional. Depending on the situation, it may raise eyebrows, but it is important to make your concerns known because some values may be imposed on the patient or you in the clinical setting, and those values may not be right. You may not agree with these values or feel that they are in the best interest of the patient.

Fourth, After a Course of Action Has Been Taken, Evaluate the Outcome. In the ICU scenario: Did improved communication occur between patients, families, and physicians? Were your efforts to advocate met with resistance or rebuff? What could you try differently the next time? What values or principles were considered most important by the decision-makers? What kind of assistance did you receive from the IEC? What role did nursing play in this situation and was it appropriate?

What Other Resources Are Available to Help Resolve Ethical Dilemmas?

Professional resources are also available to provide direction about ethical issues and behavior. The first of these is the American Nurses Association (ANA) Code of Ethics (1985). [This may be found in Chapter 3 (Table 3–3).]

The code is a statement to society that outlines the values, concerns, and goals of the profession. It should be compatible with individual nurse's personal values and goals. The code provides direction for ethical decisions and behavior by repeatedly emphasizing the obligations and responsibilities that the nurse-patient relationship details.

The eleven provisions of the Code of Ethics alludes to the ethical principles

TABLE 13–3 *International Council of Nurses Code for Nurses*

ETHICAL CONCEPTS APPLIED TO NURSING

◆ The fundamental responsibility of the nurse is fourfold: to promote health, to prevent illness, to restore health, and to alleviate suffering.

◆ The need for nursing is universal. Inherent in nursing is respect for life, dignity, and rights of man. It is unrestricted by considerations of nationality, race, creed, color, age, sex, politics, or social status.

◆ Nurses render health services to the individual, the family, and the community and coordinate their services with those of related groups.

NURSES AND PEOPLE

◆ The nurse's primary responsibility is to those people who require nursing care.

◆ The nurse, in providing care, promotes an environment in which the values, customs, and spiritual beliefs of the individual are respected.

◆ The nurse holds in confidence personal information and uses judgment in sharing this information.

NURSES AND PRACTICE

◆ The nurse carries personal responsibility for nursing practice and for maintaining competence by continual learning.

◆ The nurse maintains the highest standards of nursing care possible within the reality of a specific situation.

◆ The nurse uses judgment in relation to individual competence when accepting and delegating responsibilities.

◆ The nurse when acting in a professional capacity should at all times maintain standards of personal conduct which reflect credit upon the profession.

NURSES AND SOCIETY

◆ The nurse shares with other citizens the responsibility for initiating and supporting action to meet the health and social needs of the public.

NURSES AND CO-WORKERS

◆ The nurse sustains a cooperative relationship with co-workers in nursing and other fields.

◆ The nurse takes appropriate action to safeguard the individual when his care is endangered by a co-worker or any other person.

NURSES AND THE PROFESSION

◆ The nurse plays the major role in determining and implementing desirable standards of nursing practice and nursing education.

◆ The nurse is active in developing a core of professional knowledge.

◆ The nurse, acting through the professional organization, participates in establishing and maintaining equitable social and economic working conditions in nursing.

Reprinted with permission from International Council of Nurses (1973): ICN Code for Nurses: Ethical Concepts Applied to Nursing, Geneva, Switzerland, Inprimeries Populaires.

mentioned earlier in the text and certainly imply that fidelity to the patient is foremost. A copy of the Code with interpretive statements is available from the ANA. If you did not purchase a copy as a reference for school, consider buying it for your own use in practice.

Critics of the Code of Ethics cite its lack of legal enforceability. This is a valid criticism, because the code is not a legal document like licensure laws. However, it is a moral statement of accountability and can add weight to decisions involving legal censure. Many practicing nurses claim ignorance of the Code of Ethics or believe that it is a document for students only. However, the Code of Ethics is for all nurses and was developed by nurses. Take the opportunity to become familiar with its contents.

A second Code that addresses ethical issues is the International Council of Nurses (ICN) Code for Nurses (Table 13–3). Most recently revised in 1973, it is intended for worldwide use. Because of its international audience, this Code reflects awareness of, and respect for, cultural and religious differences. If you intend to practice in a culture different from your own, you should be familiar with the ICN Code. The development of the ICN is quite an achievement for the profession because it demonstrates the willingness of individuals from many different cultures to work together for the improvement of nursing care. Critics of the ICN code also cite its lack of legal enforceabiltiy.

In 1973, the American Hospital Association published *A Patient's Bill of Rights* (Table 13–4). This document reflects acknowledgement of the patient's right to participate in their healthcare and was developed as a response to consumer criticism of provider-controlled care. The twelve statements detail the patient's rights with corresponding provider responsibilities. Read over each statement and consider whether they seem reasonable. Less than twenty-five years ago, some of the statements were considered radical. The Bill of Rights reflects the increasing emphasis of patient autonomy in healthcare and defines limits of provider influence and control. Earlier beliefs that the hospital and physician know best (paternalism) have been challenged and modified.

Consider the settings in which you have had clinical experiences and decide how well these "rights" have been acknowledged and supported. In your future practice, keep these rights in mind. Not only are they the "right thing to do," but they have the enforceability of law.

A fourth document which you should be familiar with is the *Nuremberg Code* (Table 13–5). This code grew out of the blatant abuses perpetrated by Nazi war criminals during World War II in the name of science. Experiments were conducted by healthcare professionals without patient consent and resulted in mutilations, disability, and death. The Nuremberg Code identifies the need for voluntary informed consent when medical experiments are conducted on human beings. It delineates the limits and restrictions that researchers must recognize and respect. Because of the preponderance of research in many clinical settings, nurses have a responsibility to understand the concept of voluntary informed consent and support the patient's rights throughout the research process. After

TABLE 13–4   *Your Rights as a Hospital Patient*

We consider you a partner in your hospital care. When you are well-informed, participate in treatment decisions, and communicate openly with your doctor and other health professionals, you help make your care as effective as possible. This hospital encourages respect for the personal preferences and values of each individual.

While you are a patient in the hospital, your rights include the following:

◆ You have the right to considerate and respectful care.

◆ You have the right to be well-informed about your illness, possible treatments, and likely outcome and to discuss this information with your doctor. You have the right to know the names and roles of people treating you.

◆ You have the right to consent to or refuse a treatment, as permitted by law, throughout your hospital stay. If you refuse a recommended treatment, you will receive other needed and available care.

◆ You have the right to have an advance directive, such as a living will or health care proxy. These documents express your choices about your future care or name someone to decide if you cannot speak for yourself. If you have a written advance directive, you should provide a copy to the hospital, your family, and your doctor.

◆ You have the right to privacy. The hospital, your doctor, and others caring for you will protect your privacy as much as possible.

◆ You have the right to expect that treatment records are confidential unless you have given permission to release information or reporting is required or permitted by law. When the hospital releases records to others, such as insurers, it emphasizes that the records are confidential.

◆ You have the right to review your medical records and to have the information explained, except when restricted by law.

◆ You have the right to expect that the hospital will give you necessary health services to the best of its ability. Treatment, referral, or transfer may be recommended. If transfer is recommended or requested, you will be informed of risks, benefits, and alternatives. You will not be transferred until the other institution agrees to accept you.

◆ You have the right to know if this hospital has relationships with outside parties that may influence your treatment and care. These relationships may be with educational institutions, other health care providers, or insurers.

◆ You have the right to consent or decline to take part in research affecting your care. If you choose not to take part, you will receive the most effective care the hospital otherwise provides.

◆ You have the right to be told of realistic care alternatives when hospital care is no longer appropriate.

◆ You have the right to know about hospital rules that affect you and your treatment and about charges and payment methods. You have the right to know about hospital resources, such as patient representatives or ethics committees, that can help you resolve problems and questions about your hospital stay and care.

TABLE 13–4   *Your Rights as a Hospital Patient* Continued

◆ You have responsibilities as a patient. You are responsible for providing information about your health, including past illnesses, hospital stays, and use of medicine. You are responsible for asking questions when you do not understand information or instructions. If you believe you can't follow through with your treatment, you are responsible for telling your doctor.

This hospital works to provide care efficiently and fairly to all patients and the community. You and your visitors are responsible for being considerate of the needs of other patients, staff, and the hospital. You are responsible for providing information for insurance and for working with the hospital to arrange payment, when needed.

Your health dependent not just on your hospital care but, in the long term, on the decisions you make in your daily life. You are responsible for recognizing the effect of life-style on your personal health.

A hospital serves many purposes. Hospitals work to improve people's health; treat people with injury and disease; educate doctors, health professionals, patients, and community members; and improve understanding of health and disease. In carrying out these activities, this institution works to respect your values and dignity.

Reprinted with permission by the American Hospital Association, 1992.

reading this code, you should have increased awareness of the patient's right to autonomy and the healthcare provider's responsibility to be faithful to that right.

CONTROVERSIAL ETHICAL ISSUES CONFRONTING NURSING

Situations that raise ethical issues affect all areas of nursing practice. The following is a sampling of issues that consistently cause controversy.

Abortion

This issue has raged in the United States since the 1973 Roe v. Wade Supreme Court decision. The resolution of this case struck down laws against abortion, but left the possibility of introducing restrictions under some conditions. Efforts toward that end continue today with mixed results for both pro-choice and pro-life factions.

Historical references to abortion can be found as far back as 4,500 B.C. (Rosen, 1967). It has been practiced in many societies as a means of population

TABLE 13–5 *The Nuremberg Code*

The great weight of the evidence before us is to the effect that certain types of medical experiments on human beings, when kept within reasonably well-defined bounds, conform to the ethics of the medical profession generally. The protagonists of the practice of human experimentation justify their views on the basis that such experiments yield results for the good of society that are unprocurable by other methods or means of study. All agree, however, that certain basic principles must be observed in order to satisfy moral, ethical, and legal concepts:

1. The voluntary consent of the human subject is absolutely essential. This means that the person involved should have legal capacity to give consent; should be so situated as to be able to exercise free power of choice, without the intervention of any element of force, fraud, deceit, duress, overreaching, or other ulterior form of constraint or coercion; and should have sufficient knowledge and comprehension of the elements of the subject matter involved as to enable him to make an understanding and enlightened decision. This latter element requires that before the acceptance of an affirmative decision by the experimental subject there should be made known to him the nature, duration, and purpose of the experiment; the method and means by which it is to be conducted; all inconveniences and hazards reasonably to be expected; and the effects upon his health or person which may possibly come from his participation in the experiment.

   The duty and responsibility for ascertaining the quality of the consent rests upon each individual who initiates, directs or engages in the experiment. It is a personal duty and responsibility which may not be delegated to another with impunity.

2. The experiment should be such as to yield fruitful results for the good of society, unprocurable by other methods or means of study, and not random and unnecessary in nature.

3. The experiment should be so designed and based on the results of animal experimentation and a knowledge of the natural history of the disease or other problem under study that the anticipated results will justify the performance of the experiment.

4. The experiment should be so conducted as to avoid all unnecessary physical and mental suffering and injury.

5. No experiment should be conducted where there is an *a priori* reason to believe that death or disabling injury will occur; except, perhaps, in those experiments where the experimental physicians also serve as subjects.

6. The degree of risk to be taken should never exceed that determined by the humanitarian importance of the problem to be solved by the experiment.

7. Proper preparations should be made and adequate facilities provided to protect the experimental subject against even remote possibilities of injury, disability or death.

8. The experiment should be conducted only by scientifically qualified persons. The highest degree of skill and care should be required through all stages of the experiments of those who conduct or engage in the experiment.

Reprinted from: Trials of War Criminals before the Nuremberg Military Tribunals under Control Council Law No. 10. Vol. 2. Washington, D.C., U.S. Government Printing Office, 1949, p. 181.

control and terminating unwanted pregnancies, yet sanctions against abortion are found in both ancient biblical and legal texts. Interestingly, the sanctions against abortion generally related to fines payable to the husband if the pregnant woman was harmed. This "fine" sanction was derived from the concept of woman and fetus as male property. Greek philosophers, including Aristotle and Plato, made a distinction between an unformed vs. formed fetus. A fine was levied for aborting an unformed fetus, whereas the aborting of a formed fetus required "a life for a life." The number of gestational weeks that determine whether a fetus was formed was not stated, although the time of human *ensoulment* was understood: Aristotle believed that a male fetus was imbued with a soul at 40 days gestation (quickening) vs. 90 days for a female (Feldman, 1968). The subject of ensoulment became part of the ongoing debate regarding the time when the developing fetus becomes human. In other words—

▼

When does life begin?

▲

Judeo-Christian theologians generally came to identify the beginning of life at conception or the time of implantation. Yet, even within this tradition, the Jewish Talmud and Roman law stated that life begins at birth, because the first breath represents the infusion of life. These varied views continue to the present.

Social customs and private behavior regarding abortion have frequently differed from theological teaching. The first legal sanctions against abortion in the United States began in the late nineteenth century. Prior to that time, first-trimester abortions were not uncommon, and in fact were advertised, supporting the idea that abortion prior to quickening was acceptable.

The ethical debate about abortion today is a continuing struggle to answer the question of when life begins, as well as determining an answer to the following questions:

◆ Does the fetus have rights?
◆ Do the rights of the fetus (for life) take precedence over the right of the mother to control her reproductive functions?
◆ When is abortion morally justified?
◆ Should minors have the right to abortion without parental consent or awareness?

The struggle to answer these questions has polarized individuals into "pro-life" or "pro-choice" camps. Yet, opinion polls on the subject have found very few people to be against abortion in all circumstances, or to favor abortion as a mandatory solution for some pregnancies. The majority of Americans express views anywhere between these extremes and the legal battle to maintain or restrict abortion access continues.

The Roman Catholic church has been the religious group most frequently identified with the pro-life movement, but there are other groups religious and otherwise who support a ban on abortion. Pro-life proponents generally condone abortion only to save the life of the mother. These antiabortion groups are criticized by pro-choice as extremists, antiwoman, and repressive.

The pro-choice movement is vocal in championing the woman's right to choose and promoting the safety of legalized abortion. They cite the tragedy of past "back-alley" abortions and compare restrictions on abortion to infringements on the civil liberties of women. Within the pro-choice movement are many individuals who favor restrictions on abortions after the first trimester and oppose the use of abortion as a means of birth control. Pro-life proponents view pro-choice as antifamily extremists who do not represent the views of the majority of Americans.

How Does the Abortion Issue Affect Nursing?

Nurses are involved both as individuals and professionals. Some general guidelines are suggested:

◆ Consider what your values and beliefs are in relation to abortion and how you can best apply these values to your work and possible political action.

◆ If you choose to work in a setting where abortions are performed, review statement one of the ANA Code: "The nurse provides services with respect for human dignity and the uniqueness of the client, unrestricted by considerations of social or economic status, personal attributes, or the nature of the health problems" (ANA, 1985).

This statement outlines your responsibility to care for all patients. If you do not agree with an institution's policy or procedure regarding abortion, the patient still merits your care. If that care (i.e., assisting with abortions) violates your principles, you should consider changing your job, or developing an agreement with your employer regarding your job responsibilities. If you cannot provide the care that the patient requires, make arrangements for someone else to do so.

◆ You do not have to sacrifice your own values and principles, but you are barred by the ANA Code from abandoning patients or forcing your values on them. Such abandonment would also constitute legal abandonment and you would be subject to legal action.

◆ Some hospitals have developed conscience clauses that provide protection to the hospital and nurses against participation in abortions. Find out if your institution has such a clause.

Consider your response and possible conflict in the following situations:

You are a labor and delivery nurse working on a unit that performs second-trimester saline abortions in a nearby area. You are not a part of the staff for the abortion area, but today, because of short staffing, you are asked to care for a sixteen-year-old who is undergoing the procedure.

You work in a family planning clinic that receives federal monies. You are restricted from giving information regarding abortion services because of federal guidelines. A forty-one-year-old mother of five has expressed interest in terminating her pregnancy of six weeks gestation. She confides that her husband would beat her if he knew she was pregnant and contemplating abortion.

You are providing a class on sexuality and contraception to a group of high school sophomores. Two of the girls state that they have just had abortions. In response to your information regarding available methods of contraception, one of the girls states, "I'm not interested in birth control. If I get pregnant again, I'll just get an abortion. It's a lot easier."

You have a history of infertility and work in the neonatal ICU. You are presently caring for a twenty-four-week-old baby born to a mom who admits to taking "crack" as a means of inducing labor and "getting rid of the baby." The mom has just arrived in the unit and wants to visit the baby.

These sample scenarios are meant to illustrate the conflicts that personal values, institutional settings, and clients may create for the new graduate. In your responses, consider how you might lobby or participate in the political process to change or support existing policies regarding abortion and access to such services.

Euthanasia

Euthanasia refers to "mercy killing." It is a Greek word that means "good death" and implies painless actions to end the life of individuals suffering from incurable or terminal diseases. Euthanasia is classified as active, passive, or voluntary. Active euthanasia involves the administration of a lethal drug or other measure to end life and alleviate suffering. *Regardless of the motivation and beliefs of the individuals involved,* active euthanasia is legally wrong and can result in criminal charges of murder if carried out. In recent years, incidents of active euthanasia have become periodic news events as spouses or parents have used measures to end the suffering of their mates or children (from, for example, Alzheimer's or vegetative coma). *Passive euthanasia* involves the withdrawal of extraordinary means of life support (i.e., ventilator). *Voluntary euthanasia* involves situations when the dying individual expresses desire over the management and time of death.

As technology has advanced, patients are routinely kept alive today who would never have survived a few short years ago. Concerns regarding *quality of life* and *suffering vs. quality of life* for those individuals have resulted in a movement to have "right to die" statutes and living wills accepted (Fig. 13–1). In those states that have such statutes and recognize living wills, termination of treatment in such cases has become easier. "Right to die" statutes free health-care personnel from possible liability for honoring a person's wishes that life not be unduly prolonged (Rudy,1985).

Another document, the durable power of attorney for healthcare (DPAHC), helps ensure that a living will is carried out. The DPAHC identifies the individual who will carry out the patient's wishes in the event that he or she is incapacitated, and also discusses with healthcare providers the specific wishes of the patient regarding life-support measures.

A major impact on the availability of living wills and the DPAHC (which are referred to as *advanced medical directives*) has been the introduction of the Patient Self-Determination Act in December, 1991. Passed as part of the Omnibus Budget Reconciliation Act, advanced directives are federally mandated for all institutions receiving Medicare and/or Medicaid funds. Upon admission, all competent adults must be offered information about advanced directives. This means that all adults are told about the purpose and availability of living wills (treatment directive) and DPAHCs (appointment directive). They are then offered assistance with completing these documents if desired. The impact of advanced directives information has not yet been measured, but it certainly is influencing the communication patients have with their families, physicians, and other healthcare providers regarding detailed care. When nurses confront issues involving possible euthanasia they need to remain true to their own values and beliefs, while balancing the need to respect the patient's values as well.

Decisions to withdraw or withhold nutrition and hydration from patients is complex and the subject of ongoing debate by ethicists, healthcare personnel, and the legal system. In response to issues of hydration and nutrition, the Ethics Committee of the ANA developed guidelines in 1988. These guidelines state that there are few instances when withholding or withdrawing nutrition and hydration are morally permissible. While intended only as a guideline, this document provides direction for nurses who face such issues. Its wording has been both praised for its clarity and criticized for possible ambiguity. The primary exception to hydration and nutrition withdrawal is when harm from these measures can be demonstrated. This document is available from the ANA.

ADVANCE DIRECTIVE
Living Will and Health Care Proxy

*D*eath is a part of life. It is a reality like birth, growth and aging. I am using this advance directive to convey my wishes about medical care to my doctors and other people looking after me at the end of my life. It is called an advance directive because it gives instructions in advance about what I want to happen to me in the future. It expresses my wishes about medical treatment that might keep me alive. I want this to be legally binding.

If I cannot make or communicate decisions about my medical care, those around me should rely on this document for instructions about measures that could keep me alive.

I do not want medical treatment (including feeding and water by tube) that will keep me alive if:
- I am unconscious and there is no reasonable prospect that I will ever be conscious again (even if I am not going to die soon in my medical condition), <u>or</u>
- I am near death from an illness or injury with no reasonable prospect of recovery.

I do want medicine and other care to make me more comfortable and to take care of pain and suffering. I want this even if the pain medicine makes me die sooner.

I want to give some extra instructions: *[Here list any special instructions, e.g., some people fear being kept alive after a debilitating stroke. If you have wishes about this, or any other conditions, please write them here.]*

The legal language in the box that follows is a health care proxy.
It gives another person the power to make medical decisions for me.

I name _____ , who lives at _____

_____ , phone number _____ ,

to make medical decisions for me if I cannot make them myself. This person is called a health care "surrogate," "agent," "proxy," or "attorney in fact." This power of attorney shall become effective when I become incapable of making or communicating decisions about my medical care. This means that this document stays legal when and if I lose the power to speak for myself, for instance, if I am in a coma or have Alzheimer's disease.

My health care proxy has power to tell others what my advance directive means. This person also has power to make decisions for me, based either on what I would have wanted, or, if this is not known, on what he or she thinks is best for me.

If my first choice health care proxy cannot or decides not to act for me, I name _____

_____ , address _____ ,

phone number _____ , as my second choice.

(over, please)

LWGEN

FIGURE 13–1   *Advance Directive—Living Will and Health Care Proxy.*

Reprinted by permission of Choice in Dying (formerly Concern for Dying/Society for the Right to Die) 200 Varick Street, New York, NY 10014-4810 212/366-5540

I have discussed my wishes with my health care proxy, and with my second choice if I have chosen to appoint a second person. My proxy(ies) has(have) agreed to act for me.

I have thought about this advance directive carefully. I know what it means and want to sign it. I have chosen two witnesses, neither of whom is a member of my family, nor will inherit from me when I die. My witnesses are not the same people as those I named as my health care proxies. I understand that this form should be notarized if I use the box to name (a) health care proxy(ies).

Signature _____

Date _____

Address _____

Witness' signature _____

Witness' printed name _____

Address _____

Witness' signature _____

Witness' printed name _____

Address _____

Notary [to be used if proxy is appointed]_____

Drafted and Distributed by Choice In Dying, Inc.—the National Council for the right to Die. Choice In Dying is a National not-for-profit organization which works for the rights of patients at the end of life. In addition to this generic advance directive, Choice In Dying distributes advance directives that conform to each state's specific legal requirements and maintains a national Living Will Registry for completed documents.

CHOICE IN DYING INC.—
the national council for the right to die
(formerly Concern for Dying/Society for the Right to Die)
200 Varick Street, New York, NY 10014 (212) 366-5540

5/92

FIGURE 13–1   *(Continued)*
(Reprinted by permission of Choice in Dying Inc.)

Ethicists generally agree that while prolongation of life by extraordinary means is not always indicated, clarifying the circumstances when such care may be stopped (withdrawn) or possibly never begun (withheld) frequently creates controversy, particularly when the quality of life (coma, persistent vegetative state) is likely to be questionable.

Opponents of the right to die movement believe that it represents the erosion of the value of human life and may encourage a movement toward the acceptance of suicide. They caution that the lives of the weak and disabled may come to be devalued as society concentrates on the pursuit of "quality life." If passive euthanasia achieves societal acceptance, who will speak out in favor of protecting incompetent or dependent individuals who are not living society's view of a "quality life"?

Proponents of the right to die movement believe that it provides a more natural control of living and dying to the individual and family by removing the artificial prolongation of life through technology.

Consider your response and possible conflict in the following situations:

A twenty-two-year-old quadriplegic repeatedly asks you to disconnect him from the ventilator. His family rarely visits and he believes that he has nothing to live for.

The spouse of an advanced Alzheimer's patient states that he can no longer watch his wife of forty-three years suffer. "She would not have wanted to live this way." His wife is presently being treated for dehydration, malnutrition, and a urinary tract infection. She is confused and is frequently sedated to manage her combativeness. Use of a feeding tube is being contemplated because of her refusal to eat.

The attending physician for a terminal AIDS patient refuses to order increasing doses of pain medication because of her concern that it may cause a repeat episode of respiratory depression. The patient's pain is unrelieved and he begs you for medication. "Please help me. I know I'm dying."

The parents of a twenty–nine-week old premature infant with Downs syndrome and tracheoesophageal fistula request that no extraordinary care be provided. They want the baby kept warm and nurtured but refuse to sign the consent form for surgery.

For each of these scenarios, consider what both your reaction and the possible resources you would utilize to resolve the conflicts.

The Use of Reproductive Technology

Depending upon the source, 10–20% of all couples in the United States are identified as infertile. Because of this, and the legalization of abortion, the development and use of reproductive technology is a subject of considerable interest and controversy.

What Is the Ethical Consideration in Artificial Insemination?

Artificial insemination (AI) involves the use of husband (AIH) or donor (AID) sperm in cases of infertility or when a single woman wishes to be artificially impregnated.

The ethical arguments surrounding the issue involve beliefs about the use of reproductive interventions both inside and out of marriage. For example, the Roman Catholic church opposes AI, including the use of AIH, under all circumstances because it is an unnatural act and reduces people to objects (Berger,1987).

Proponents of AI cite the ability of a woman to achieve pregnancy with a relatively simple intervention. The use of AIH allows a woman to achieve pregnancy with her own husband's genetic material and is generally supported because it is within a committed relationship. The issue is more controversial when donor sperm is used, and the woman is single. The way in which we define family and parenthood may be challenged, particularly when lesbian couples are involved.

What Are the Ethical Issues Surrounding Surrogate Motherhood?

The flip side to AI is surrogate motherhood. Unlike simple AI, there is no anonymity of the donor uterus. The surrogate mother is known, having been selectively chosen and contracted for the purpose of carrying a pregnancy for another couple to claim as their own. To date, some genetic fathers and artificially inseminated surrogate mothers have fought bitter legal and emotional wars to gain custody of the offspring. Concern for the well-being and rights of the newborn, genetic father, and surrogate mother have been discussed at great lengths in the courts, media, and ethical circles. Efforts have been made to remove any financial incentive for surrogate motherhood (New York Advance Legislative Service, 1992) because carrying a pregnancy for the purpose of making money has been likened to selling a human being. Contracting for the "sale"of a human being has raised disturbing issues; for example, the refusal of the biological mother to relinquish the child in spite of a "contract" (Baby M), and the birth of a grossly deformed child to a surrogate mother, resulting in the refusal of anyone to accept the child as his or her own. This latter case was most damning because the child is likened to "damaged goods" abandoned by both the buyer and seller.

What Is the Ethical Issue Regarding the Use of Fetal Tissue?

Fetal tissue from elective abortions has been identified as a potentially beneficial treatment for Parkinson's disease and other degenerative disorders because of its unique embyronic qualities. Proponents argue that it is available tissue that can be put to some beneficial use in patients who at the present time do not have any other hope of significant improvement or cure.

Critics who assail the use of fetal tissue as a further erosion of respect for the unborn were successful in causing a federal ban on the use of fetal tissue for research in the United States during the 1980s. They believe that the limited research which already has occurred regarding fetal tissue has created the mentality that pregnancy can be used as a means of providing parts and tissues for others. This ban was removed in early 1993 after President Clinton took office. A similar line of thinking has been used regarding the use of anencephalics as organ donors.

What Are the Ethical Issues Regarding In Vitro Fertilization?

This procedure involves fertilization of a mother's ovum with the father's sperm in a glass laboratory dish followed by implantation of the embryo in the mother's uterus.

Since the birth of the first successful in vitro fertilization baby in 1978, the procedure has gained popularity as a last-chance method for some infertile couples to have a child. The availability of the technique has created a new subspecialty practice in obstetrics and raised ethical issues for consideration. Opponents of the procedure argue that is an unnatural act and removes the biological act of procreation from the intimacy of marriage. The cost of the procedure is also a source of criticism, calling into question whether insurance should cover the cost, and whether the procedure should be available to all couples, regardless of ability to pay. Questions concerning informed consent for the procedure merit attention as well. Many infertility clinics offer this service but have not been "up front" about reporting their success rate or qualifications. Standardized methods of reporting this information are now being established. To be ethical, all such clinics should define "success" the same way, i.e., success equals pregnancy, or success equals live birth. The two definitions are very different. Qualifications of the staff should be available to patients and the subspecialty should lobby for standards of practice that are enforceable and available to the public. Possible side effects, from the drugs used to induce hyperovulation as well as from anesthesia, or from surgical injury during the laparoscopy, should be explained.

Should anyone who desires the procedure have access or should the procedure be limited to those in a heterosexual marriage? Most clinics have limited their services to heterosexual couples to avoid adverse publicity but this policy is starting to change as single and lesbian women seek out avenues of becoming biological parents.

Most importantly, who does the embryo belong to and what are his or her rights? There have been court cases involving marital disputes regarding the custody of the frozen embryos. What are the rights of the embryo in such instances? Can a "parent" choose to destroy the embryos over the objection of the estranged spouse, or, on the other hand, should one "parent" be able to obtain custody of the embryos when their spouse wants them to be thawed out and destroyed?

How Should the Ability to Diagnose Genetic Defects Prenatally be Utilized?

At the present time, genetic disorders, such as Tay-Sachs, cystic fibrosis, Huntington's chorea, and retinoblastoma, can be diagnosed early in pregnancy. As this technology advances, how should it be used? Should screening remain voluntary, or as some have suggested, should it be mandatory to detect fetal disorders that could be aborted or possibly treated? Should the results of such genetic screening be made available to insurance companies? Critics argue that this information could be used as a means of coercion for couples regarding reproductive decisions if future insurance coverage is then limited. As this technology advances, safeguards need to be applied in order to prevent invasion of privacy and any move toward a societal interest in eugenics.

Allocation of Scarce Resources

When the subject of scarce resource allocation is mentioned, justice is the core issue. What is fair and equal treatment when healthcare financing decisions are made? Who should make such decisions and on what basis? Critics argue that healthcare is not a scarce resource in this country, but that it is the access to such care which is scarce for many. They believe that this scarcity of access could be eliminated if our priorities in governmental spending were altered. However, as of 1991, more than 11% of our Gross National Product (GNP) was spent on healthcare, an alarming amount because the cost of healthcare has continually skyrocketed in the last ten years without signs of leveling off (Ward, 1990). Yet, over thirty-seven million citizens are without health insurance or reasonable means of accessing any but stopgap emergency care (Cohen, 1990). Is national health insurance on the horizon as a solution? The answer is unclear, but some fundmental change in healthcare policy is likely as our society struggles to control costs while maintaining or expanding access to healthcare.

Allocation also raises a number of questions. For example, do all individuals merit the same care? If your answer is an immediate "yes," would you change your mind if the patient was indigent with no chance of paying the bill? If you still say "yes," should this same indigent patient receive a liver transplant as readily as someone who has insurance or cash to pay for it? These and other questions are being asked by individuals, government, and ethicists as well as healthcare providers. Perhaps at the core of this subject is a more fundamental question: Is healthcare a right or a privilege that comes with the ability to pay? If access to healthcare is a right that should be provided to all citizens, are we as a society prepared to pay the bill? And, is there a level of healthcare that is essential for all, and beyond which becomes a matter of private financing?

The type of care that is provided and supported is another aspect of the debate. For example, should health promotion and prevention receive as much or more emphasis as illness-oriented and rehabilitative care? It is widely acknowledged that each dollar spent on preventive care (i.e., prenatal care) saves three or more dollars in later intervention (i.e., neonatal ICU), yet our national and state healthcare expenditures (i.e., Medicare and Medicaid) are weighted in favor of an illness model for reimbursement.

What Are Some of the Possible Solutions Being Debated?

In recent years, some individuals, including former Governor Richard Lamm of Colorado, have proposed the idea of healthcare rationing for the elderly, specifically as it relates to the use of expensive technology that often prolongs the last few weeks of life and suffering (Lamm, 1986). He believes that such 11th hour expenditures are unwanted by many elderly, and consume disproportionate amounts of health care resources. He has been criticized for his views, but defends his ideas as an example of acknowledging the finite resources of society.

Governor Lamm believes that other more vulnerable groups, such as uninsured children, be given a more equitable portion of healthcare services (i.e., well-baby clinics). Others argue that healthcare is already being rationed and that we should recognize this fact and articulate our priorities.

The state of Oregon has gone one step further, imposing guidelines on the type of care that its Medicaid funds will cover. Deciding that preventive care affects a majority of its citizens, funding for such care as immunizations and prenatal care was made a priority, whereas extraordinary care that benefits only a few individuals, such as a bone marrow transplant, will not be covered (Rooks, 1990). This utilitarian approach, emphasizing the greatest good for the greatest number, is not without its critics, but it is an effort to provide direction for healthcare priorities. Oregon's plan was initially vetoed by the federal government and has undergone some revision, still emphasizing preventative care and treatment for disorders which affect a majority of citizens. Other states are now looking at the Oregon model as they plan healthcare reform.

Healthcare Rationing

You may have already experienced situations of healthcare rationing or limited access. As a nurse you may feel powerless and frustrated when patients do not receive care because they cannot afford it or, on the other hand, feel angry because indigent patients are placing heavy burdens on both private and public facilities. Consider your values and professional responsibilities as you think through this issue. As an individual and a nurse, you need to take a stand regarding health resource allocation and support efforts to improve access, while determining in your mind what type of healthcare you believe to be ethically justifiable.

As medical technology advances, ethical issues and concerns will continue to play an ever-increasing role in your nursing practice.

The general public, healthcare professions, religious traditions, as well as the legal system, will all have influence in the attempts to resolve the ethical issues affecting healthcare in the twenty-first century. Keeping an open mind to these controversial dilemmas is difficult, but it is hoped you will examine your personal values and continue to make decisions that are based on the welfare of the patient.

REFERENCES

American Nurses Association. (1985): *Code for Nurses with Interpretative Statements.* Kansas City, MO, ANA.

Bandman, E. L., Bandman, B. (1990): *Nursing Ethics Through the Life Span.* 2nd ed., East Norwalk, CT, Appleton & Lange.

Banja, J. D. (1990): Nutritional discontinuation: Active or passive euthanasia? *J Neurosci Nurs* 22(4):258.

Berger, J. (1987): Vatican official assails method of fertilization. *New York Times,* October 8, B6.

Cohen, S. (1990): The politics of Medicaid: 1980-1989. *Nurs Outlook* 38(5):229.

Edwards, B. S. (1990): Does the DNR patient belong in the ICU? *Crit Care Nurs Clin North Am* 2(3):473.

Editorial (1988): *New York Times,* June 4, 26.

Erickson, J. R. (1990): Making choices: The crux of ethical problems in nursing. *AORN J* 52(2):394.

Ericksen, J. (1989): Steps to ethical reasoning. *Canad Nurse* 85:23.

Erlen, J. A. (1990): In my opinion . . . Anencephalic infants as a source of organs: The need for caution. *Child Health Care* 19(3):187.

Feldman, D. M. (1968): *Marital Relations, Birth Control and Abortion in Jewish Law.* New York, Schocker Books.

Fiesta, J. (1990). The Cruzan case—No right to die. *Nurs Manag* 21(9):22.

Fletcher, J. F. (1966): *Situation Ethics.* Philadelphia, Westminster Press.

Hall, J. K. (1990): Understanding the fine line between law and ethics. *Nursing 90* 20(10):34-39.

Kjervik, D. K. (1990): Ethical and legal dilemmas of battered women. *J Profess Nurs* 6(5):253.

Kozier, B., Erb, G. (1988): *Concepts and Issues in Nursing Practice.* Menlo Park, CA, Addison-Wesley.

Lamm, R. (1986): Rationing of health care: The inevitable meets the unthinkable. *Nurse Practitioner* 11(5):57.

New York Advance Legislative Service (1992): Regular Session, Ch. 308, S.B. 1906.

Noddings, N. (1992): In defense of caring. *J Clin Ethics*. 3(1):15.

Nuremberg Code (1949): Trials of War Criminals Before the Nuremberg Military Tribunals under Control Council Law No. 18. Vol. 2. Washington D.C., U.S. Government Printing Office.

Oddi, L. F., Cassidy, V. R. (1990): Participation and perception of nurse members in the hospital ethics committee. *Western J Nurs Res* 12(3):307.

Parker, R. S. (1990): Nurses' stories: The search for a relational ethic of care. *Adv Nurs Sci* 12(1):31.

Pederson, C., Duckett, L. Maruyama, G. (1991): Using structured controversy to promote ethical decision-making. *J Nurs Educ* 29(4):150.

Pinch, W. J., Spielman, W. L. (1990): The parent's perspective: Ethical decision-making in neonatal intensive care. *J Adv Nurs* 15(6):712.

Rast, A. M. (1990): Anencephalic infants and organ procurement. *Imprint* 37(3):61.

Rooks, J. (1990): Let's admit we ration health care—then set priorities. *Am J Nurs* 90(6):39.

Rosen, H. (Ed.) (1967): *Abortion in America*. Boston, Beacon Press.

Rudy, E. B. (1985): The living will: Are you informed? *Focus Crit Care* 12(6):51.

Shannon, T. A. (1990): Ethical issues involved with in vitro fertilization, *AORN J* 52(3):627.

Smerke, J. M. (1990): Ethical components of caring. *Crit Care Nurs Clin North Am* 2(3):509.

Steele, S. M. (1983): *Values Clarification in Nursing*. 2nd ed. East Norwalk, CT, Appleton-Century-Crofts.

Uustal, D. B. (1990): Enhancing your ethical reasoning. *Crit Care Nurs Clin North Am* 2(3):437.

Ward, D. (1990): National health insurance: Where do nurses fit in? *Nurs Outlook* 38(5):206.

Zorb, S. L., Stevens J. B. (1990): Contemporary bioethical issues in critical care. *Crit Care Nurs Clin North Am* 2(3):515.

14

Legal Issues

Sarah Stark, J.D., R.N.

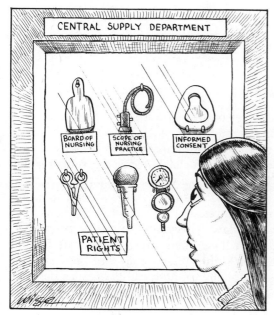

Knowledge regarding legal aspects is the best defense a nurse can have.

Men stumble over the truth from time to time, but most pick themselves up and hurry off as if nothing happened.

—Sir Winston Churchill

After completing this chapter, you should be able to:

- Describe the purpose of the nurse practice act.
- Identify the parameters of the nurse practice act in your state.
- Describe functions of a Board of Nursing.
- Identify sources for standards of nursing practice.
- Describe the process for obtaining and maintaining your license.
- Identify legal risks and defenses in nursing practice.
- Discuss the nurse's role in risk management.
- Describe the role of a nurse as a witness.
- Describe the nurse's role in dealing with nurses who are impaired.
- Discuss at least two controversial legal issues.

As you begin your nursing career, you will be expected to understand and function within certain legal responsibilities. Failure to understand these responsibilities and effectively defend yourself in certain situations will result in exposure to legal risk. It is important for the nurse to understand legal responsibilities as they relate to nursing, specifically to the nurse, the client, and the institution. This chapter will present some helpful hints on how you can significantly increase your protection against being sued as well as deal effectively with a legal situation if necessary. Knowledge is the most important defense a nurse can have. With it you can avoid the embarrassing position of the new graduate in the cartoon. Knowledge will assist you to avoid the most common legal pitfalls. But the *most important* thing for the nurse to remember is that the client's safety comes first. If you are doing what is best and *safest* for the client, your chances of having legal trouble decrease remarkably. Let's begin with a quick introduction to where our laws come from.

SOURCES OF LAW

What Are the Sources of the Law?

Our legal system is based on several types of law. The first and best known is *statutory* law. These are the laws that are passed by each state legislature and by our federal Congress. These written codes are hard to read because of the legal terminology and format used in them. These laws cover the rules for our relationships with each other. The nurse practice acts are examples of state statutory law and the Federal Food, Drug and Cosmetic Act is an example of a statutory law produced by the Federal Congress.

The next type of law is *constitutional* law. This refers to rights, privileges, and responsibilities that were stated in or have been inferred from the United States Constitution, including the Bill of Rights. States may not pass laws or institute rules that conflict with constitutionally granted rights or rules because the Constitution is the highest law of our country. The right to privacy is an example of Constitutional law.

Another type of law to consider is *administrative* law. This body of law refers to the rules and rulings made by administrative agencies that have been granted the authority by statute (legislatively passed law) to act in this manner. An example of this type of law are the rules and regulations passed by boards of nursing to control nursing practice in each state.

Another type of law is *common* law. This type of law refers to the decisions made by judges in court cases or established by rules of *custom and tradition*. The first, or case law, is the result of a legal principle, *stare decisis*, which means that once an issue has been decided all other cases concerning the same issue should be decided the same way. Another word for this is *precedent*. Each state

TABLE 14–1 *Good Samaritan Statutes*

◆ Care must be provided in good faith.

◆ Care must be gratuitous, no compensation is made for the care rendered.

◆ A higher standard of care may be required of healthcare workers because of their higher level of expertise.

◆ Nurses will be expected to provide care at the level of an ordinary nurse in a similar circumstance.

◆ Does not cover a person who is soliciting business or representing an agency.

◆ Does not cover the care rendered in an emergency department situation.

◆ Care provided should not be willfully or wantonly negligent.

has its own case law. Each state's body of case law may differ since it is based on an individual judge's decisions and, as you are well aware, not all judges think alike. If there is no existing legal principle, which often happens with the rapidly expanding nursing and medical practice issues, the court may expand an existing rule from another case to fit the circumstances. The court may look at custom and tradition, which means the way it has always been done, or the court may develop a new rule to resolve the problem.

The *Good Samaritan Law* is enacted by the individual state to protect and encourage healthcare professionals to provide care in an emergency situation. This law provides immunity from civil liability when a person provides assistance in an emergency. There are several conditions regarding protection under the Good Samaritan Law (Table 14–1). The nurse will be evaluated by how a reasonable and prudent nurse would have responded in the same situation. The Good Samaritan Law does not provide immunity when a nurse is providing care as an employee of an agency or hospital. Now let's look at some specific examples of these types of law that will be very important to you. (Table 14–2 has a listing of definitions of common terms.)

LEGAL ASPECTS OF NURSING

How Is Nursing Practice Controlled?

Nurse Practice Acts

Nurse practice acts are enacted by each state (statutory law) and are based on the police power granted each state from the federal government to protect the safety of its residents. Because of this, each state's practice act may be different from any other state's act. The only practice act you need to worry about is the

TABLE 14–2 *Common Legal Terms*

Torts: Civil (not criminal) wrongs committed by one person against another person or property. Includes the legal principle of *assault and battery*.

Deposition: An oral investigation done under oath and taken in writing. Purpose is to answer questions related to a specific issue. May include expert witnesses, or those directly related to the case. May be included in the trial phase of the case.

Plaintiff: The person who files the lawsuit and is seeking damages for a perceived wrongdoing.

Defendant: The person who is being accused of the wrongdoing. The person then must defend himself against the charges.

Defamation: A civil wrong in which an individual's reputation in the community, including the professional community, has been damaged.

Expert witness: A person who has specific knowledge, skills, and experience regarding a specific area. May be asked to provide information regarding the standards of care and whose testimony will be allowed in court.

Good Samaritan Law: Provides civil immunity to professionals who stop and render care in an emergency. Care provided must be within the expertise of the individual.

Interrogatory: A process of discovering the facts regarding a case through a set of written questions exchanged through the attorneys representing the parties involved in the case.

Malpractice: Improper performance of professional duties; a failure to meet the standards of care that resulted in harm to another person.

Negligence: Failure to act as an ordinary prudent person (nurse); a person is harmed as a result of the failure to act.

Proximate Cause: A legal concept referring to the cause and effect; an injury would not have occurred but for a specific cause.

Reasonable Care: The level of care or skill that is customarily used by a competent healthcare worker of similar education and experience in caring for an individual in the community in which the person is practicing.

one for the state in which you practice. Even if you are licensed in another state, but not currently practicing there, you must practice in accord with the rules of the state where you are working. Because these acts are different from state to state, you must always investigate the practice act for the state in which you are planning to work. You can obtain copies of a state practice act from the board of nursing or licensing agency for nurses in that state (See Appendix A for addresses of State Boards of Nursing). You must be licensed in each state in which you work.

Some practice acts regulate practice by controlling who may use the titles registered nurse (RN) and licensed practical nurse (LPN)/licensed vocational nurse (LVN). Others regulate by controlling the scope of practice and determining the specific activities for each level of nursing, that is, who can perform what functions. Most state nurse practice acts include the following information:

◆ Describes how to obtain licensure and enter practice within that state.

◆ Defines the educational requirements for entry into practice.

◆ Definitions of and scope of practice for each level of nursing practice.

◆ The process by which individual members of the board of nursing are selected and the categories of membership.

◆ Identify situations that are grounds for discipline, i.e., circumstances in which a nursing license can be revoked or suspended.

◆ The appeal steps if the nurse feels the disciplinary actions taken by the board of nursing are not fair or valid.

Some practice acts are very specific and detailed, others simply grant the board authority to declare the rules and regulations (administrative law), and to establish the details. In order to understand the scope of practice within a specific state in which you are practicing or you wish to practice, you must obtain a copy of the rules and regulations the board or administrative agency has established in that state.

▼

WHAT ARE THE DUTIES OF THE BOARD OF NURSING?

Licensure
Scope of practice
Approve education programs
Discipline licensed nurses

▲

Boards of Nursing

Each state sets up a board of nursing, sometimes called a board of examiners, to enforce the provisions of the nurse practice act for that state. Sometimes these boards control all levels or scopes of nursing practice within the state and sometimes there is a different agency for each level, i.e., RN, LPN/LVN. These agencies also belong to the National Council of State Boards of Nursing, Inc., so some decisions and directions for the profession can be made with input from the whole nation instead of each state acting as an island. This is helpful, as nurses are a very mobile group and it is important that they be able to travel from state to state without losing the ability to practice their profession.

The boards of nursing make and enforce the rules for practice in their individual states. Some function more in an advisory capacity to some other agency that has the authority to enforce the law, however, some boards of nursing function autonomously. The most common powers and duties of the board of nursing include the following:

1. Examination and licensure of new candidates.
2. Responsible for the definition of scope of practice.
3. Approval of nursing education within the state.
4. Discipline of nurses for infraction of the board's rules or the nurse practice act.

Types of discipline are usually at several levels depending on the severity of the problem. The board of nursing has the authority to censure, suspend, revoke, or deny licensure. Each of the nursing boards has the authority to determine if the disciplinary measures are temporary or permanent. Some measures may have conditions of behavior attached. A new trend in discipline is for the boards of nursing to require treatment of impaired nurses. For example, an impaired nurse may be required to participate in a specific rehabilitation program, or a nurse who has had his or her license suspended for providing unsafe care may be required to take and pass a refresher course. If the stipulated behaviors and conditions of the disciplinary measures are met then the nurse will be allowed to have the suspension removed.

Most of the boards of nursing are composed of members of the professions they control. Some states also have consumers included on their boards. Members become part of the nursing board as a result of an appointment by some governmental person or group. Specific governmental groups or individuals (i.e., governor) are given authority to make these appointments by the practice act of that specific state. Political affiliation and activities may be considered in making the appointments.

Licensure

Receiving a license to practice nursing is a privilege, not a right. Even the successful completion of an educational program in nursing does not give you

TABLE 14–3 *Protect Your License*

◆ Do not let anyone else borrow it.
◆ Do not let anyone copy it unless you write "copy" across it. In some states it is illegal to copy your license.
◆ If you lose it, report it immediately and take the necessary steps to obtain a duplicate.
◆ Be sure that the board of nursing knows whenever you change your address, whether you move across the street or across the nation.
◆ Practice nursing according to the scope and standards of practice in your state.
◆ Know your state law so you will not do anything that could cause you to be disciplined by the removal of your license.

the right to have a license. A license is granted by a state after a candidate has successfully met the requirements in that particular state. Examples of these requirements include high school education, successful completion of a nursing education program, application to the appropriate national and state agencies, fee payment, not being a felon (having criminal record), and passing the national examination for the appropriate level of licensure (NCLEX-RN or PN). Since the license is only supposed to guarantee the public safety, the level of expertise necessary to pass the test is the minimum level needed to provide safe care.

Because you have gone to a great deal of expense and work to obtain this license you should guard it carefully (Table 14–3).

MALPRACTICE

What About Malpractice?

Another area of legal concern is malpractice. *Malpractice* can be defined as behavior by a professional nurse that fails to meet the standard of acceptable care, or misconduct by a professional in the performance of professional duties. Although you will be a professional nurse as soon as you receive your license, not everything you do from then on relates to performance as a professional. For example, when you are shopping, or driving, or doing any of many other activities, it is possible for you to be guilty of negligence by being careless and causing injury; but that is not malpractice. In order for you to be accused of malpractice, you must have been acting in a professional role as a nurse.

Malpractice cases have four basic components that must be proved by the *plaintiff*, the person who files the law suit. The *defendent* is the person who is being accused and must defend himself against the charges made. These elements include:

◆ A duty owed to the plaintiff by the defendant.
◆ A breach of that duty by the defendant.
◆ Harm caused to the plaintiff (damages).
◆ A cause and effect relationship between the breach and the harm caused.

Failure on the part of the plaintiff to prove any one of these elements may result in dismissal of the case. In most situations a nurse owes a duty to clients to whom he or she has been assigned. A breach of duty may be either doing something the nurse should not have done (commission) or not doing something the nurse should have done (omission). Each is equally significant. Not challenging an incorrect order is just as serious as giving the wrong drug to a client.

▼

WHAT ARE THE ELEMENTS OF A MALPRACTICE CASE?

Own a duty
Breach a duty
Damage
Cause and effect

▲

There are also additional or surrounding circumstances that will be considered during a case. These include the difficulty of the nursing function involved, the foreseeability that harm would occur from incorrectly performing the procedure or function, the nurse's known or presumed skill in performing the function, and the urgency of the situation. It is important to remember that nurses are presumed to be safely skilled in all ordinary nursing functions. In order to prove that all of the elements or components necessary for a case are present, the plaintiff must establish the standard of care. The most common way to establish the standard of care is to consult an expert witness to review the case. The expert would then be available to testify regarding the standard of care applicable for that specific case.

What Is Expert Testimony?

Expert testimony is the written or verbal evidence given by a qualified expert in an area. Nurses are the best experts on what is appropriate nursing care. In order to be qualified, the nurse's education and experience are presented to the court to prove that he or she is knowledgeable about current standards and practice. These are the standards that a reasonably prudent nurse would follow in order to provide safe nursing care.

What Are Standards of Practice?

Standards of practice are the boundaries by which the knowledge and skill levels of a professional nurse are determined. The most common rule is the *reasonable person rule*. This rule is based on the assumption that a nurse is expected to use a reasonable level of skill, knowledge, and care that is possessed by other nurses of similar education and background. There have been many cases that have tried to identify the specific standards, but in reality the best way to identify them is to look at the resources most often used to prove whether the standards have been adhered to or not.

What Are the Sources of Proof of Standard of Care?

When the standard of care must be proved in a court of law, certain resources are frequently used. The first is an expert witness. This individual should be a member of the profession in question who is qualified to identify what a reasonable member of the profession would do under circumstances like th question. Another resource is documentary evidence. Examples of this ir textbooks, journal articles, professional treatises, and standards publishe national organizations such as American Nurses Association. Statutes and ministrative rules and regulations, as well as agency (hospital) policies a regulations, may be used. It is very important for each nurse to be aware of tl policies and procedures of their respective agency or hospital.

What Are Defenses to Malpractice Claims?

Common defenses to malpractice claims include demonstrating that one of the essential elements is not present or did not occur. One way to provide this defense is to prove that the nurse acted reasonably under the circumstances. The second common area of defense is to prove that the client assumed the risk of harm or that the client contributed to the harm by his actions. *Assumption of the risk* means that the client willingly and knowingly agreed to the action that caused harm. An example would be a mentally competent client who has been told that failure to take insulin will cause a serious reaction but refuses to take the insulin anyway. That client cannot sue the nurse for not giving the insulin since the client had the knowledge to understand the risk and the right to refuse the insulin. *Contributory negligence* means that the client, through his own actions, contributed to or was partially responsible for the damage that occurred. This does not release the nurse from being held responsible for negligent care, it simply means that because the client's behavior caused an unreasonable risk of harm, the nurse defendant should not be held totally responsible. In some states, using a *comparative negligence* theory, the courts may try to decide how much o the harm was caused by the client's action and how much by the nurse's actior The client can then recover only the amount based on the nurse's error.

▼

LEGAL DEFENSES

Elements not proven
Assumption of risk
Contributory negligence
Statute of limitations

▲

Another defense is the *statute of limitations*. Each state has its owr of limitations. These statutes define the length of time following the ever which the plaintiff may file the lawsuit. After this specific time has pa plaintiff loses the right to bring suit for the event. Some circumstances the passage of time on a statute of limitations, including the compete client and the age of the client. In most situations the time frame for of limitations does not pass for children until they reach the age of their state. In considering incompetent clients, the statute of limitations may never run out. However, if a lawsuit has been brought on behalf of such clients, the issue will be resolved and cannot be brought up again. You should know what this statute of limitations is in your state.

What Things Are Nurses Most Often Sued For?

Some areas in nursing practice seem to be involved in more lawsuits than others. One of these areas is client *falls*. This may include falls out of bed, falls on something spilled on the floor, or falls because a nurse has not provided adequate supervision for the client.

Another common problem area is *drug administration*. The most common errors include failure to administer the right drug to the right client, in the right amount, by the right route, at the right time; failure to recognize side effects or contraindications; or failure to know client allergies.

Newer areas of concern are *failure to obtain needed medical assistance* for a client whose condition is changing and *failure to challenge an inappropriate order*. These areas are uncomfortable for many experienced nurses as well as for the new graduate because they often involve challenging a physician about care or lack of care. They require that the nurse have current and accurate information. They also require the nurse to use assertiveness techniques well. It is not enough to identify problems. The nurse must identify the problems, and contact the physician and/or other resources to get appropriate care. Let's look at an example:

Mrs. Hayes, sixty-seven, with chronic obstructive pulmonary disease, is having increasingly difficult respirations, increased cyanosis, and increased anxiety. She tells you she just can't breathe. You have done all the measures for which you currently have orders, without her getting relief. It is 2 AM. You call the physician. She orders Valium 10 mg IM now. Even as a new graduate you know that Valium is contraindicated by the respiratory status. You call your supervisor, who tells you that Dr. Jones is a good physician and must know what she is doing. You do not go ahead and give the medication. You must try the physician again. If that is not successful you must go over the supervisor's head. You may not simply not give the medication without notifying your chain of command. You must continue to try to get effective help for the client.

The nurse also has a responsibility to evaluate the quality of nursing care given. If nursing care is below standard or another nurse is functioning under the influence of an inappropriate substance, such as alcohol or drugs, you must protect the client from the impaired nurse and report your concerns to the supervisor. In some states this responsibility has been added to the state law or rules and regulations making failure to report an offense an area of discipline by the board of nursing.

Floating is a problem that can put even the most experienced nurse at an increased risk. According to the Joint Commission on Accreditation of Health Organizations (JCAHO) Standards for Nursing Care 2.3.3, "If a nursing staff member is assigned to more than one type of nursing unit or patient, the staff member is competent to provide nursing care to patients in each unit and/or to each type of patient." Another standard that protects the nurse who is required to "float" to another unit is JCAHO Standard NC. 2.3.3.1, which states, "Adequate and timely orientation and cross-training are provided as needed." (JCAHO, 1990) When asked to float to another area of patient care where the nurse does not feel qualified to provide safe care, the nurse should tactfully and objectively state why he or she feels unable to deliver safe patient care in that area.

Good documentation is one of the best definitive actions a nurse can take. By recording the care administered, the client's response, and the overall status of the client's condition, the nurse can demonstrate that the standard of care was met. There is more on documentation in the section of this chapter on how to decrease risk factors for both the nurse and the client. Check Tables 14–4 and 14–5 for more defensive behaviors that will help protect you from making the errors that commonly result in lawsuits.

TORTS

Torts are *civil* (not criminal) wrongs that are done to clients. When a criminal act has occurred, the court seeks to punish the person responsible. In civil cases or tort actions, the person who is filing the suit seeks compensation for damages he feels he suffered as a result of the action or activity in question. This section will discuss some of the most common torts or civil actions.

What Is Assault and Battery?

Consent to treatment issues have provided many cases. Consent cases are usually based on the legal principle of *assault and battery*. The legal issue involved is whether the client agreed to the touching that occurred. Consent forms are required whenever an invasive procedure will be done. Remember that it is ultimately the responsibility of the physician to do the basic explanation of the procedure, its risks, and alternatives. This responsibility is considered a duty that cannot be delegated by the physician. The nurse witnesses the signature, and validates and documents the client's understanding. Documentation of the client's level of understanding or the client's refusal to receive information necessary to ensure an informed consent is critical. This action is considered nec-

TABLE 14-4   *Guidelines for Defensive Charting*

◆ All entries should be accurate.

◆ Make corrections appropriately and according to agency or hospital policies. Do not obliterate any information that is in the chart.

◆ If there is information that should have been charted and was not, then the nurse should make a "late entry" noting the time the charting actually occurred and the specific time the charting reflects. Example: 10/13/92, 10:00 late entry, charting to reflect 10/13/92 . . . .

◆ All identified client problems, nursing actions taken, and the client responses should be noted. Do not describe a client problem and leave it without including the nursing actions taken and the client response.

◆ Be as objective as possible in charting. Rather than charting "the client tolerated the procedure well," chart the specific parameters checked to determine that conclusion. Example: "ambulated, tolerated well" would be more effective if charted "ambulated complete length of hall, no shortness of breath noted, pulse rate at 98, respirations at 22."

◆ Each page of the chart should contain the current date and time. Frequently chart forms are stamped ahead of time. Each time you enter information on a new page, make sure it reflects the current time of charting.

◆ Follow through with who saw the client, and what measures were initiated. Particularly note when the doctor visited; if you had to call a doctor for a problem, what was the doctor's response, the nursing actions, and the client response. This is especially important if you had to make several calls to the doctor.

◆ Make sure your notes are legible and clearly reflect the information you intended. It is a good idea to read over your nurse's notes from the previous day to see if they still make sense, and accurately portray the status of the patient. If the notes do not make sense to you the next day, imagine how difficult it would be to decipher the information at a later date.

essary to ensure client safety, and is included in entry-level examinations for LPNs and LVNs as well as RNs. Activity number 30, in the Job Analysis of Newly Licensed Registered Nurses is "Verify that the client or family has information needed for informed consent" (Yocum, 1989). A client decision is usually considered to be informed when she or he understands the basics of the procedure, the important risks involved, the alternatives to it and what is likely to happen if the procedure is refused.

▼

WHAT ARE THE ELEMENTS OF INFORMED CONSENT?

The client must know:
1. **The procedure**
2. **The risks**
3. **Alternatives**

▲

TABLE 14–5   *Tips for Being at Your Best*

◆ Be very careful if you have been interrupted during a task. This is very common in nursing. But many accidents happen because the nurse did not remember what he or she had been doing or where he or she was in a task.

◆ If you are fatigued you are more likely to make mistakes. Follow all the steps thoroughly when you are tired. This is one of the reasons that double shifts may not be wise.

◆ Listen to your clients. Often they will tell you if what you are planning to do is different or unusual. Being able to take the time to do a second check may save you and your client trouble.

◆ Never do a procedure you do not know how to do at the appropriate standard of performance. It is better to be embarrassed by admitting you need help or supervision than to risk hurting someone.

◆ Never be afraid to admit you made a mistake. Corrective action may stop or at least reduce harm.

◆ Keep current and up to date in your practice knowledge base. An article in a professional journal may keep the lawsuit away.

◆ Do not rush when you are extra busy. Set priorities on what *must* be done and do it carefully.

If the nurse finds that the client does not have adequate information to meet this criteria he or she should not let the client sign the form and should notify the physician immediately. Consent is not informed if the client is under the influence of mind-altering medications, such as preoperative medications. Since most preoperative medications contain a narcotic, the consent form must be signed prior to the administration of the medication. The consent form is invalid if it is signed after the procedure has already occurred. Informed consent is not required if the procedure is necessary to save a life and is done in an emergency.

What Is Meant By Confidentiality?

Many states have physician-client *privilege* laws, which protect communications between care givers and client. Many states extend physician-client privilege to nurses and sometimes to other healthcare givers as well. Even where there are no specific statutes to provide the privilege, there is a legal presumption that clients should be able to give information to healthcare givers so they can receive proper care, without concern that this information will be shared with others. This privilege belongs to the client, not the healthcare giver, which means that only the client can decide to give it up. The privilege is usually extended to the medical record and any information it contains. As a professional, it is important to observe confidentiality when

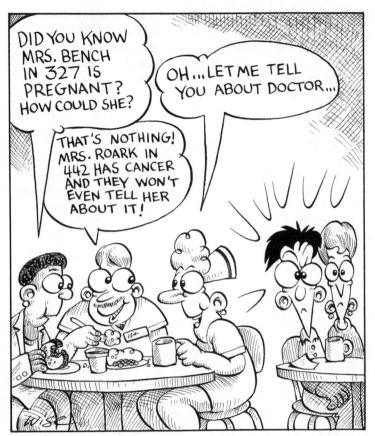

FIGURE 14–1   *Maintaining confidentiality is both an ethical and a legal consideration in nursing.*

talking about clients at home and at work. You must be very careful to keep information about the client or from the client to yourself and to share it only with healthcare workers who must know the information to plan or give proper care (Fig. 14–1).

There are a few exceptions to this. Disclosure to protect public health is usually required, but it is rarely the nurse who is required to do the disclosure. There may be specific statutes that require disclosure. Child, elderly, or spouse abuse, gunshot wounds or violent injury, contagious diseases, ongoing criminal activity, and occupational injuries are examples. Since each state is different it is important to know the laws on this matter in your own state. You also need to know whose responsibility it is to do the reporting and to whom the reporting should be done.

What Is Invasion of Privacy?

A similar cause of action is for *invasion of privacy*. This cause of action can be used in several ways, like photographing a procedure and showing it without the client's consent, going through a client's belongings without consent, or talking about a client's private life publicly. The most important and frequently violated area of this client right is failure to treat the client with respect by preventing unnecessary exposure of the body and by limiting the number of individuals to whom the client is exposed. Even minor infractions of this legal responsibility can have major consequences. It is easy to forget that nurses have an ethical as well as legal responsibility in this area, as our culture holds the right of privacy in high regard. As you become even more accustomed to dealing with clients, it can be harder to remember that what you consider commonplace and normal may seem extremely difficult and demeaning for the client.

What Is Defamation?

Defamation refers to causing damage to someone else's reputation. If the means of transmitting the damaging information is written, it is called *libel*; if it is oral or spoken, it is called *slander*. The damaging information must be communicated to a *third* person. Action cannot be taken if the information in question was said to the individual about whom the nurse is making the statement. The actions likely to result in a defamation charge are giving out inaccurate or inappropriate information from the medical record or speaking negatively about your co-workers (supervisors, doctors, other nurses).

The defenses to defamation accusations are truth and privilege. If the statement is true it is not actionable under this doctrine. If it is privileged as discussed above, and appropriately shared within the scope of that privilege, no action can be taken under defamation. This does not mean it may not be actionable under another doctrine, such as invasion of privacy. As a general rule you should avoid sharing private information or gossiping about your clients or your coworkers.

What Is False Imprisonment?

The final area of concern in this section is *false imprisonment*. False imprisonment means that you make someone wrongfully feel that she or he cannot leave a place. The use of physical restraints or threatening physical or emotional harm without legal justification constitutes false imprisonment. The most common example of this tort is telling a client that she or he may not leave the hospital until the bill is paid. Another example is using restraints or threatening to use them on competent clients to make them do what you want them to do against their wishes. There are many restrictions on the appropriate use of restraints, both hard and soft. You must be aware of policy in your agency as well as state restrictions.

RISK MANAGEMENT

How Do I Protect Myself and My Client From All These Risks?

Risk management refers to the process of reducing or financing the cost of predictable losses. The term was originally used in the insurance industry and is now applied to healthcare as well. It can be used formally at the institutional level as well as informally at your personal level. Risk management includes identification, evaluation, and treatment of possible risk situations to reduce the chance of loss.

At the institutional level this may include an employee whose job is to review all the problems that occur in the institution to try to identify the most common features and eliminate them. One of the tools often used for this is the *incident report*. When you make or identify an error, you are usually required to make out an incident report so the event can be studied and hopefully prevented from occurring again. This means that you must fill out the report as honestly and completely as possible. For the institution it means that incident reports should never be used to punish the nurse or as a basis for determining firing or pay raises. To use the incident report in this manner increases the risk of dishonesty in filling out the form and in identifying situations where the form should be completed. Most authorities agree that you do not mention the completion of an incident report in the medical record. You *do* document the event in objective language if it is appropriate to do so.

The risk manager reviews the incident reports to obtain an overall picture of problems within the agency and to identify methods for reducing these risks. The most common method used to reduce risk is providing inservice teaching sessions for staff. Sometimes policies or procedures need to be changed to provide safer care. Agencies also carry insurance to protect against claims that have not been prevented.

Individually, you can also do your own risk management:

◆ Identify situations hardest for you to cope with safely.
◆ Set goals to help manage these problems.
◆ Use behavior tips.
◆ Get personal malpractice insurance!

What Else Can I Do to Protect Myself and the Client?

There are several things you can do to cut down the risk of a successful lawsuit. One is *documentation*. Your care and the client's condition should be carefully and thoroughly documented (Fig. 14–2). Do not do your charting ahead. Keep

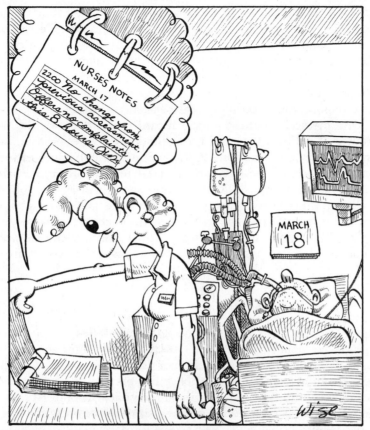

FIGURE 14–2 *It is critical that the nurse's notes reflect the current condition of the patient.*

notes for yourself when you are too busy to do it at the time events occur. Understand the principles involved in the type of charting your agency uses and use it correctly. Never falsify your charting. If you have not done something either do it now or do not chart it as done! Be clear, accurate, and complete. Use the client's own words whenever possible. Do not put in your opinions about the client or his care unless you are using problem-oriented record charting and are in the assessment statement. Date and time every entry, including day, month, and year. Do not pre- or postdate entries. If someone has put a note in that causes your note to be out of order, identify the cause and sequence your note correctly. If you have forgotten something in your notes, add it when you remember it, but note that you had forgotten to add it at the correct time and label it a "late entry." Never delete something that you have accurately charted because someone else does not like what you said. Do not fight with other healthcare workers in the chart by making statements about the quality of their care. Never recopy someone else's notes. If you make an error, put a single line through it and write "error" and your initials. Do not use correction fluid to make corrections. Write legibly and sign your name correctly. After a lawsuit has been filed, do not ever add or delete something to make yourself or someone else look better. Courts and attorneys are not stupid and doing the wrong things will be making the opposition's case easier.

The medical record is a legal record that stands for the truth of what is written in it without the need for testimony to corroborate it. What is omitted from it is considered undone. Other important behaviors include *knowing and following the policies and procedures* of your institution, and *thinking* before you speak or do anything. A little common sense will help a lot. Before you say something, think how you would feel if it were said about you. Consider what is truly safest for the client, not what will necessarily make you or the client happiest. It is important to carry your own malpractice insurance! Remember, the clients have the right to file a lawsuit whether your care was negligent or not.

How Do I Know What Type of Malpractice Insurance I Need?

Malpractice insurance usually comes in two varieties, the *claims made* policy and the *occurrence* policy. In the claims made policy the nurse is covered only if the suit or claims are filed during the period actually covered by the policy. This covers the time from when the policy begins until the policy ends. If the claim is not filed during this period of time, the policy will not pay. In the occurrence policy the nurse is covered if a suit or claim arises during the term of the policy. The occurrence policy will cover claims for damages that may be filed after the policy terminates. As you can see, the occurrence policy is more useful because you do not have to continue to carry it if you are not working. Read the policy carefully: does the policy cover you unequivocally or is there a "reservation of right," which means the insurance company may decide not to cover the incident in question.

Many nurses think that they do not need to carry their own insurance because their agency or hospital carries insurance that covers them. It is true that the agency carries insurance but it covers the nurse as an employee of that agency not as an individual. This means that the insurance is basically to protect the agency, not the individual nurse. If a nurse is sued and does not have his or her own policy, the nurse will have only minimal control over how the suit is handled. The nurse's reputation is at stake and he or she will not be able to determine whether the case is settled or fought in the courts. If the nurse has his or her own policy, then she or he will have her or his own attorney to represent his or her best interests in the case. There has been a recent series of cases that have held the nurse liable to the agency for money paid by the agency or its insurer as a result of the nurse's malpractice. In these cases, nurses without insurance have been required to pay back those monies to the agency.

There are a few attorneys who feel that nurses should not carry their own policy because they are more likely to be sued if they have those resources. This is a dangerous game as the current trend is to sue anyone who may have had any contact with the event the suit is based on. The situation requires the nurses to get themselves excluded if they were not actually involved. This process costs a great deal of money. An individual insurance policy will protect against this risk.

When you get your policy, be sure to read it. There is a lot of fine print, but get out your magnifying glass and read through it anyway. It will be a real education for you as well as help you know what your protection is and under what circumstances the policy will pay.

What Happens When I Go to Court?

Sometimes in spite of all your efforts, you find yourself in court as a defendant. You may even choose to go as an expert witness. There are some things about how you handle yourself in the court room that will make a big difference in how effective you are there.

1. You need to look and act like a professional. That means that you must be prepared. Know the case; review the record ahead of time.

2. Be clear, accurate, and concise. If you do not know an answer, say so, do not guess.

3. Never give opinions unless asked for them. Stick to the facts!

4. Speak slowly and in a well-modulated tone of voice. Do not allow yourself to be rattled by the opposing attorney.

5. If you do not remember a question or do not understand it, ask for it to be repeated or clarified. Many attorneys use long, many-part questions to confuse you. Do not get caught in this trap.

6. If you have stated an opinion, stick to it. Do not get confused by other questions or comments. Do not over-react to statements by other witnesses. Be cool, calm, and collected!

7. Do not allow yourself to be goaded into angry or disdainful responses. Speak to the judge, jury, or your questioner. Do not look around the room blindly or at someone in the audience.

8. Avoid the use of "always" and "never" and vague comments like "maybe," "I think" or "possibly."

9. Do not answer more than is asked for by the question. In other words, don't discuss other events that were occurring on the unit at the same time as the incident in question. If you feel other circumstances have a bearing on your case, tell your attorney so the information can be used for your defense.

The nurse will meet with the attorney that represents him or her before going to a deposition or into court. Many attorneys will role-play situations with you ahead of time so you will not be surprised by how cross-examination is conducted by the opposing attorney.

Under many circumstances, going to court is a frightening and unpleasant event. If you choose to go as an expert witness, try to talk to someone who has already served in that role so you will have some idea what to expect. Your effectiveness in this role may play a significant part in the outcome of the case. Do not accept the role unless you feel sure that you can provide the necessary information and you are comfortable with the standards of nursing care required in the situation in the hypothetical question.

What Is an 'Impaired Nurse'?

Impaired nurses are nurses who are unable to function effectively because of some type of substance abuse. More attention is currently being given to this area because of the heightened awareness in our society as a whole as well as the increasing recognition of the severity of the problem in healthcare workers. High stress and easy access seem to contribute to the problem. Boards of nursing are increasingly concerned about this issue as it has significant impact on rendering safe client care. Because of the impact on safe patient care, some states will discipline the nurse who fails to report a nurse who works in an impaired condition as well as the impaired nurse. Many states have programs set up to allow nurses to meet specific behavior criteria, such as blood or urine testing, ordered evaluations, and attendance at rehabilitation programs, while disciplinary action is being taken. The primary concern is to assist the impaired nurse back to full and appropriate nursing practice. State boards often work closely with national and state organizations such as the American Nurses Association to develop effective programs for dealing with this problem. It is always best for a nurse who has developed an impaired status to voluntarily take steps to ensure client safety and get rehabilitative assistance. If this must be done through the state boards, the discipline will remain on the nurse's record for the rest of his or her career. The nurse should have legal assistance or advice when dealing with the state board in disciplinary hearings or actions.

CONTROVERSIAL LEGAL ISSUES AFFECTING NURSING

Because developments and advances in medical and nursing care occur constantly, there are many areas of practice that do not have firm rules to follow when making decisions. Changes in healthcare delivery have sparked controversy about a variety of issues.

Third-Party Reimbursement

One example is *third-party reimbursement*, the right of an individual nurse, usually a nurse practitioner, to be paid directly by insurance companies for care given. Although on the surface this seems simple, there are many political and turf battles being fought over it. The growth of the field of independent practice for nurses is an important step in providing alternatives to the high cost of healthcare for many people. If such nurses cannot be paid for through third-party reimbursement, many clients will be unable to afford to use them, and this cost-effective, quality form of healthcare may not be available. Institutions and agencies need third-party reimbursement to stimulate the use of specialists within the agency, thus providing a cost-effective alternative delivery system for the agency. Sometimes other healthcare workers, whose services can be reimbursed, have been hired to do jobs nurses could have done as well or better.

Legislative changes will be necessary to alter these policies. Your support will be important when your state decides these issues. Professional behavior includes concern with and participation in the direction healthcare will take in the future.

Peer Review

Another recent new direction is *peer review*. This is often referred to as *quality assurance*. It means that you, as a professional nurse, will be involved in evaluating the care that you and other nurses provide. This can be done by various activities. Some examples of quality assurance include:

1. A nursing audit or evaluation of what nurses do for clients.
2. Policy and procedure development.
3. Staff preparation and skill documentation.
4. Continuing education and certification.
5. Employee evaluation.
6. On-going monitoring such as infection control and risk management systems.

Accreditation of hospitals now requires that the activities chosen for peer review be documented and demonstrated within the agency (JCAHO, 1990). This is a very positive development in nursing as it ensures that practice will be scrutinized and evaluated and that guidelines for nursing care delivery will be available.

Right to Life/Death

Biomedical advances have also brought controversy to nursing practice. Reading the newspaper or watching television will demonstrate the current legal concerns. When can a person decide to die? When can the machines be turned off? How much care must be given? Although the right of a client to refuse treatment has been well established, there seem to be some times when that right may not exist. When refusal of treatment means death, some special rules may apply. For pregnant clients, the right may not include refusal of treatment if death of the fetus will occur (Raleigh Fitkin-Paul Morgan Memorial Hospital v. Anderson, 42 N.J. 421, 201A, 2nd 5 37 (1964)). Cases continue to be decided both ways on the right to death issue. Cruzan v. Director, Missouri Department of Health, 110 S. Ct. 2841 (1990), a landmark case decided by the United States Supreme Court, said that if a person had expressed the wish not to live as a vegetable, mechanical assistance could be withdrawn. Medical science cannot even agree on one acceptable definition of death. Definitions range from the Harvard Definition of absence of awareness of external stimuli, no movements or spontaneous breathing, no reflexes, and a nearly flat brain wave repeated twice in 24 hours, to the Uniform Definition of Brain Death (Uniform Laws Annual, 1981), which requires irreversible cessation of all functioning of the brain.

Living Will and Durable Power of Attorney

In response to the confusion in cases about the right to die, the use of the *living will* and the *durable power of attorney* have been developed. Many states now have statutes or common law cases that establish whether these legal tools will be accepted and how they must be worded and timed. The living will is used to allow a competent, adult individual to state that he does not want any unusual medical procedures or life-saving equipment used to prolong life. He may also include instructions for decisions to remove such equipment once it is in place. Often used in conjunction with the living will is the durable power of attorney. This allows the competent adult to appoint a specific person to authorize care after incompetence of that individual occurs. Unlike most powers of attorney, which only allow someone else to do what you could do yourself, the durable power of attorney does not become effective until the disabled person cannot make decisions for himself/herself. This also allows the designated person to enforce the terms of a living will, which in many states is still advisory and can be ignored by choosing the care that would result in the same outcome as a living will might have. Your responsibility as a nurse is to know of the existence of such legal forms and the agency policy concerning them, to put copies on the chart, and to assist with appropriate care based on the patient's wishes. The nurse is not always involved in decisions about when and how to enforce the terms of these tools, but should be prepared to assist in these decisions. If a nurse becomes aware of family or patient conflict concerning them he or she will need to bring this to the attention of the physician, and assist in a resolution, if possible.

There are other areas of concerns, such as reproductive healthcare, organ donation, transplantation of foreign devices such as the Jarvik heart, and genetic engineering, and, as time goes on, new areas will arise that nursing will have to address. Continuing education, critical thinking, and an open mind will help you to learn about and deal with the conflicts inherent in this field. Take the opportunity to visit the hearings conducted by the board of nursing in your state. By becoming involved with the legal and disciplinary process you will be much more aware of how you can protect yourself and your patients.

REFERENCES

Bernzweig, E.P. (1987): *The Nurse's Liability for Malpractice,* 4th ed. New York, McGraw-Hill.

Creighton, H. (1986): *Law Every Nurse Should Know,* 5th ed. Philadelphia, W.B. Saunders.

Hogue, E. *Nursing Case Law Reporter: Cases and Commentary,* National Law Publishing.

Joint Commission on Accreditation of Health Organizations (1990): *Nursing Care Scoring Guidelines. 1991 Standards.* Oakbrook, IL.

Northrop, C., Kelly. M., (1987): *Legal Issues in Nursing,* St. Louis, C.V. Mosby.

Pence, G.E. (1990): *Classic Cases in Medical Ethics.* New York, McGraw-Hill.

Yocom, C.J. (1989): *Job Analysis for Newly Licensed Registered Nurses.*

IN SEARCH OF EMPLOYMENT: FINDING YOUR NICHE IN THE WORK WORLD

15

Employment Considerations: Opportunities and Resumes

Kathleen M. Speer, P.N.P., Ph.D., R.N.

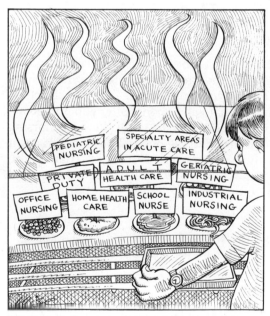

There is a smorgasbord of opportunities in nursing. You can always go back and make another selection.

The world is all gates, all opportunities.
                                        —Ralph Waldo Emerson

There are two things to aim at in life:
first, to get what you want;
and, after that, to enjoy it.
Only the wisest of mankind achieve the second.
                                        —Logan Pearsall Smith

After completing this chapter, you should be able to:

◆ Assess trends in the job market.

◆ Describe the various settings in which a nurse is employed.

◆ Describe the important parts of the resume.

◆ Review all aspects of obtaining employment.

According to Barbara Redman PhD, RN, FAAN, executive director of the American Nurses Association, "The demand for nurses has been outstripping the supply for some time and will continue to do so for the forseeable future." She goes on further to state, "Nursing remains a growth field as well as an exciting and demanding profession" (Birk, 1992). Resources on job hunting and trends in employment support Redman's optimistic view. However, in some geographic locations, especially in metropolitan areas with large numbers of nursing graduates, the job opportunities for the graduate nurse are declining. More people are entering nursing and fewer people are leaving because of the profession's stability and flexibility. It is important to take geographic location into consideration as you are planning your job search. Resources are available each year in the career directories of many of the national journals. Be sure to refer to them for a current assessment of the job market.

Seeking Employment

How to Find the Job That's Right for You

As your schooling nears completion, it's time to focus on your interests and set your sights on your first job. It will be important for you to prioritize those options that are significant and to determine your specific career goal or objective. It is important to take time to select the job that will not only offer you immediate satisfaction, but will also give you the opportunity to grow. Because nursing offers so many options, it is exciting to think of all the possibilities that can occur along your career path. So, the first thing to do is to "think big." That's right, let yourself dream. Envision yourself moving in any direction in a career that fascinates you with possibilities that you can hardly imagine to exist.

I am walking in the door of the corporate office of the UCLA's Medical Center. I feel a sense of energy and vitality as I see my name on the door— Vice President of Nursing Operations.

Does this sound far-fetched to you? It's up to you to select the type of nursing you like to do and what you are best suited for. The first key to making the right career decision is self-understanding. Through self-understanding, you can determine who you are and what you like, and that will assist you in setting an appropriate career goal that will increase your negotiating power by focusing your job search. Also, it will provide criteria with which you can weigh job offers and options. (Chapter 16, on interviewing, discusses self-assessment strategies in detail.)

Why Set a Career Goal?

The answer to this question is simple. Each time you succeed in meeting a career goal, you increase your self-confidence and self-esteem. A career goal defines who or what you wish to be professionally. In addition, it will help tie together the elements of your job search—the resume writing, researching, contacting employers, and the interviewing process—by giving you a direction.

Just remember, knowing what you want is the key to researching jobs, comparing offers, and choosing a satisfying career position. So don't rush through this process. Forming your career goals and objectives is essential to landing that first job.

What Employment Opportunities Are Available?

There are a number of areas in which a nurse may be employed. The largest employers are hospitals or acute care facilities. In hospitals there are a wide variety of positions, although often new graduates are placed in staff nurse positions. If it is a general hospital, you need to first choose what areas interest you most. Table 15–1 lists some of the hospital areas from which you might select.

Possible opportunities for nurses in the hospital may include staff, charge positions, management, and advanced clinical practice. In many hospitals staff positions may be made up of different levels, especially if the hospital participates in clinical or career ladders. Charge positions may involve responsibility for a particular staff or a particular day or it may involve managing staff for an entire unit. There are a variety of opportunities for nurses in management as their experience level increases. Management positions may include head nurse, di-

TABLE 15–1 *Hospital Areas*

Pediatrics	Cardiology
Oncology	Intensive Care
Medical	Surgical
Rehabilitation	Neurological
Orthopedic	Neonatal
Maternal/Child	Women's Healthcare
Emergency	Operating Room
Dialysis	Psychiatric
Geriatrics	Outpatient
Nutrition Services	Infection Control
Urology	Transport
Intravenous Therapy	Burns

rector, or assistant over several units. The term "director of nursing" is becoming a title of the past. Many institutions now refer to the person charged with the management of all of nursing as vice-president. It will depend on the organizational structure of the institution as to job titles.

Advanced nurse practitioner (ANP) is a broad title that may encompass many specialties. These specialties may include clinical nurse specialists, practitioner, nurse anesthetists, and educators. These nurses practice in an expanded role in nursing. The ANP may have a master's or doctoral degree. ANPs function differently in each state depending on the nurse practice act for that respective state.

Clinical nurse specialists usually specialize in a particular specialty area, often even a subspecialty of that specialty area. Examples of this might be a pediatric clinical nurse specialist with a focus on nutrition or cardiovascular surgery. Clinical nurse specialists are the clinical experts for that area. The clinical nurse specialist may also oversee education for staff, research, and provide consultation. To use the title clinical nurse specialist the nurse must have a master's degree in nursing and be qualified to take the certification exam in that particular clinical area.

Nurse practitioners may be used in both hospital and community health settings. The primary focus of nurse practitioners is health promotion and maintenance. Their functions may include assessments, treatment of acute minor illnesses, and health maintenance. The nurse practitioner also provides continuity of care for patients. Nurse practitioners function either independently or interdependently with other healthcare providers. Often a nurse practitioner may be in practice with a physician. As of 1992 in order to be able to take a certification exam all nurse practitioners must have graduated from a master's program in nursing. Another issue that has affected nurse practitioners in the past few years has been the use of malpractice insurance. Malpractice insurance rates have risen and it has been difficult to find insurance companies to provide coverage. (See Chapter 14 for more information regarding malpractice insurance.)

Nurse anesthetists work in the operating room or day surgery area providing anesthesia for patients. Although most of these patients do not require complicated care or physician's immediate attention, nurse anesthetists do work under the direction of a physician. Preparation for the position includes advanced education in nursing at a school of anesthesiology. These programs provide certification in anesthesia.

Nurse educators help to coordinate and assess the education needs of nurses in the institution. This position is especially important in states that have mandatory continuing education requirements for nurses. With areas becoming more specialized, many times new graduates do not have all the education needed to prepare them to function in specific areas. Nurse educators coordinate internship and orientation programs to assist in this transition.

Entry-level positions in the hospital are usually *staff nurse* positions. Working in the community, in such positions as occupational health, school health, and the military, may require a bachelor's degree in nursing (BSN) and/or at least one year of hospital nursing. Other areas that nurses may also find employment may be in community health, home health care, and nursing agencies. To assist you in choosing the right job and in planning for your future career, the following are examples of job qualification, expectations, and responsibilities for a variety of nursing positions:

Staff nurse

◆ Some areas of the country may require a BSN or may make title differences between levels of educational preparation (diploma, ADN, and BSN).

◆ Directs, organizes, and plans patient care.

◆ Emphasis on technical skills.

◆ Often rotates shifts.

Charge nurse

◆ May require a BSN.

◆ Responsible for making staff assignments, management, and monitoring staff care.

◆ May also assume direct patient care.

Nurse manager

◆ May require a master's degree or previous experience.

◆ May be directly responsible for the overall management of a unit or area.

◆ Monitors quality of care delivered.

◆ Responsible for budget and hiring/firing of staff.

House supervisor

◆ Previous experience required, usually as charge nurse or nurse manager.

◆ Provides direction and management to all the units or areas of the hospital.

◆ Frequently utilized on 3–11, 11–7, and weekend shifts.

◆ May also help to coordinate staffing and patient admissions.

Infection control nurse

◆ Monitors infectious diseases throughout the institution.

◆ Identifies trends and potential causes or sources of infection.

◆ Establishes policies for infection control on nursing care units.

Inservice education

◆ May require a master's degree and previous experience.

◆ Provides and coordinates education for staff in the institution.

◆ May be asked to do public speaking.

◆ Coordinates and plans with specialty areas for internship programs.

Director of nursing/Vice-president of nursing

◆ May require a master's degree; sometimes a doctoral degree may be required along with previous management experience.

◆ Responsible for overall management of all nursing staff and nursing care provided.

◆ May determine type of nursing care delivery system.

◆ Involved with budget, goal-setting, and determining philosophical beliefs of the institution.

◆ Has responsibility for hiring/firing of management personnel.

Military nurse

◆ Responsibilities often correspond to staff nurse, charge nurse, and nurse manager positions.

◆ May have opportunity to travel.

◆ Has excellent retirement and benefits.

◆ Often higher level of rank for BSN or higher educational level.

Nurse practitioner

◆ May require master's degree and certification as a practitioner.

◆ Responsible for primary care and health promotion.

◆ Frequently works with a physician.

◆ May conduct physical exams, teach health, treat minor acute illnesses, and write prescriptions (depending on state regulations).

Home health care

◆ Frequently required to have a year's previous experience, often in a hospital setting.

◆ Provides direct care to patients at home.

◆ Requires independent thinking and judgment.

School health nurse

◆ May require a BSN and/or practitioner certification, along with previous experience.

◆ Oversees the general health and well-being of children in a certain school or district.

◆ May provide health screening, teaching, minor acute care, and first aid.

RESUME WRITING

How Do I Write a Resume?

▼

IN DESIGNING YOUR RESUME, PLAY IT <u>SAFE</u>! THAT IS—

<u>S</u>imple,
<u>A</u>ppropriate,
<u>F</u>unctional, and
<u>E</u>conomical (Hanks and Belliston, 1976).

▲

Resumes are often your first introduction to an employer. Your resume tells your potential employers who you are, and gives you the chance to sell yourself. This is your opportunity to tell them about your strengths. Take the time to make it neat and presentable. You need to include information that is important (not frivolous or fluff), and will make them want to call you for an interview. Your resume should tell the employer (a) exactly who you are, (b) the type of job you are looking for, and (c) your qualifications. A resume is a concise factual presentation of your educational and employment history (Table 15–2).

What Is the Necessary Information for a Resume?

The following is a brief description of each suggested component of a resume. It is very important that your resume and letter be neatly typed with correct spelling and grammar.

TABLE 15–2   *Resume Guidelines*

- ◆ Always typed
- ◆ 1–1½-inch margin on all four sides
- ◆ 8½ × 11-inch paper
- ◆ White, off-white, light blue, light grey paper (no bright colors such as red or green; they are not professional)
- ◆ High-quality bond paper
- ◆ Plain lettering, no elaborate scroll
- ◆ NO errors and no correction fluid
- ◆ Neat
- ◆ Underlined, capitalized, or boldface type to highlight important categories
- ◆ One to two pages in length

Demographic Data—That's All About You As a Person

At the top of the page, put your name and address. Make sure this is an address where you will receive information quickly, especially if you are finishing school and your future address is unknown. Telephone numbers, especially during the daytime hours, are also important to include.

Career/Professional Objective—Where Do You Want to Go?

There is a wide variety of ways to address your career objective. You may wish to state the type of job that you desire (e.g., staff nurse in pediatrics, charge nurse in geriatrics). You may also write a short-term and long-term objective (e.g., staff nurse in pediatrics—short-term objective, or management position in pediatrics—long-term objective). Be specific and brief when writing career objectives. Avoid being vague or nebulous, because the employer will not know what type of position you desire.

Experience—What Do You Know How to Do?

This section can be developed in a variety of ways. It is an overview of your work history and any special talents or skills you may possess. Often it is written in chronological order, beginning with your most recent job. You need to include your job title, where you worked, and the time you were employed. You may wish to stop there or you may include actual responsibilities that you performed. You may also highlight certain skills or abilities that you feel are important to the job. Highlighting skills and abilities is especially important if you are seeking a job that will have others competing for that position. Be sure to pull out and identify all your strengths (organization, technical ability, etc.).

Education—Where Did You Go to School, High School to Present?

Again, most of you will see this section presented in chronological order. Be sure to include the following:

- Name of institution.
- Location (city, state).
- Degree—major, minor.
- Date completed.
- Certifications or specialized education.
- Date received.

Licensure—What Can You Do and Where Can You Do It?

This area is especially important for a nurse. Because of the possibility of some disreputable person obtaining your license number, the actual number many times is not included on your resume. Do include the state where you are licensed, and when you will be taking the licensure examination.

Honors and Awards—Who Gave You a Pat on the Back?

This is an optional section. If you are newly graduated or will be applying for a job that may have a number of competitors, it may be one you wish to include. This section shows that you have been recognized for special skills and/or abilities. You may include high school awards and volunteer work, if you are a new graduate. Avoid awards that are frivolous, such as "best legs" awards. You should also include any scholarships that you may have received. If you have not received any honors or awards, do not include this section on your resume.

Professional Organizations—What Do You Belong To?

You may list any organizations in which you are a member and/or have held an office. They may be professional or community groups. This is an optional section.

References—Who Knows About You?

It is usually best to put the statement "provided upon request," because this section can become too lengthy and take up valuable space. Usually you can provide references on the application form.

Look at the examples of resumes and adapt what works well for you (Figs. 15–1 and 15–2). You have probably seen many examples have other headings, but do not include these sections unless they apply. These sections may include honors, presentations, publications, and workshops attended. Some people include age, health, and marital status on resumes. This information is not usually relevant and should be omitted.

What Else Is Included With the Resume?

Along with your resume you should also enclose a cover letter that gives a brief introduction (Fig. 15–3). You can summarize the important areas in your resume, but remember to keep the letter fairly short, about one-half page. Try to find out the actual name of the person who is hiring and address your letter to this person. Letters sent to the "Nurse Recruiter" or to the "Director of Nursing" or "Vice-President of Nursing" are more likely to be tossed aside.

In your letter, state why you want to work at this particular place. Then summarize your accomplishments. End your letter by asking for an interview. Be sure you enclose how you may be reached (Table 15–3).

After a reasonable period of time, one week to ten days, call the person to whom you sent your resume and make sure that your resume was received. Also ask if there are any questions regarding your resume. Keep track of this on your record of contacts and resumes sent (Fig. 15–4).

Now that your resume is ready, and you've identified your needs and the kind of environment where you'd like to practice, you're ready to track down information on specific employers. Exactly how do you find out what you want to know?

Resume of Linda Smith

Personal Information

200 Any Place Avenue
Dallas, TX 77777
214-555-5555

Professional Objective	A staff nurse position on a pediatric unit.
Education	June, 1994 Baccalaureate Degree in Nursing University of Texas @ Arlington Arlington, Texas

Experience

9/90–Present	Pediatric Nurse Technician Children's Medical Center of Dallas Dallas, Texas
1/89–8/90	Nurse's Aide Richmond Memorial Hospital Richmond, Virginia
Licensure	NCLEX taken July 13 and 14 in Dallas, Texas
Honors	Children's Medical Center Scholarship Sigma Theta Tau Clinical Award, University of Texas @ Arlington
Professional Organizations	Texas Student Nurse Association
References	Upon Request

FIGURE 15–1 *Resume Example #1.*

Linda Smith
Anywhere Street
Dallas, TX 77777
Home—214-555-3333
Work—214-555-4444

Licensure   Will take NCLEX CAT on June 15, 1994.

Experience   Pediatric Nurse Technician
Children's Medical Center of Dallas
Dallas, Texas
9/90–Present
Responsibilities: taking vital signs, weighing patients, patient care, charting, technical procedures

Nurse's Aide
Richmond Memorial Hospital
Richmond, Virginia
1/89–8/90
Responsibilities: General patient care—vital signs, I & O, bathing

Education   Associate Degree in Nursing
El Centro College
Dallas, Texas
May, 1991

References   Provided upon request

FIGURE 15–2   *Resume Example #2.*

One of the first things you can do is *network.* Networking is contacting everyone you know and even some people you don't know to get information about their specific organization or institution. Places that you can network are at your facility during clinical, at student organization programs, at career days at colleges, and at job opportunity fairs. Keep track of all this information on your record of contacts and resumes sent so that you will have easy access to the information. It will be important to document your follow-up actions and results—don't forget to keep copies of correspondence and notes on any conversations with potential employers in a file. Remember to date all entries—

November 1, 1994

Linda Smith
101 Anywhere Street
Dallas, Texas 77777
214-555-5555

Ms. Katherine Ryland
Nurse Recruiter
Children's Medical Center of Dallas
1935 Hospital Street
Dallas, Texas 75235

Dear Ms. Ryland:

I am interested in applying for a position at your hospital. I became acquainted with your hospital when I attended the Texas Nurse's Association Job Fair. I have always wanted to work with children.

I have completed my ADN in nursing from El Centro College in Dallas. I maintained a 3.6 on a 4.0 scale, and received a clinical award my last semester.

I would like to set up an appointment sometime during the week of March 24 when I will be out for spring break. Please let me know a convenient time. My phone number is 214-555-5555.

I look forward to meeting you. Please feel free to contact me if you have any questions.

Sincerely yours,

Linda Smith

FIGURE 15–3   *Example of a Cover Letter.*

TABLE 15–3 *Reminders for Cover Letters*

◆ 8½ × 11-inch paper, white, off-white, light blue
◆ Typed with no mistakes
◆ No smudges
◆ 1½–2-inch margin on all sides
◆ Signed, usually with black ink
◆ No abbreviations
◆ Use business letter format

---

briefly put information received, interviews requested and granted, resumes sent, and job offers given. Nurse recruiters and managers are always impressed with an organized person.

Table 15–4 presents a summary of the steps to finding a job.

EMPLOYMENT CONSIDERATIONS

How Do You Decide on an Employer?

Salary, job responsibilities, and facility location are not the only important major considerations for determining an employer—don't forget to consider the total compensation package, that is, your benefits.

Often benefits are overlooked because their cost tends to be more invisible than the exciting new salary that you'll be receiving. Some organizations spend as much as 40% of their total employee payroll to provide this extra compensation. You should consider them your "hidden paycheck."

Most employers offer similar types of benefits in their total compensation packages. Whether you are a full or part time employee, your benefits will be prorated depending on the number of hours you work. Usually you can mix and match benefits around a few selected items (Table 15–5). For example, most employers have some type of specific traditional plan. Some may even have a flexible plan that offers a number of options from which to choose.

Regardless of the package you decide on, don't forget that there is usually a waiting period before the coverage is effective. Check with your institution—coverage with some health plans begins on one's first day of employment, but not always. Sometimes waiting periods may be as long as three to six months. Pension plans may require an even longer time before an employee is eligible to participate. Check with your employer to see what their program offers (Newby, 1990).

Employer Address and Phone Number	Interviewer and Title	Date Resume Sent	Date and Time of Interview	Inquiry or Application Letter	Application Submitted	Thank You Letter Sent After Interview	Job Offer Received	Confirmation or "No Thank You" Letter Sent	Comments or Notes

FIGURE 15–4   *Record of Employer Contacts and Resumes Sent.*

TABLE 15–4 *Your Checklist for Finding a Job*

√ Define your goals.

√ Develop your resume.

√ Identify potential employers.

√ Send your resume and cover letter.

√ Return a follow-up phone call.

√ Schedule an interview.

√ Send a follow-up letter.

√ Keep record of employer contacts (Fig. 15–4).

√ Make an informed decision where to work.

Let's take a few minutes to look at some of the basic benefits that you'll need to decide on.

Health, Dental and Vision Insurance

The most common type of coverage is health insurance. Health insurance claims are generally covered at 80% by such companies as Blue Cross/Blue Shield, Prudential, Metropolitan Life, and Mutual of Omaha, to name just a few. With this kind of plan, you or your family simply receive healthcare from the physician and facility of your choice and the insurance company pays for it on a *fee-for-service* basis. Usually, major insurance companies won't pay for well visits or

TABLE 15–5 *Benefit Package Options*

◆ Health and life insurance

◆ Accidental death and dismemberment coverage

◆ Sick or short-term disability pay

◆ Vacation pay

◆ Profit sharing and retirement plan

◆ Long-term disability leave

◆ Dental and/or vision care

◆ Parking

◆ Tuition reimbursement

◆ Loan programs

◆ Dependent care programs

◆ Health and wellness programs

physical examinations. All of this is subject to the conditions of each individual plan. Vision plans generally cover regular eye exams and provide for corrective lenses. Most often dental care includes x-rays and prophylactic dental hygiene at 100% reimbursement. Usually all other dental work is covered at 80%. As you might know, with any policy there are certain out-of-pocket expenses such as deductibles that have to be met. You may choose or have the option for supplemental insurance to take care of paying for the deductible. Whatever plan you choose, be sure to determine whether or not you want to arrange coverage for your dependents and/or spouse. After you terminate your employment at that facility, don't forget that the institution is required by law (COBRA) to offer you continued coverage at your expense for your health insurance for a specified period of time (Newby, 1990).

Some healthcare plans offer reimbursement for prescription drugs. Other

TABLE 15–6 *Health Insurance Terms You Need to Know*

TERM	DEFINITION
Coinsurance	The portion of your medical bills that you are responsible for paying after you have met the deductible. A ratio of 80/20 is standard, with you paying 20%.
Exclusions	Specific items not covered under your policy. Some policies exclude physical examinations, and health carriers can now legally exclude the treatment of AIDS.
First-dollar coverage	This policy pays all medical bills without a deductible. Almost impossible to find because coverage is so expensive.
Precertification	Some carriers require preapproval for receiving nonemergency treatments. These carriers may not cover certain treatments or will pay only partial benefits if precertification is not acquired. Your doctor should be aware of this when choosing treatment methods for you.
Pre-existing condition	An illness or condition you have before your policy is issued. Some pre-existing conditions are never covered. Most companies will not pay for the treatment of a pre-existing condition for at least a year after your policy is effective.
Preferred provider organization (PPO)	Under a PPO system, the list of healthcare providers from whom you can choose is limited. Your physician may not be included on that list.
Reasonable and customary	The rates generally charged for specific treatments in your area. If a doctor's fees are considerably higher than the fees charged by most doctors, your insurance company may cover only partial fees.
Waiting period	The period of time at the start of your coverage during which your carrier will not pay for certain treatments.

plans give you the opportunity to go to health maintenance organizations (HMOs). In this situation, your family must go to a group of physicians or other healthcare professionals to get benefit coverage for the service. These services are covered on a *prepaid* basis. Usually your out-of-pocket expenses in HMOs are less because the physician is paid monthly by the plan whether you need his or her services or not (Green, 1991). Table 15–6 provides a description of various health insurance terms that you need to know.

Another example is a preferred provider organization (PPO), in which your employer or insurance company arranges for *fee-for-service* healthcare with a specific provider on a *predetermined* rate. With a PPO you are free to select a physician or facility for insurance coverage, however, you must go to one of the preferred providers within the organization in order to obtain the lowest cost for healthcare (Green, 1991).

Life Insurance and Death and Dismemberment

Check to see what type of basic life insurance is offered by your employer. The amount of the coverage could be fixed at an amount of $10,000 or $20,000, or it might even be based on a percentage of your salary. Often this life insurance is available upon employment and may not cost you a penny. An added plus is that you might be eligible for this coverage without having to have proof of good health if you enroll within a stated period of time. Take advantage of this. This is a smart decision. Here's a tip: it's certainly easier and often less expensive to purchase life insurance when you're just starting your career. What type of life insurance should you consider? Basically, there are two types: *employer-sponsored* and *individually purchased* life insurance (Green, 1991). Table 15–7 summarizes types of employer sponsored life insurance.

Disability Coverage

Short- and long-term disability coverage becomes effective if you're unable to work either temporarily or permanently. This is helpful to you because you can collect a major percentage of your salary while disabled.

Vacation and Sick Leave

Time off, in days or hours, is accrued during pay periods. These plans often give you a certain number of days based on your length of employment. Some institutions may give you a percentage of pay or a dollar amount, if you don't use your accrued or allocated leave.

Education Assistance

Employers often offer incentives for you to go back to school, ranging from the provision of a flexible work schedule to tuition reimbursement for continuing education credits or degree completion.

TABLE 15–7   *Types of Employer-Sponsored Life Insurance*

Group term life insurance	◆ Known as "straight life": offers basic coverage for a short period of time at a low premium. ◆ You'll have protection with a cash value. ◆ The coverage ceases when you terminate employment.
Permanent life	◆ It builds a cash value, dividend, or interest. ◆ May have to prove you're in good health by taking a physical. ◆ Coverage is continued if you change jobs or are terminated.
Paid-up plans	◆ A combination of accumulating whole life and decreasing amounts of group life. ◆ May be offered at retirement.
Universal life	◆ Cash value or your investment income is deposited into a fund. ◆ May use this cash to pay your premium. ◆ Interest earned doesn't have to be reported for tax purposes.
Credit life	◆ Very expensive. ◆ Often difficult to cancel the policy. ◆ Usually offered by a bank.

Adapted from Green, L.A. (1991): Life insurance: Vital protection for your vital signs. *Healthcare Trends Transition,* April: 69.

Pensions, Tax-Deferments, Annuities, and Savings Plans

You're never too young to think about retirement. Usually a percentage of your paycheck is automatically deducted and placed into your retirement fund each pay period. Some of these plans allow taxes to be deferred until you make a withdrawal from these funds. The deduction may be a contribution to Medicare or to a tax-sheltered optional retirement program.

Reimbursement Accounts ("Cafeteria Plans")

"Cafeteria plans" are reimbursement spending accounts that operate under Section 125 of the Internal Revenue Service Code. In this situation, employers may offer employees two different types of accounts: healthcare and dependent daycare. Each item is paid for with *pre-tax dollars*. This obviously translates into a big savings for you, because with a cafeteria plan you have more money to spend as the amount of income that is taxed is reduced.

Dependent Care for Children and Elderly

Be sure to check with your employer to see what kind of on-site care or financial assistance would be available to your children and/or elderly family members.

Health-Wellness Program

You may wish to participate in a health-wellness program, which might include instruction in smoking cessation, weight reduction, and fitness as well as em-

November 1, 1994

Linda Smith
101 Anywhere Street
Dallas, TX 77777
214-888-5555

Ms. Joan Winter
Assistant Vice President
Children's Medical Center of Dallas
1935 Hospital Street
Dallas, TX 75235

Dear Ms. Winter:

It is with regret that I must submit my resignation. I have been offered a position with Hancock Hospital. My period of employment at
Children's has been very positive. I feel I have gained much experience that will be of great benefit to me in my career. My last day of
employment will be November 20, 1994.

Thank you for the opportunity to work at your facility and your kind
consideration.

Sincerely,

Linda Smith

FIGURE 15–5 *Letter of Resignation*.

ployee assistance programs. These are all available to promote a healthy lifestyle, which reduces employee absence and increases productivity.

When doing your job search, reviewing benefits is a major part of your decision. So, as a new graduate, be sure to familiarize yourself with all the options that are available to you. Often the personnel department or, in large organizations, the employee benefits person will be available to you to answer your questions. The decisions you make soon after graduation as well as in the early months of employment will have a far-reaching effect on your future.

What If It Is Time for You to Change Positions?

If you think it is time to change positions or explore other options, it is best to submit a letter of resignation. Give at least two weeks notice. Check your contract to see if you agreed to give more than two weeks notice and, if possible, give four weeks notice. If you are leaving on less than amiable terms, it is best not to express this in your letter. You can always take grievances to personnel or the human resources department. Figure 15–5 is an example of a letter of resignation.

Finding your niche in the workplace can certainly be a confusing, frustrating, and stressful experience. Having a basic understanding of the process of job hunting can go a long way to minimize the drawbacks that might be encountered. Determining your career objective and writing your resume are key aspects to the employment process. Be sure to keep track of all your potential employer contacts, as this will help organize and assist you in the employment decision-making process.

REFERENCES

Allen, D., Callein, J., Peterson, M. (1988): Making shared governance work. *J Nurs Admin* 18:37.

Birk, S. (1992): Mapping out the job market. *Directions*—Supplement to *Am Nurse*, p. 12.

Conley-Ferrey, M., Holland, L. (1992): The quest for the right job. *Healthcare Trends Transition* October:30.

Green, L.A. (1991a): Health insurance benefits: Vital to both body and pocketbook. *Healthcare Trends Transition* February:36.

Green, L.A. (1991b): Life insurance: Vital protection for your vital signs. Part II: Individually purchased plans. *Healthcare Trends Transition* May:50.

Green, L.A. (1991c): Life insurance: Vital protection for your vital signs. Part I: Employer-sponsored policies. *Healthcare Trends Transition* April:69.

Hanks, K., Belliston, L., Edwards, D. (1977) *Design Yourself.* Los Altos, CA, William Kaugmann, Inc.

Huey, F. Your first job, in *The AJN Guide.* New York, American Journal of Nursing.

Newby, P.K. (1990): Pack up your benefits in your old kit bag . . . . *Benefits Rev* Nov/Dec:35.

Michalek, M. (1992): Fall forward or spring behind. *Graduating Nurse* Fall:22.

Nursing Career Opportunities (1990): New York, American Journal Nursing.

Philbrick, M. (1991): Sink or swim: Staying afloat amidst a sea of job offers. *Healthcare Trends Transition* March:22.

Porter-O'Grady, T. (1987): Shared governance and new organizational models. *Nurs Econ* 281.

Recruiters on resumes (1992): *Graduating Nurse* Fall:26.

The AJN Guide 1991 (1990): New York, American Journal of Nursing.

The 1991 Job Market (1991): Oradell: N.J., Registered Nurse.

Werning, S.C. (1990): How far from home will you roam? *Healthcare Trends Transition* Nov/Dec:14.

16

Interviewing For Employment

Alice Pappas, Ph.D., R.N.

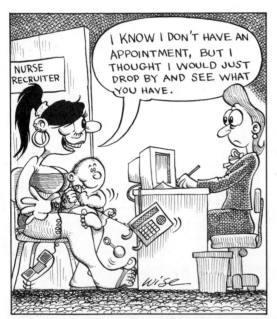

The first impression is a lasting one—
make it count for you, not against you.

"Ok world, here I come ready or not!"
—Unknown

After completing this chapter, you should be able to:

◆ Describe the essential steps involved in the interviewing process.
◆ Discuss typical questions asked by interviewers.
◆ Analyze your own priorities and needs in a job.
◆ Identify short-term career goals.

The process of interviewing involves a major transitional step between school and the real nursing world. With graduation in sight you are eager, but probably a little anxious about moving into the workplace, looking for the perfect match to your hard-earned diploma or degree.

As you consider possible employment opportunities, approach the upcoming interviews as you would any graded class assignment: *Do your homework!* Careful preparation is the key to a successful interview. Despite claims to the contrary, most worthwhile job offers do not happen to someone who just walks in the personnel or nursing office. The continued expansion of the healthcare field has created a vast array of opportunities for new graduates. You have developed marketable skills that are in demand, but you must prepare to sell yourself successfully to prospective employers.

▼

Plan your campaign each step of the way to enhance your chances for success!

▲

Give yourself ample time to consider what type of position you want and need, as well as the possibilities and limitations of the job market under consideration. You can compare the process to the selection of a marriage partner, car, home, or any other major life choice. After all, this position will help define who you are, and influence your career path. Become informed and selective in the process. Too often, new graduates accept their first position without sufficient knowledge of their own needs or the organization they select. Days or weeks into the job, surprise and disappointment sets in, as the reality of the situation becomes obvious: *"I'm not happy in this position," "I can't believe I took a job like this,"* or *"They never said anything about this during the interview."* Although there is no guarantee that a job will be heaven sent and wonderful, job dissatisfaction and turnover can be decreased if careful consideration is given to possible job selection before embarking on the actual interview.

The following steps are suggested as a guide to thorough background preparation. (Refer to Chapter 15 for more information on job opportunities and resume writing.)

SELF-ASSESSMENT

What Are My Clinical Interests?

Box 16–1 will help you identify your clinical interests and the possible reasons why. Hint: This will also help you answer interview questions about your choices.

Assess Your Wants and Desires/Likes and Dislikes

Identify your interests and the possible reasons why.

Interests	Reasons

1. I prefer to work with clients whose age is _____ _____

2. I prefer to work in a small hospital vs. a large medical center _____ _____

3. I prefer rotating shifts vs. straight shifts _____ _____

4. I prefer an internship vs. general orientation _____ _____

5. I prefer to have a set routine or constantly changing environment _____ _____

6. I prefer these areas (e.g., pediatrics, community health, medical, etc.) _____ _____

BOX 16–1

Assess Your Wants and Desires/Likes and Dislikes Continued

---

7. Which of my religious beliefs
   or values might impact
   where I work? _____

_____

_____

_____

_____

_____

_____

Next, start writing down possible settings where you could pursue these interests. For example, if you thrive in a fast-paced environment with high acuity, a critical care unit or emergency department may be for you. Within this category, however, are many specialties. Do you enjoy the medical or surgical aspects more? Cardiac or general medicine? Depending on your interests, there may be a number of possible paths to pursue (Fig. 16–1).

As you identify areas of clinical interest, try to prioritize your interests. This step may seem like a nonissue if you "eat, sleep, and drink" one specific specialty, but many people have two or more strong interests and this step helps to outline some possibilities. Believe it or not, some senior students confess to liking every clinical rotation, and are up in the air about which direction to take. If that description fits you, hang in there—you are not alone! There is a "smorgasbord" of job opportunities in nursing. You may want to taste of several before you find the one that really fits your needs. That's what is so nice—if you really get into an area you don't like, you have the option to change. All nursing experiences, both negative and positive, contribute to your experience in a productive way. The more areas you sample, the broader your knowledge base.

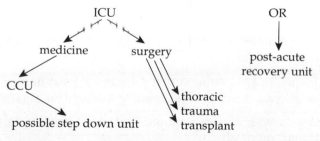

FIGURE 16–1   *The environment I would like to work in.*

Recruiters like flexibility in new graduates, but let's try and narrow your interests just a bit. Perhaps you can identify what you liked about each rotation and then prioritize possible interests or identify common experiences.

....

Peds—*enjoyed the children and opportunity to teach families.*

Med/Surg—*diabetic patients were challenging, staff were friendly, opportunties for teaching postop patients.*

Psych—*increased communication skills and self-confidence.*

OB—*teaching opportunities, enjoyed challenge of caring for high-risk OB population.*

ICU—*increased technical skills, opportunity to work with complex patients, supportive environment with staff.*

Community—*working with families, opportunity to enhance teaching and communication skills.*

....

From the above example, you can see that teaching, communication skills, working with families, a challenging environment, and a supportive staff are common themes. Remember these characteristics; they are important starting points for identifying your areas of interest. Depending on how you prioritize them, they can be applied in a variety of settings. The specific job market you are looking at may then narrow your interest to a more manageable list. For example, communication skills and family teaching may be your priority. As a result, community health may be a strong interest, but job inquiries reveal that staff positions require at least one year's experience in an acute care setting. Knowing this fact eliminates a nonproductive search, but may be useful information for later career planning. Where could you work in order to obtain the experience to promote your interest in community health?

What Are My Likes and Dislikes?

Another way to approach self-assessment involves identification of your likes and dislikes. This is related to interests, but on a more personal level. The job you eventually select may have some drawbacks, but it should meet many more of your likes than dislikes in order to be a good "fit." Write out your responses to the following questions:

1. **Do you enjoy an environment that provides a great deal of patient interaction, or do you thrive in a technically oriented routine?**

   Think back to your clinical rotations and see if you can find a pattern to being "turned on or off."

   ◆ I liked opportunities for doing many technical skills.

◆ I was uncomfortable with slower-paced routine (i.e., postpartum, nursery).

◆ I liked to see results of care as soon as possible (i.e., postop recovery).

2. **Do you enjoy working closely with other staff or prefer a more autonomous role in patient care?**

    This question may influence a setting with primary care or team nursing. Why did you like or dislike one type or the other? Talk over your responses with some friends who may have had other experiences and get their opinions as well.

3. **Do you learn best in a highly structured environment, or in more informal, on-the-job training?**

    Knowing your learning style can guide your interest in, and selection of, an internship or orientation program. For example, internships range from formal classes with lengthy preceptorships to more informal orientations of fairly short duration. Remember that a program that meets your needs may not be the answer for your best friend. Write down what you would like from an orientation or internship program. Look over your list and prioritize what you need and want.

4. **Do you really like making autonomous decisions, or do you want and need more direction and supervision at this point in your professional development?**

    You will shortly have completed nursing school, backed up by employment in an ICU throughout your senior year. Are you ready to be a 3–11 charge nurse in a small rural hospital, or do you want a slower transition to such responsibility? If this situation were offered, would you be flattered, frightened, or flabbergasted? Write down your reaction and consider how you would respond to the recruiter who offers you such a position.

5. **How much physical energy are you capable and willing to expend at work?**

    Running eight to twelve hours a day may or may not act as a tonic. Think back to the pace of your clinical rotations and consider how your body reacted (minus the anxiety associated with instructor supervision, if you can!). Would you prefer a unit that has some predictable periods of frenzy and pause, or do you thrive on the unpredictable?

6. **Are you a day, evening, or night person?**

    In other words, are there certain times of the day when you are at your best? How about your worst? Be honest and realistic with your answers. Very few people are equally efficient and effective twenty-four hours a day. If your body shuts down at 10PM or you resist all efforts to wake up before 9AM, certain shifts may need to be eliminated.

7. **Do you like rotating shifts, or perhaps more realistically, can you work rotating shifts?**

One aspect of reality shock for some new graduates is the realization that straight days ended with the last clinical rotation in school. Hospital staffing is twenty-four hours a day, seven days a week—a possibly unpleasant aspect of nursing, but real. Assess your ability to work certain shifts and try to strike a flexible approach. Identify a possible rotation pattern (i.e., days/evenings, or evenings/nights) or your willingness to work a straight evening or night position.

Consider the impact of your choices on family, social, and recreational needs. If there are certain shifts you must rule out, recognize that this may limit your job choices and plan accordingly. Giving some thought to your flexibility ahead of time will help you avoid committing to any and all shifts during an interview, and will facilitate your job hunt.

8. **Can you work long hours (i.e., twelve-hour shifts) without too much tension and fatigue?**

The twelve-hour staffing option offers flexibility (three days on, four days off) but leaves some people exhausted and irritable. Consider your personal needs outside of work when you respond to this item. Can you climb into bed or put your feet up after a nonstop twelve-hour shift, or do you need to pick up family responsibilities when you walk in the door? The four days off may well compensate for three days of fatigue, but map out your needs before you interview.

9. **Do you like making decisions quickly, or generally favor a more relaxed approach to clinical problems?**

In general, ICU and Telemetry require more immediate reactions than Adolescent Psych and Orthopedics. Does the ICU environment excite or bewilder you? Would you prefer a slower pace? *Don't criticize yourself for your likes or dislikes.* Slower-paced units require different strengths, not less knowledge. You have nothing to gain by working in an ICU if you dislike the setting. *Meet your own needs, not someone else's.*

10. **What do you need in a job to be happy?**

This does not mean money or benefits, but rather the sense that the job is worth getting excited about. Think about past employment you've had, whether healthcare related or not. Why did you like the job? What made you stay? Possible answers include opportunities for growth, advancement, working with people you respect, or collegiality. Remember, *your answers should address things which are important to you.* You may want to compare your answers with others whose opinions you value to gain a broader perspective.

What Are My Personal Needs and Interests?

A third aspect of self-assessment focuses upon personal needs and interests. *How much time and effort are you willing and able to give to your career at this point in time?* Will work be a number one priority in your life, or does family or continued education take precedence?

Is relocation a possibility? If so, what are the possibilities? If you are considering relocation, decide how you will gather information on possible job opportunities in the area(s) under consideration. Include newspapers, professional journals, and possible family or other personal contacts as sources of information. Develop a list of pros and cons for each location under consideration if this is a voluntary move. Include your personal interests in the decision (i.e., cost of living, access to recreational activities, opportunities for advanced education).

How much are you willing to commute? The job opportunity may be terrific but can you live with a one-hour commute each way? Find out the probable commuting time for the hours and days you want to work and add this piece of information to your collection of facts about various institutions. If you are remaining in the same locale this may be common knowledge, but if you are relocating this will determine the need for housing arrangements.

What salary range are you willing to consider? Although starting salary for new graduates is generally nonnegotiable, differentials for evenings, nights, and weekends create a range of salary possibilities. If you want an extended internship, a lower starting salary may be offered. Are you willing and able to trade this off for the benefits of an extended internship? Some areas of the country offer considerably higher salaries than others, but factor in the cost of living before you move out of town, or you may be unpleasantly surprised by a monthly rent that swallows up your salary.

Is overtime desirable in your life? Can it be reasonably juggled with other interests and time demands? The extra money may sound great and look impressive on your paycheck, but do not put unreasonable demands on yourself. A nursing shortage creates a need for overtime in many settings, but give some thought to what kind of overtime you can and cannot do when the question is asked.

What Are My Career Goals?

The final step of your self-assessment is the development of career goals. Yes, you really do need to have some goals. You are the architect of your professional future, so take pen to paper and start designing. Consider your answers to the following questions.

What do you want from your first nursing position? Possible answers might include developing confidence in decision-making, more proficiency with technical skills, and increased organizational abilities.

What are your professional goals for the first year? Third year? Fifth year? If you cannot imagine your life, let alone your career, beyond one to two years, relax. Many people feel uncertain planning beyond their initial position. Close your eyes and try to imagine yourself one year out of school. Compare yourself to recent graduates you have seen during your rotation and try to imagine the roles they are developing. Possible answers might include:

◆ **First-year goal:**

Becoming a competent staff nurse in Pediatrics or ICU.

◆ **Third-year goal:**

Achieving certification in your speciality area.

Involvement in a professional organization.

Possibly moving into a charge position on your unit or,

Returning to school for advanced education.

◆ **Fifth-year goal:**

Completing an advanced degree or moving into a management position.

If you honestly do not think you will return to school at this point in your life, don't feel as though you should fake your answer. Develop a comfortable response to a question regarding your goals for the first year, and consider what you might want to be doing after that time. Remember, it is far easier to gauge how your career is progressing if you have established goals that you can refer to. This is also a favorite question posed during interviews, so spend some time thinking about it!

RESEARCHING PROSPECTIVE EMPLOYERS

How Do I Go About Researching Prospective Employers?

Media Information

NEWSPAPERS.   Its time to start reading the Sunday employment section to get specific information about current openings in your area. Scan the ads to see if any are targeted specifically for graduating seniors or graduate nurses. Focus on these initially because they will include information on possible internships or specialized orientations, as well as specific openings for graduate nurses. The ads will also give you a name and number to contact for further information. Clip the ads which interest you and start a file for each potential employer.

JOB FAIR/OPEN HOUSE.   You may have the opportunity to attend a nursing job fair or hospital "open house" as a "soon-to-be graduate nurse." Take advantage of this opportunity to collect information about specific employers and possibly make initial contacts for later interviews. Leave your jeans and tennis shoes at home on these occasions though. Take some time with your appearance because first impressions are important! (See strategies for interview success for specifics regarding physical appearance and grooming.)

If you plan to formally interview at the institution in the future, take home their brochure and become familiar with the information it contains. Recruiters appreciate applicants who know some basic facts about their institution. It will also help you respond to one of their favorite lines of questioning: "Why do you want to work for our institution?" or "In what way(s) do you feel you can contribute to our organization?"

Employee Contacts

If you have friends or family, or simply know someone who works at an institution you are considering for employment, make an effort to speak with them about the job environment. As "insiders" they may be able to give you a perspective about the employer that the ads, recruiter, or interview cannot. Possible questions you may want to ask them include: "Why do they enjoy working there?" "What was orientation like?" "How is employee morale?"

Personnel/Recruitment Contacts

LETTER-WRITING CAMPAIGN.   If you plan to send your resume with cover letter, triple-check both for grammatical errors. You can obtain addresses through ads or telephone contact. Make sure you include your phone number in the mailing so that they can contact you if needed, as well as the probable date you would like to begin employment.

TELEPHONE CONTACT.   Before you pick up the phone, get out your calendar and start planning likely dates for possible interviews, as well as the approximate date you want to begin working. Armed with this information, you can comfortably answer questions beyond the fact that you would like them to send you a brochure. Depending on the institution you contact, personnel or nurse recruitment may want you to send a resume, or may press you to set up an appointment for an interview. Be prepared!

PERSONAL CONTACT.   If you plan to just stop by personnel or nurse recruitment for brochures and an application, make sure you give some thought to your appearance. Tee shirts, shorts, and jeans are not appropriate and have caused otherwise well-qualified applicants to be passed over for further consideration.

THE INTERVIEW PROCESS

How Do I Plan My Interview Campaign?

Set Up Your Schedule

Keep the following points in mind:

- ◆ Identify when you want to begin employment and mark your calendar.
- ◆ Work backward from this date to plan dates and times for interviews.
- ◆ Plan no more than two interviews in one day. If you do, beware of information overload and the risk of being late for at least one interview. Have two or three possible dates available on your calendar before you call the personnel office or nurse recruitment. Advance planning will keep you from fumbling on the phone when they tell you your first choice is unavailable!

While you are on the phone, ask some questions about their interview process. How much time should you plan for the interview? It may range from under one hour to a half a day.

What does the interview process involve? It may involve a tour and multiple interviews including personnel, nurse recruitment, one or more clinical managers, and possibly staff. If you are applying for an internship, it is not unusual to be interviewed by a panel of three or four people. Knowing this ahead of time may increase your anxiety, but it is less stressful than being surprised by this fact at the door.

Will more than one interview be required? Some institutions will use the first interview as a screening mechanism. You may be asked to come back for a follow-up interview.

How do you get to the personnel or nurse recruitment office? Ask for directions ahead of time if you are unfamiliar with the area. Have a good idea of the time involved for travel.

Will you be able to meet with clinical managers from different areas on the same day? Are there new graduates in the area you can talk with? This is important if you are interested in more than one area.

Will a tour of the unit(s) be included? If this is not a standard part of the interview process, express interest in having one so you can get a more realistic idea of the setting and possibly meet some of the staff.

Prepare to Show Your Best Side

Develop your responses to probable interview questions. (See Table 16–1 for some examples of responses.) If you don't plan possible responses, you run the risk

TABLE 16–1   *Key Points to Remember About Your Responses During the Interview*

◆ Answer honestly.

◆ Do not brag or gloat about your achievements, but do show yourself in a positive light.

◆ Remember that you are your best salesperson!

◆ Do not criticize past employers or instructors. It is more likely to reflect unfavorably on you than on them.

◆ Do not dwell on your shortcomings. Turn them into areas for future development: "I need to improve my organization skills. Managing a group of patients will be a challenge, but I am looking forward to it."

of looking wide-eyed as you fumble for an answer, or ramble on around the subject.

In Box 16–2, you will find examples of interview questions that you should be familiar with.

Rehearse the Interview

If you role-play a possible interview, it will probably increase your comfort level for the real thing. The following are some suggestions for a rehearsal:

◆ Dress for the part. It will add some authenticity to the situation.

◆ Choose a supportive friend or family member to role-play the interviewer.

◆ Practice your verbal responses to sample questions.

◆ Ask for constructive feedback regarding your appearance, body language, and responses.

Many applicants say they have no questions at the end of the interview. This may be true, or may reflect the urge to end the interview and relax! Some words of advice: *Prepare a few questions!* This will be *your opportunity* to gather important details and possibly impress the interviewer with your interest. The following is a sampling of possible questions:

◆ What is your evaluation process like? Who will evaluate me and how can I get feedback about my performance?

◆ I'd like some more information about your preceptorship program. How long will I have a preceptor, and what can I expect from the preceptor?

◆ What is the nurse:patient ratio on each of the shifts I may be working?

BOX 16–2

Sample of Interview Questions

The following is a sampling of interview questions you should be familiar with. Prepare your responses.

1. What area(s) of nursing are you interested in and why?

   _____

   _____

   _____

2. Tell me about your clinical experiences. Which rotations did you enjoy the most? Why?

   _____

   _____

   _____

   _____

3. Which one did you enjoy the least? Why?

   _____

   _____

   _____

   _____

4. What do you feel are your strengths? Why?

   _____

   _____

   _____

   _____

   _____

5. How about your weaknesses? Why?

   _____

   _____

   _____

   _____

BOX 16–2

Sample of Interview Questions Continued

---

6. Why do you want to work for our organization?

   _____

   _____

   _____

   _____

7. What qualifications do you have that make you believe that you will be successful in this staff position?

   _____

   _____

   _____

   _____

8. What skills do you feel you have gained from your past work experiences that may help you in this position?

   _____

   _____

   _____

   _____

9. Tell me a little about yourself. How would others describe you?

   _____

   _____

   _____

10. What are your future career plans? Where do you expect to be in two or three years? Five years?_____

   _____

   _____

   _____

Continued.

BOX 16–2

Sample of Interview Questions Continued

11. What turns you on about nursing? On the other hand, what turns you off? Why?

_____

_____

_____

_____

12. What is your philosophy of nursing?

_____

_____

_____

Spend some time looking over your answers. Do they describe you accurately? Rework your answers until you feel comfortable with them, but don't try to memorize the words. They should serve as a guide for the upcoming interview.

TABLE 16–2 *The Do's and Don't of Interviews*

DO'S	DON'TS
◆ Look over your wardrobe and select a conservative outfit. *Ladies, if you own a suit consider wearing it, but don't blow your budget buying an outfit you will never wear again.* Other acceptable outfits include a business-type dress or skirt with coordinated top.	◆ Flashy clothes that would be better suited to a social event.
◆ **Accessories:** Conservative makeup and hairdo. Minimal jewelry and hosiery.	◆ Casual clothes such as tee shirts, jeans, tennis shoes or sandals. *They may reflect the "real" you, but this is not the place to show that aspect of your personality.*
Gentlemen should consider a suit or jacket with coordinated slacks, shirt, and tie.	◆ Poor grooming or hygiene.
Take a few minutes to look yourself over in the mirror.	◆ Brand new shoes, which may turn your day into a "painful" experience.

◆ How often will I have to rotate shifts?

◆ What is your policy regarding weekend coverage?

Look over the recruitment brochures for additional ideas on questions. This shows that you are interested in the institution and have done your homework.

Strategies for Interview Success

One of the most important strategies for successful interviewing is to *dress for success*. (See Table 16–2 for a list of do's and don'ts.)

Watch your interviewing etiquette. Mom taught you to mind your manners, and this is an opportunity to put that education to good use.

Make sure you know the name of the individual who is scheduled to meet with you.

▼

CRITICAL FIRST 5 MINUTES!

The initial five minutes of an interview are critical. Research shows that the decision to continue interest or possibly hire is made during this time.

▲

Arriving early may give you a chance to look over additional information about the institution, or possibly give you more time for your interview. If you are delayed or cannot keep the appointment, call the interviewer to reschedule.

Be aware of your body language; that is, establish eye contact with the interviewer and maintain reasonable eye contact during the interview. *Try to avoid or minimize distracting nervous mannerisms.* Keep your hands poised in your lap, or in some other comfortable position. If you "talk with your hands," try not to do this continually. If you cross your legs, don't shake your foot. If offered coffee or other drink, decide whether this will relax you or complicate your body language. Show enthusiasm in your voice and body language. Do not smoke or chew gum. Give a winning smile when you are introduced and offer to shake hands. Women sometimes have a problem with shaking hands. Practice it at home to become more comfortable.

Demonstrate interest in what the interviewer has to say. Do not contradict or argue with the interviewer! Do not ask about salary and benefits until all other aspects of the interview have been completed, including your other questions! If you want to take some notes during the interview, ask the interviewer if he or she minds. This is generally quite acceptable. Bring along your list of questions and if you can't recall them when given the chance, ask to take out your list. Do not check off information during the interview like you are grocery shopping!

Phases of the Interview

The interview is generally divided into three areas, each of which serves a particular purpose. The first is the *introduction*. This is a "lightweight" section that should help to put you somewhat at ease. Some effort to "break the ice" will be made and the communication may focus on the traffic, weather, or the excitement you probably feel about your upcoming graduation. Take some slow deep breaths and make a conscious effort to relax. Remember that you are making an initial impression with your verbal and nonverbal behavior.

The second phase is *fact-finding*. Depending on the skill and style of the interviewer, you may be unaware of the subtle change in conversation, but questions about you will most likely now be asked. Remember the answers you rehearsed and make an effort to use that information. Your resume may be used as a source of questions, so make sure you can speak to its contents. Be prepared to offer your references and possibly explain why you have selected these particular individuals. If you have a tendency to give short responses or avoid answering the question, a skilled interviewer will reword the question, or possibly note that you do not answer questions well.

The *closing* is the last phase of the interview process. The interviewer may summarize what has been discussed and give you some ideas about the next step in the process (i.e., tour, meeting with clinical manager(s), or a follow-up interview). This is your time to ask questions. However, if you feel full of facts and unable to ask any questions at this time, "leave the door open" to future contacts by saying, "I believe you answered all my questions at this time, but may I contact you if I have some questions later on?"

After the initial interview, you may tour the area(s) in which you will work. Show interest when this tour is offered and use it as an opportunity to observe the surroundings for such things as professional behaviors and organizational and environmental factors. If you have the chance, interact with the staff, especially new graduates. Ask what they enjoy about their unit and job position. Before leaving, make sure you thank the interviewer for his or her time and interest.

How Do I Handle Unexpected Questions or Situations?

Ok, you did your homework and you're prepared for anything, but out of the blue you are asked a question you never expected. What should you do? Saying "No fair" is not a good answer! Take a deep breath, pause, and consider saying something like this: "That's an interesting question. I'd like to think about my answer for a minute if you don't mind. Can we come back to that subject later in the interview?" Given a temporary break, you will have time to develop your thoughts on the subject. Don't blow the question off, however, because the interviewer will most likely bring it up again. Suppose you answer the question, but feel your response was incomplete or off the mark. Look for an opportunity at the end of the interview to bring up the subject again, saying something like,

"I've had some time to think about an earlier question and want to add some additional information, if you don't mind."

Job Offers and Possible Rejection

Let's consider a positive outcome first. If you are offered a position during or at the end of the interview, three possible reactions are likely:

◆ You are not ready to say yes or no. This is your first interview and you have two more interviews scheduled.

◆ You would like very much to work here. The job offer is just what you're looking for.

◆ You don't want the position. It is not what you thought it would be, or something about the institution turns you off.

Whichever decision you make about the job offer, the following are helpful tips for your response:

1. Be honest. If you have other interviews to complete, say so. Be prepared to tell the interviewer when you will make your decision about the job offer.

2. Avoid being pressured to say "yes" if you are not ready to commit to the job, or feel that the position does not meet your needs.

3. Be polite. Ask for some time to consider the offer if you are unsure of what you want to do at the present time.

4. If you know the offer does not interest you, decline the offer graciously, and express appreciation for their interest in you.

5. Accept the offer and smile!

Suppose you receive a rejection or no job offer for the position, despite your interest and preparation. Before you leave in a state of dejection, scrape up the courage to ask for a possible explanation if it hasn't been made clear at this point. If you do not find out about the rejection until later, consider calling the interviewer for this information. Common reasons for rejection include the following. See if any of these factors might apply to you!

Lack of opening for your interests and skills. They liked you, but couldn't find a spot right now, or a more qualified candidate was selected for the position.

Poor personal appearance, including inappropriate clothes. You stopped by for the interview on your way to work out.

Lack of preparation for the interview. You were unable to answer questions intelligently, or showed lack of knowledge of, or interest in, the employer.

Your answers were superficial or filled with "I don't know."

376 CHAPTER 16 ◆ INTERVIEWING FOR EMPLOYMENT

Poor attitude, dominated by "What's in this for me?" instead of "How can I contribute to the organization?" Your first question focused upon salary and perks.

Answers and behavior reflected conceit, arrogance, poor self-confidence, or lack of manners or poise. They should hire you just because you showed up! Or a resume and responses that did not reflect initiative, achievements, or a reliable work history.

You have no goals or future orientation. After all you just want a job.

Perceived lack of leadership potential. You like being a follower in all situations and do not want to make decisions.

Poor academic record without a reasonable explanation. You worked as hard as you could in school, but the teachers didn't like you; you lacked appropriate references; or your references were not available or did not reflect favorably upon you.

Look over the possible reasons and decide which ones you have some control over and plan some remedial action in these areas. Fortunately, the job market for GN's and RN's is in your favor. You have the opportunity to spruce up your interviewing skills or etiquette and try again.

▼

If at first you don't succeed, try, try again.

▲

POSTINTERVIEW PROCESS

Now that the interview is over, you may want to relax, celebrate, or jump in your car to make your next interview appointment. *Stop for a few minutes* and jot down some notes about the interview. This is particularly important if you have other interviews to go. First of all, critique the interview. Consider these questions:

1. What do you think were your strengths and weaknesses?
2. Is there anything you wish you had or had not said? Why?
3. Were there any surprises?
4. How do you feel you handled the situation?
5. What can you do differently the next time?

Also be sure to write down details about the job, which will help you decide on its relative merits and/or drawbacks. If you do not do this, you may not be able to distinguish job A from job B by the time the interviews are finished. You may experience information overload after a number of interviews, but if you have taken notes about each, the sorting process will be easier. (Chapter 15 includes an employer contact record keeping chart for this process.)

After the interviews are over, rank your job offers against your personal list of priorities in order to make an informed choice. This may be an unnecessary step for you if you were sold on a particular interview. However, it is a good idea to consider interviewing at least two institutions, if only to strengthen your decision about the first interview. It will help eliminate possible doubts about your choice later on. If there is a job you think you are really interested in, do a couple of other interviews first. This will give you some experience in interviewing and you may be able to conduct a more positive interview for the position in which you are really interested. It may also "open your eyes" to other possibilities.

Follow-Up Communication

Remember how nice it is to get a thank you note in the mail or phone call of appreciation? Well, the same idea carries over to the work world: write those letters!

FOLLOW-UP LETTER.   Take a few minutes to write a note of thanks to the interviewer for the time and interest spent on your behalf. You may want to include additional information in the note: your continuing interest in the position if you hope an offer will be made, the date you will be making your job decision, additional thanks for any special efforts extended to you (lunch, individualized tour), and any change in phone numbers and appropriate times when they may be able to contact you.

LETTERS OF REJECTION.   As soon as you make up your mind regarding job offers, notify other prospective employers of your decision. Decline their job offer graciously and include an expression of appreciation for their interest in you. Remember, you have accepted a position elsewhere, but your career could take a turn in the future that may bring you back to the institution you are now declining. Leave a positive impression.

TELEPHONE FOLLOW-UP.   Based on the interview(s), you should have a pretty clear idea of the "how" and "when" of further contact. A phone call may be appropriate when you haven't heard from a recruiter by an agreed-upon-date. You can contact a recruiter or interviewer by phone to decline a job offer, but a personal letter is preferable to leaving a phone message.

▼

Good luck with your interviews!

▲

REFERENCES

Aiserstein, T.J. (1990): Taking charge—how to land the job you want. *RN* 53(2):15-18.

Davidhizar, R. (1989): How to find the perfect job. *Today's OR Nurse* 11(7):15-20.

Flanagan, L. (1988): Entering and Moving in the Professional Job Market: A Nurse's Resource Kit. ANA Pub. #ECO-146 American Nurses Association p. 1-34. Kansas City.

Glasser, G. (1990): Your mama taught you better . . . discourteous applicants. *RN* 53(6):120.

Kelsey, K.L. (1989): An open letter to a graduate nurse. *Imprint* 36(5):9.

McAlvanah, M.F. (1988): Interviewing 1988 style. *Pediatr Nurs* 14(4):332.

Tyler, L. (1990): Watch out for "red flags" on a job interview. *Hospitals* 64(14):46.

Washington, R. (1990-91): A practical guide to interviewing. *Imprint* 37(5):38.

Weis, D. (1990): 10 questions recruiters will ask. *Nursing* 20(3):116-118.

THRIVING . . .
NOT
JUST
SURVIVING

17

Self-Care Strategies

Barbara Michaels, Ed.D., R.N.

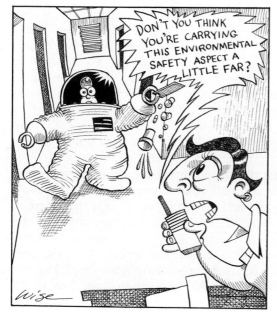

Nurses must be aware of the potential threats to their well-being.

"I will use words which emanate power, strong words to guide me. My words today will be strong and powerful. I will choose words that convey a sense of mastery, competence, and ability: I can. I will. I am. I do . . . "

—Rochelle Lerner, 1985

After completing this chapter, you should be able to:

- Identify potential threats to your health and well-being.
- Describe how impediments to your health and well-being affect you personally and professionally.
- Discuss the implications of caring for the self.
- Identify strategies for self-care.
- Formulate a plan of care for yourself that is based on identified deficits in self-care.

In order for nurses to effectively take care of their clients, they must first take care of themselves. As a new graduate in your first year of practice you need to make "taking care of yourself" a top priority. The work environment will be demanding; you will be exposed to learning opportunities and be introduced to a whole new area of professional responsibilities. How you perceive yourself often determines how effective you are as a nurse. The way you feel about yourself will be influenced by your values, actions, successes, and failures during your first year after graduation. Self-care is the foundation that will assist you in thriving in nursing instead of just surviving.

EMPOWERMENT AND SELF-CARE

Learning about self-care is really about empowerment. The word "power" comes from the French word, "pouvoir," which means "to be able." To *empower* means to enable—enable self and others to reach their greatest potential for health and well-being. In current literature on co-dependency, however, the concept of enabling is seen in a negative light because it refers to doing things for others that they can do for themselves. Actually, preventing friends and loved ones from dealing with consequences for their behavior is very *disempowering*.

With empowerment comes a feeling of well-being and effectiveness. There are times and situations in our lives when we feel more or less powerful. Examples of occasions when one feels powerful or powerless are given in Table 17–1. You may find as you read through the list that there are some situations in your life where you do feel powerful and some where you don't. Self-assessment of our sense of well-being and self-esteem helps us to know where to begin. Because change is a constant and all of us are in varying states of emotional, physical, and mental change at any given time, it is important to assess ourselves on a regular basis. As a matter of fact, knowing oneself is the very first step in learning to care for one's self. Empowerment in all spheres of our being is very important. Examine the Holistic Self Assessment Tool (Box 17–1), which includes measures of our emotional, mental, physical, social, spiritual, and choice potentials.

"Emotional wholeness" is what I term our "feeling" reality. The ability to express a wide range of emotions is indicative of good mental health. Nurses are often very good at helping their patients "feel" their feelings, but often have a difficult time feeling and expressing their own.

Experiencing "mental wholeness" implies that we maintain our childlike ability to dream and fantasize about the future. Nurses frequently have an overabundance of concrete knowledge of the practice of nursing. We appreciate the challenge of a difficult patient. However, because of the mental demands of the nursing profession, we often don't take time out to learn other disciplines.

TABLE 17–1 *Examples of Times One Feels Powerful or Powerless*

I FEEL POWERLESS WHEN:

- ◆ I'm ignored
- ◆ I get assigned to a new hospital unit
- ◆ I can't make a decision
- ◆ I'm exhausted
- ◆ I'm being evaluated by my instructor
- ◆ I have no choices
- ◆ I'm being controlled or manipulated
- ◆ I have pent-up anger
- ◆ I don't think or react quickly
- ◆ I don't speak loud enough
- ◆ I don't have control over my time

I FEEL POWERFUL WHEN:

- ◆ I'm energetic
- ◆ I get positive feedback
- ◆ I know I look good
- ◆ I tell people I'm a nurse
- ◆ I have clear goals for my career
- ◆ I stick to decisions
- ◆ I speak out against injustice
- ◆ I allow myself to be selfish without feeling guilty
- ◆ I tell a good joke
- ◆ I work with supportive people
- ◆ I'm told by a patient or family that I did a good job

Adapted from Josefowitz, N. (1980): Paths to Power. Menlo Park, CA, Addison-Wesley, p. 7.

Nurses frequently neglect their physical health. We make certain that our patients receive excellent health education and discharge instructions, and worry when they are noncompliant. However, as nurses we do not always follow through when it comes to such things as physical exams, mammograms, and dental health for ourselves. We work long hours and don't plan adequate time for physical recuperation.

Because our profession is such a demanding one, we often don't take the

BOX 17–1

Holistic Self-Assessment Tool

Emotional potential

_____   I push my thoughts and feelings out of conscious awareness (denial).

_____   I feel I have to be in control.

_____   I am unable to express basic feelings of sadness, joy, anger, and fear.

_____   I see myself as a victim.

_____   I feel guilty and ashamed a lot of the time.

_____   I frequently take things personally.

Social potential

_____   I am overcommitted to the point of having no time for recreation.

_____   I am unable to be honest and open with others.

_____   I am unable to admit vulnerability to others.

_____   I am attracted to needy people.

_____   I feel overwhelmingly responsible for others' happiness.

_____   My only friends are nurses.

Physical potential

_____   I neglect myself physically—overweight/underweight, lack of adequate rest and exercise.

_____   I feel tired and lack energy.

_____   I am not interested in sex.

_____   I do not engage in regular physical and dental check-ups.

_____   I have seen a doctor in the past six months for any of the following conditions: migraine headaches, backaches, gastrointestinal problems, hypertension, or cancer.

_____   I am a workaholic—work is all important to me.

Spiritual potential

_____   I see events that occur in my life are controlled by external choices.

_____   I find the world a basically hostile place.

_____   I lack a spiritual base for working through daily problems.

_____   I live in the past or the future.

_____   I have no sense of power greater than myself.

Mental potential

_____   I read mostly professional literature.

_____   I spend most waking hours obsessing over people, places, or things.

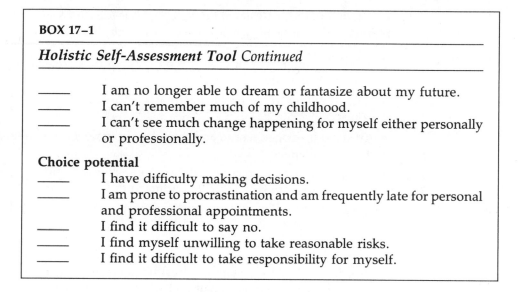

BOX 17–1

Holistic Self-Assessment Tool Continued

_____ I am no longer able to dream or fantasize about my future.
_____ I can't remember much of my childhood.
_____ I can't see much change happening for myself either personally
or professionally.

Choice potential
_____ I have difficulty making decisions.
_____ I am prone to procrastination and am frequently late for personal
and professional appointments.
_____ I find it difficult to say no.
_____ I find myself unwilling to take reasonable risks.
_____ I find it difficult to take responsibility for myself.

time to cultivate our social potential. When we do spend time with friends, it is because they "need" us. When we get together with friends who are nurses, we spend the time together talking about work.

"Spiritual potential" simply means that we have a daily awareness that there is something more to living than mere human existence. Nurses with spiritual potential see that life has meaning and direction.

The ability to know that we have choices in life is the final area of the assessment tool. Nurses without choice power see life as black and white, with little gray in the middle. Awareness of our choices eliminates the black and white extremes and enables us to act rather than react in situations. Nurses with choice power are able to make decisions and take risks and feel good about it.

If you found yourself answering in the affirmative in any of the areas on the self-assessment, be aware that a perfect score in life is impossible and unrealistic. Perfectionism (needing to be perfect) is an excellent way to sabotage personal and professional growth. Use the tool not only to assess the negatives in your life, but also to look at the areas where you are experiencing growth. You can't survive nursing school, for example, and not experience growth in all areas.

Suggested Strategies for Self-Care Based on the Holistic Self-Assessment Tool

Not having our life in a state of balance and not having a vision for the future often reflects a state of poor self-esteem. Nathaniel Branden, often referred to as the "father of the self-esteem movement," has identified several factors found in individuals with healthy self-esteem. A few of these are:

- A face, manner, way of talking, and moving that project the pleasure one takes in being alive.
- Ease in talking of accomplishments or shortcomings with directness and honesty.
- An attitude of openness to and curiosity about new ideas, new experiences, new possibilities of life.
- Open to criticism and comfortable about acknowledging mistakes because one's self-esteem is not tied to an image of "perfection."
- An ability to enjoy the humorous aspects of life, in oneself and others. (Branden, 1992, p. 43)

Our responses in only one or two of the six assessment areas may reflect healthy self-esteem. The key to developing healthy self-esteem is to become aware of the areas that need the most repair and work on them. However, it is essential to maintain a sense of balance; going overboard in one or two areas is counter-productive. For example, a nurse who exercises five times a week, follows a healthy diet, and sleeps well, but is emotionally numb and does not have a clear vision for her future, is out of balance. It is a good idea to use this tool every six months to one year—similar to taking an inventory at home or in a business.

Am I Emotionally Healthy?

Being emotionally healthy means that you are aware of your feelings and are able to acknowledge them in a healthy way. Nurses who have good emotional health know when they are feeling fearful, angry, sad, ashamed, happy, guilty, or lonely and they are able to distinguish between these feelings. They have found appropriate ways to express their feelings without offending others. When feelings are not expressed or at least acknowledged, they frequently build up, which results in emotional bingeing. Sometimes our bodies take the brunt of unacknowledged feelings in the form of headaches, gastrointestinal problems, anxiety attacks, and so on.

It is important to remember that feelings or emotions are neither good or bad. They are indications of some of our self-truths, our desires, and our needs. Box 17–2 is an exercise to help access and acknowledge feelings.

What About Friends and Fun? How Do I Find the Time?

An occupational hazard of nurses is overcommitting, both personally and professionally. As a result, they frequently have difficulty in meeting their social potential. Michaels (1990) found that student nurses were very remiss in engaging

---

BOX 17–2

Exercise to Help Access and Acknowledge Feelings

1. Turn your attention to how you are feeling. What part of your body feels what?

2. Recognize to yourself that this is how you are feeling, and give it a name. If you hear an inner criticism for feeling this way, just set it aside. Any feeling is acceptable.

3. Let yourself experience the sensations you are having. Separate these feelings from having to do anything about them.

4. Ask yourself whether you want to express your feelings now or some other time. Do you want to take some other action now or later? Remind yourself that you have choices.

---

in recreational activities. However, the findings indicated that students who did engage in recreational activities on a regular basis were less depressed and scored lower on tools used to measure depression, burnout, and co-dependency.

Student nurses often say they do not engage in recreational activities because they cost money and that all their money goes into living expenses. First of all, it is important to include some money in your monthly budget for fun. Depriving yourself of time for recreation on a regular basis may lead to impulsive recreational spending such as a shopping binge using credit cards or money allotted for something else. There are many things to do and places to go that will give you pleasure. Several examples are enclosed in Table 17–2.

Another area in the social arena where many nurses have difficulty is in forming relationships outside of nursing. If you spend all your free time with nurses, chances are that you will talk "shop." Nursing curricula are very science-intensive because there is so much to learn in such a short period of time. Cultivate some friends who have a liberal arts or fine arts background. Also choose friends who have different political opinions, come from a different part of town, a different culture, or a different socioeconomic class.

POTENTIAL OCCUPATIONAL THREATS TO HEALTH AND WELL-BEING

There are many potential threats to health and well-being that nurses encounter on a daily basis. Some of these potential threats, such as mental and physical

TABLE 17–2 *Some Pleasurable Activities*

Go on a picnic with friends.

Invite friends over for potluck dinner.

Go to a movie.

Plan celebrations after exams or completing a project.

Introduce yourself to three new people.

Visit a museum.

Call an old friend.

Play with your children.

Borrow someone else's children for play.

Volunteer for a worthwhile project.

Get active in religious activities.

Spend some time people-watching.

Take up a new hobby.

Invite humor into your life.

fatigue associated with rotating work schedules and work-related injuries, have been a part of nursing practice for many years. Others, such as exposure to HIV infection, are relatively new. In either case, nurses must learn to deal with these threats—or deal with the consequences of chronic back pain, sleep deprivation, or contracting communicable diseases, such as AIDS and tuberculosis.

Am I Really in Danger of Contracting AIDS?

AIDS is a very real threat to health professionals. Prior to the late 1970s, AIDS was not to be found in the professional literature. Today articles about AIDS not only are found in nursing literature, but appear almost on a regular basis in the daily papers. Of recent concern has been the number of cases where patients have contracted AIDS from a health professional who was careless in the use of universal precautions. To prevent transmission of HIV nurses and healthcare workers must adhere to universal precautions. In an editorial in *The American Nurse* by Barbara Fassbinder, who is one of the first three healthcare workers known to have contracted the HIV virus through a non-needlestick injury in 1986, wanted to share the following message with all healthcare workers:

▼

"Listen to the experts and take universal precautions seriously. Your life depends on it."
(Fassbinder, 1992, p. 4)

▲

. . . That is my message. It is a simple message, and yet one that is too often ignored in the workplace for a variety of reasons, including inconvenience and denial that anything bad can ever happen. A few moments of inconvenience may save your life. And if you think nothing bad can ever happen to you, I'm living proof that that can be a fatal attitude. (Fassbinder, 1992, p. 4)

When universal precautions are correctly implemented, contracting AIDS from a patient is highly unlikely. (An additional comment by the editors: all of the nurse educators who reviewed this chapter expressed increasing concern regarding the graduate nurses' adherence to and understanding of universal precautions.) Nurses who work in emergency departments and surgery are in areas of high risk of exposure to HIV. Another area of increasing concern about exposure to blood and body fluid contamination is in labor and delivery. The American Nurses Association (ANA) does not promote mandatory testing of patients, nor do the Centers for Disease Control. Both organizations believe that the transmission of AIDS is halted by strict adherence to universal precautions and infection control practices, as well as education of both consumers and healthcare professionals. Mandatory testing for HIV status may be required by some institutions, however, you must give written valid consent for the test to be performed. The results of the test cannot be used to determine employment. If an employer discriminates based on HIV status, two federal laws are violated, the Rehabilitation Act and the Americans with Disabilities Act. It is recommended that employers not require testing, but encourage employees to determine their HIV status. To obtain more information regarding employment rights of HIV + healthcare workers, contact the Centers for Disease Control in Atlanta, Georgia for their document, "HIV/AIDS Surveillance Report," November, 1991. Another source of information is the ANA's "Compendium of HIV/AIDS Position Policies & Documents," ANA, September, 1992, Pub. No. PR 8.

Is Substance Abuse Really a Problem for Nurses?

The incidence of substance abuse among nurses is very high. Available data indicates that there are between 40,000 and 70,000 chemically impaired nurses in the workforce (Robbins, 1987). Researchers have found that nurses in recovery from chemical dependency were likely to have been in the upper one-third of their graduating class and were considered very able by their nurse colleagues (Bissell, 1981; Brennan, 1983; and Reed, 1989).

There is considerable stigma associated with the diagnosis of chemical dependency or alcoholism. The nursing profession has chosen to use the term "impaired professional" for nurses who are impaired because of the use of alcohol or other drugs, or psychological dysfunction. If you suspect a nurse of chemical dependency, do not ignore it. Programs to help impaired nurses have been in place since 1982. There are many state-run programs that provide intervention and subsequent support and monitoring during the recovery of an impaired nurse. In this way a practicing nurse does not need to lose his or her license. When the program is successfully completed (after approximately two years), the nurse is deemed successfully treated. Programs for identifying and monitoring the impaired nurse vary from state to state. Find out how your state handles this issue by contacting your state board of nurse examiners, which can be found in Appendix A of this book.

SELF-CARE

How Do I Take Care of My Physical Self?

Nurses are great when it comes to patient education. As a matter of fact, it is one of our strengths as a profession. Sometimes we have difficulty applying this information to ourselves. Taking care of ourselves physically is very important. Our profession is both mentally and physically challenging. Taking care of ourselves physically entails proper nutrition, getting adequate sleep, and exercising on a regular basis.

The United States Surgeon General's 1988 report on Nutrition and Health recommends the following:

- ◆ **Fats and Cholesterol:** Select low-fat/low-cholesterol foods such as lean meats, fish, poultry, and low-fat products. Avoid butter, foods that are deep-fried, marbled meats, and processed cheeses.

- ◆ **Complex Carbohydrates and Fiber:** Choose whole-grain bread and cereal products, pastas, vegetables, and fruits naturally high in complex carbohydrates. Avoid desserts and canned fruits that contain refined sugars.

- ◆ **Sodium:** Select food naturally low in salt and cut down the amount of salt added during food preparation and at the table. Reduce intake of foods such as ham, bacon, salted snacks, and other highly processed foods.

- ◆ **Alcohol:** Consume no more than two drinks a day: alcohol contains only empty calories.

- ◆ **Exercise:** Incorporate some form of exercise, such as walking, into your weekly schedule.

A good exercise program is one that includes activities that foster aerobic activity, flexibility, and strength. A very important part of an exercise program is that it be a regular habit. To be effective, the program should take three to six hours a week. And it doesn't have to cost money. You don't have to belong

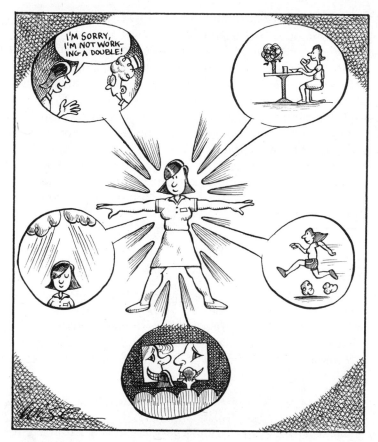

FIGURE 17–1   *Learn how to take care of yourself.*

to a gym or invest in exercise equipment. Aerobic activities include walking, jogging, swimming, bicycling, and dancing. Minimal fitness consists of raising your heart rate to 100 and keeping it there for thirty minutes.

Strategies to Foster My Spiritual Self— Does My Life Have Meaning?

Having a sense of spiritual well-being or good spiritual health is defined by Ellison (1983, p. 331) as a feeling of being "generally alive, purposeful and fulfilled." People who have a sense of spiritual well-being find their lives to be a positive experience, have a relationship with a power greater than themselves, feel good about the future, and believe there is some real purpose in life. If we find that our life lacks meaning and our spiritual health is lacking, how do we go about finding spiritual well-being?

Daily prayer and meditation are very important in maintaining a spiritual self. M. Scott Peck (1978) states that the process of spiritual growth is an effortful and difficult one because it is conducted against a natural resistance, against a natural inclination to keep things the way they were, to cling to the old maps and old ways of doing things, to take the easy path. Reading religious material or studying the great religions are two examples. There are many spiritual books, enough reading for a lifetime.

In addition to reading what others have written about the subject, many people access their spiritual selves with the practice of meditation. Meditating allows us time to become quiet, heal our thoughts and bodies, and be grateful. A sample meditation on gratitude and healing is included in Table 17–3.

How Do I Increase My Mental Potential? It's Okay to Daydream . . .

Nursing students get considerable opportunity to exercise their mental potential while they are in nursing school. However, this activity is primarily in the form of formal education. There are many other ways to exercise this potential. One of the first ways is to concentrate on removing negative thoughts or self-defeating beliefs from our mind. Examples of statements that nursing students frequently make are:

◆ "I must make A's in nursing school."

◆ "I must have approval from everyone and if I don't, I feel horrible and depressed."

◆ "If I fail at something, the results will be catastrophic."

◆ "Others must always treat me fairly."

◆ "If I'm not liked by everyone, I am a failure."

◆ "Because all my miseries are caused by others, I will have no control over my life until they change."

If you relate to any of these statements, you have some work to do on your belief systems. You are setting yourself up for failure by having extremely high expectations of yourself. In addition, you are giving other people power over your own destiny. Remember, you can't change others. The only person you can change is yourself.

One way that we can change these internal beliefs is to learn how to give yourself daily affirmations. Simply put, affirmations are powerful, positive statements concerning the ways in which we desire to think, feel, and behave. Some examples are, "I am a worthwhile person"; "I am human and capable of making

TABLE 17–3   *A Meditation on Gratitude and Healing*

Take a deep breath and gently close your eyes. Give a few big sighs . . . sighs of relief . . . and see if your body wants to stretch a little . . . or yawn . . . (pause).

Now pay attention to the rhythm of your breathing . . . . Feel your body rise gently as you breathe in, and relax as you breathe out . . . (pause for several breaths) . . . every outbreath is an opportunity to let go . . . to feel the pleasant warmth and heaviness of your body . . . a little more on each outbreath . . . (pause).

Now, as you breathe in, imagine your breath as a stream of warm, loving light entering through the top of your head. Let it fill your forehead and eyes . . . your brain . . . your ears . . . and nose . . . feel the light warm and relax your tongue, your jaws, and your throat. Let your whole head float in an ocean of warm light . . . growing brighter and brighter with each breath . . . (pause) . . . . Thank your eyes for the miracle of sight . . . your nose for the fragrance of roses and hot coffee on cold mornings (or whatever you like) . . . your ears for the richness that sound is . . . your tongue for the pleasure of taste . . . and let the light fill and heal every cell of your senses . . .

Breathe the light into your neck . . . let it expand gently into your shoulders . . . and breathe it down your arms . . . and into your hands . . . right to the tips of your fingers . . . . Thank your arms and hands for all you have created and touched with your life . . . . All the people you have hugged and held to your heart . . . . Rest in the warmth and love of the light . . . light that grows brighter with every breath . . . .

And breathe the warm light into your lungs and your heart . . . feeling it penetrate your entire chest, filling every organ, every cell with love. As you breathe, send gratitude to your lungs for bringing in the energy of life—and to your heart for sending life to all the cells of your body for serving you so well for all these years . . . rest in the gratitude and love . . . in the light that continues to grow brighter with each breath . . . (pause).

And breathe the light into your belly, feeling it penetrate deeply into your center, into the organs of digestion and reproduction . . . and sense the miracle of your body . . . the mystery of procreation and of the ability to beget life . . . let the light expand through your torso and down into your buttocks . . . growing warmest and brighter . . . balancing and healing all the cells of your body . . . .

Breathe the light into your thighs . . . into bone and muscle, nerve and skin, alive with the energy of light . . . comforted in your caring and your love . . . and let the light expand into your calves . . . and your feet . . . right to the soles of your feet . . . feeling gratitude for the gift of walking . . . letting the lovelight grow brighter and brighter . . . .

Rest in the fullness of the light . . . enjoying the lifeforce . . . and, if there is any place in your body that needs to relax or to heal, direct the light there and hold that part of yourself with the same love you would give to a hurt child . . . (pause).

Now, as you breathe, sense how the light radiates out from your body . . . just as a light shines in the darkness, surrounding you in a cocoon of love . . . and you can sense that cocoon extending all around your body, above and below you, and to all sides, for about three feet . . . like a giant cocoon . . . a place of complete safety where you can recharge your body and your mind . . . (pause).

Table continued on following page

TABLE 17–3   *A Meditation on Gratitude and Healing Continued*

And you can imagine the light around other people . . . surrounding them with the same radiance of love, gratitude, and healing . . . see your loved ones in the light . . . see those who you think of as your enemies in the light . . . then let the light expand until you can imagine the entire world as an orb of light . . . (pause) . . . amidst a universe of light (pause) all connected . . . all at peace . . . and feel the wonder and majesty of creation . . . (pause). Now for a minute or two just rest . . . just breathe . . . returning to the warm, comfortable feelings within you . . . (long pause).

Begin fading out the music now, and then read the instructions for reorientation.

And now, begin to reorient yourself to the room . . . slowly and at your own pace . . . bringing the peace and gratitude back with you.

Reprinted with permission from Borysenko J. (1987): Minding the Body, Mending the Mind. Menlo Park, CA, Addison-Wesley.

mistakes"; and "I am able to freely express my emotions." Always begin affirmative statements with "I" rather than "you." This practice keeps the focus on self rather than others and encourages the development of inner self-worth.

▼

The power of affirmation exercises lies in consistency—repetition encourages ultimate belief in what is being said.

▲

Begin each day with some affirmations. Try some of the examples in Table 17–4. These enable us to feel better about ourself and consequently raise our self-esteem. Stand in front of a mirror and tell yourself that you are a special person and worthy of self-love and the love of others. Another suggestion would be to record some positive affirmations on your telephone answering machine and call your phone number in the middle of the day or when you are having a slump or attack of self-pity; hearing your own voice say you are okay can have a very positive effect.

What Are My Choices and How Do I Exercise Them?

Many of us negotiate our way through life, never realizing that we have many choices. We remain victims, waiting for life to happen, rather than taking a proactive stance. In his best-selling book, *The Seven Habits of Highly Effective People,* Stephen Covey (1989) states that the very first habit we must develop is to be *proactive.* We stop thinking in black and white and come to realize that in every arena of our lives, we have choices about how to respond and react. Covey differentiates between people who are proactive versus people who are reactive. Examples of proactive versus reactive language are included in Table 17–5. Pay

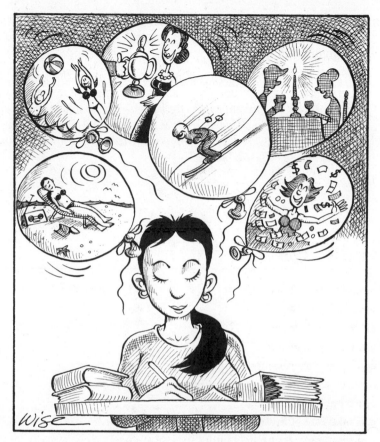

FIGURE 17–2   *Daydream—send up your brain balloons!*

attention to your own language patterns for the next few weeks. Are there times when you could say "I choose"? You can choose to respond to people and situations, rather than react. Exercising our choice potential also entails that we act responsibly toward others. We recognize that other people have the right to choose for themselves and to be accountable for their own behavior.

Before we can act responsibly toward others, we must first act responsibly toward ourselves. This involves self acceptance and self love. In his most recent book, Leo Buscaglia (1991) states this very eloquently:

....

BEING WHO WE ARE

People who feel good about themselves are not easily threatened by the future. They enthusiastically maintain a secure image whether everything is falling apart or going their way. They hold a firm base of personal assuredness and self-respect that remains constant. Though they are concerned about what others think of them, it is a healthy concern. They find external forces more challenging than threatening.

Perhaps the greatest sign of maturity is to reach the point in life when we embrace ourselves—strengths and weaknesses alike—and acknowledge that we are all that we have; that we have a right to a happy and productive life and the power to change ourselves and our environment within realistic limitation. In short, we are, each of us, entitled to be who we are and become what we choose. (Buscaglia, 1991, p. 7)

TABLE 17–4 *Affirmations*

◆ I am a worthwhile person.
◆ I am a child of God.
◆ I am willing to accept love.
◆ I am willing to give love.
◆ I can openly express my feelings.
◆ I deserve love, peace, and serenity.
◆ I am capable of changing.
◆ I can take care of myself without feeling guilty.
◆ I can say "No" and not feel guilty.
◆ I am beautiful inside and out.
◆ I can be spontaneous and whimsical.
◆ I am human and capable of making mistakes.
◆ I can recognize shame and work through it.
◆ I forgive myself for hurting myself and others.
◆ I freely accept nurturing from others.
◆ I can be vulnerable with trusted others.
◆ I am peaceful with life.
◆ I trust the process of life.
◆ I am free to be the best me I can.
◆ I love and comfort myself in ways that are pleasing to me.
◆ I am automatically and joyfully focusing on the positive.
◆ I am giving myself permission to live, love, and laugh.
◆ I am creating and singing affirmations to create a joyful, abundant, fulfilling life.

TABLE 17–5 *Examples of Proactive Vs. Reactive Language*

REACTIVE LANGUAGE	PROACTIVE LANGUAGE
There's nothing I can do.	Let's look at our alternatives.
That's just the way I am.	I can choose a different approach.
He makes me so mad.	I control my own feelings.
They won't allow that.	I can create an effective presentation.
I have to do that.	I will choose an appropriate response.
I can't.	I choose.
I must.	I prefer.
If only.	I will.

Reprinted with permission from Covey, S. (1989): Seven Habits of Highly Effective People. New York, Simon & Schuster, p. 78.

REFERENCES

American Nurses Association (1984): *Addictions and Psychological Dysfunction in Nursing: The Profession's Response to the Problem.* Kansas City, ANA.

Beattie, M. (1987): *Co-dependent No More.* Minnesota, Hazelden Foundation.

Beattie, M. (1989): *Beyond Co-dependency.* New York, Harper & Row.

Bissell, L. (1981): The alcoholic nurse. *Nursing Outlook* 29:100-105.

Bissell, L, Haberman, P.W. (1984): *Alcoholism in the Professions.* New York, Oxford University Press.

Borysenko, J. (1987): *Minding the Body, Mending the Mind.* Menlo Park, CA, Addison-Wesley.

Borysenko, J. (1990): *Guilt is the Teacher, Love is the Lesson.* New York, Warner Books.

Branden, N. (1992): *The Power of Self-Esteem.* Deerfield, FL, Health Communications.

Brennan, L. (1983): *The recovering alcoholically impaired nurse: a descriptive study.* Unpublished master's thesis, Rutgers University.

Buscaglia, L. (1991). *Born for Love,* Thorofare, NJ, Slack, Inc.

Compton, P. (1986): Drug abuse: A self-care deficit. *J Psychosocial Nurs* 7:20.

Covey, S. (1989). *Seven Habits of Highly Effective People.* New York, Simon & Schuster.

Cronin-Stubbs, D., Schaffner, J.W. (1985): Professional impairment: Managing the troubled nurse. *Nurs Admin Quart* 9:44.

Edelwich, J, Brodsky, A. (1980): *Burnout: Stages of Disillusionment in Health Professionals.* New York, Human Sciences Press.

Eller, R.A., Bernadine, L.I. (1989): Responding to the chemically dependent student. *J Nurs Educ* 28:87.

Ellsion, C.W. (1983): Spiritual well-being: conceptualization and measurement. *J Psy and Theology.* 11:330-40.

Fassbinder, B. (1992): Time to face the enemy—together. *The American Nurse*, Nov-Dec, 24:4.

Fehring, R.J., Brennan, P.F., Keller, M.L. (1987): Psychological and spiritual well-being in college students. *Res Nurs Health* 10:391.

Firth, H., McIntee, J., McKewon, P., Britton, P. (1986): Burnout and professional depression: Related concepts? *J Adv Nurs* 11:633.

Fischer, K.E. (1987-1988): Adult children of alcoholics: Implications for the nursing profession. *Nurs Forum* 4:159.

Flood, M. (1989): Addictive eating disorders. *Nurs Clin North Am* Philadelphia, W.B. Saunders.

Freudenberger, H.J., North, G. (1985): *Women's Burnout.* Garden City, NY, Doubleday.

Friehl, J.C., Friehl, L.D. (1985): Co-dependence assessment inventory. *Focus on Family*, 3:20.

Friehl, J.C., Friehl, L.D. (1987): Uncovering our frozen feelings: The iceberg model of co-dependence. *Focus on Family* 6:10.

Friehl, J.C., Friehl, L.D. (1988-1989): Excellent word, lousy diagnosis? *Focus on Family* 6:30.

Gordon, V.C., Ledray, L.E. (1985): Depression in women. *J Psychosocial Nurs* 23:26.

Green, P. (1989): The chemically dependent nurse. *Nurs Clin North Am* Philadelphia, W.B. Saunders.

Grissim, M., Spangler, C. (1976): *Womanpower and Health Care.* Boston, MA, Little, Brown.

Haack, M. R. (1987): Alcohol use and burnout among student nurses. *Nurs Health Care* 12:239.

Haack, M.R. (1988): Stress and impairment among nursing students. *Res Nurs Health* 11:125.

Haack, M., Hughes, T. (1989): *Addiction in the Nursing Profession.* New York, Springer Publishing Co.

Hall, S.F., Wray, L.M. (1989): Co-dependency: Nurses who care too much. *Am J Nurs* 11:1456.

Hamilton, J.M., Keifer, M. (1986): *Survival Skills for the New Nurse.* Philadelphia, J.B. Lippincott.

Hill, L., Smith, N. (1985): *Self-Care Nursing.* East Norwalk, CT, Appleton-Century Crofts.

Hingley, P., Cooper, C. (1986): *Stress and the Nurse Manager.* New York, John Wiley.

Hutchinson, S.A. (1986): Chemically dependent nurses: The trajectory toward self-annihilation. *Nurs Res* 35:196.

Hutchinson, S.A. (1987a): Chemically dependent nurses: implications for nurse executives. *J Nurs Admin* 17:23.

Hutchinson, S.A. (1987b): Toward self-integration: The recovery process of chemically dependent nurses. *Nurs Res* 36:399.

Hutchinson, S.A. (1987c): Self-care and job stress. *Image: J Nurs Scholarship* 19:192.

Josefowitz, N. (1980): *Paths to Power.* Menlo Park, CA, Addison-Wesley.

Lawrence, R.M., Lawrence, S. (1987): The nurse and job related stress: Responses, Rx, and self-dependency. *Nurs Forum* 2:34.

Legal Questions (1993): HIV testing: Condition of employment. *Nursing 93.* p. 67.

Lerner, H.G. (1985): *The Dance of Anger.* New York, Harper & Row.

Lerner, H.G. (1988): *Women in Therapy.* New York, Harper & Row.

Lerner, R. (1985): *Daily Affirmations.* Pompano Beach, FL: Health Communications.

Malasch, C. (1982): *The Cost of Caring.* Englewood Cliffs, NJ: Prentice-Hall.

Marram van Servellen, G., Soccorso, E.A., Palermo, K., Faude, K. (1985): Depression in hospital nurses: Implications for nurse managers. *Nurs Admin Quart* 9:74.

Marriner, T.A. (1988): *Guide to Nursing Management.* St. Louis, MO, C.V. Mosby.

Michaels, B. (1990): Antecedents to professional impairment: burnout, depression, codependency and alcohol use in community college nursing students. Major applied research project, Nova University.

Murphy, S.A. (1989): The urgency of substance abuse education in schools of nursing. *J Nurs Educ* 28:2147.

O'Quinn-Larson, J., Pickard, M.R. (1985): The impaired nursing student. *Nurse Educ* 14:36.

Peck, M. (1978): *The Road Less Travelled*. New York, Simon & Schuster.

Powell, J. (1985): *Will the Real Me Please Stand Up?* Allen, TX, Tabor.

Reed, M. (1986): Descriptive study of chemically dependent nurses. *J Psych Nurs Res*, New York, John Wiley and Sons.

Reed, P.G., Leonard, V. (1989): An analysis of the concept of self-neglect. *Adv Nurs Science* 12:39.

Rippere, V., Williams, R., eds. (1985): *Wounded Healers: Mental Health Workers' Experiences of Depression.* New York, John Wiley.

Robbins, C. (1987): A monitored treatment program for health care professionals. *J Nurs Admin.* 17:17-23.

Schaef, A.W. (1987): *When Society Becomes an Addict*. San Francisco, Harper & Row.

Smythe, E.M. (1984): *Surviving Nursing*. Menlo Park, CA, Addison-Wesley.

Steinem, G. (1992): *Revolution from Within: A Book of Self-Esteem*. Boston, Little, Brown, and Co.

Subby, R. (1987): *Co-Dependency: Lost in the Shuffle*. Pompano Beach, FL, Health Communications.

"Toward a State of Self Esteem." The Final Report of the California Task Force to Promote Self-Esteem and Social Responsibility, January, 1990.

Tavris, C, ed. (1984): *Every Woman's Emotional Well-Being*. Garden City, NY: Doubleday.

Tubesing, D.A. Tubesing, N.L. (1983): The Caring Question. Minneapolis, Augsburg.

Wegscheider, D. (1979): *If Only My Family Understood Me*. Minneapolis.

Wegscheider-Cruse, S. (1985): *Choicemaking*. Pompano Beach, FL, Health Communications.

Woods, N. (1989): Conceptualizations of self-care: Toward health-oriented models. *Adv Nurs Sci* 12:1.

Zerwekh, J, Michaels, B. (1989): Co-dependency: Assessment and recovery. *Nurs Clin North Am* Philadelphia, W.B. Saunders.

18

NCLEX-RN and the New Graduate

Jo Carol Claborn, M.S., R.N.

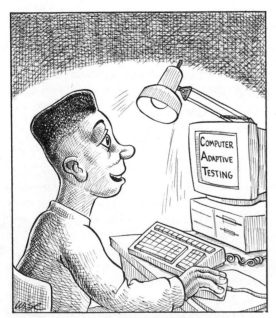

The NCLEX-RN goes computer.

"The way I see it, if you want the rainbow, you gotta put up with the rain."

—Dolly Parton

After completing this chapter, you should be able to:

◆ Discuss the role of the National Council of State Boards of Nursing.

◆ Discuss the implications of computer adaptive testing (CAT).

◆ Identify the process and steps for preparing to take the NCLEX-RN.

◆ Identify criteria for selecting a review book and a review course.

Planning and preparing for the National Council Licensure Examination for Registered Nurses (NCLEX-RN) is an essential component of the transition process. As with other aspects of transition, planning begins before you graduate. Planning ahead will assist you in a more comprehensive preparation, as well as decrease your anxiety about the examination. Being prepared and knowing what to expect will help you to maintain a positive attitude.

THE NATIONAL COUNCIL LICENSURE EXAMINATION for REGISTERED NURSES (NCLEX-RN)

Who Prepares It and Why Do We Have to Have It?

The National Council of State Boards of Nursing is the governing body for the committee that prepares the licensure examination. Each member board or state determines the application process and deadlines in their state, as well as the mechanics of administering the examination. In 1982 the National Council implemented an integrated approach to the design of the paper and pencil test. The same examination was given across the nation on the same day under very similar conditions. Research for the computer administration of the NCLEX began in May 1985 (NCSBN, 1993). The introduction of computer adaptive testing (CAT) in April 1994 changes the way the test is administered. Every state continues to require the same passing level, as this represents a national examination with standardized scoring.

The NCLEX is NOT designed to determine everything you know, nor to determine if you are a capable clinical specialist. Your performance on NCLEX will not influence entry into a baccalaureate or graduate program. The NCLEX is used to regulate entry into nursing practice in the United States. The purpose of the examination is to determine if the candidate is competent to perform safe effective nursing care (NCSBN, 1991). Upon successful completion of the examination, you will be given a license to practice nursing in the state in which you applied for licensure. If you wish to practice nursing in another state, you must contact the state board of nursing in that state for specific directions for licensure. This process is called "licensure by endorsement." You cannot practice nursing in a state without a current license from that state.

The content of the examination is based on a test blueprint that is determined by the National Council. The current blueprint reflects entry level nursing practice as identified by research and the Job Analysis Study of Newly Licensed Registered Nurses, 1989. This research study is conducted by the National Council about every 3 years. The job analysis research in 1984 and 1988 indicated the majority of new graduates were working within a general medical-surgical environment and that is reflected in the current blueprint for the NCLEX (Yocom, 1990). The preliminary findings from the job analysis study completed in October

1992 continue to support the predominance of the medical surgical work environment for the newly licensed registered nurse. The information obtained in the 1992 study will be analyzed with possible impact on future examinations. The current test plan, discussed below, will continue to be implemented with CAT (Yocom, 1993).

The NCLEX-RN Test Plan

The examination is made up of questions that are designed to test the candidate's ability to apply the nursing process and to determine appropriate nursing responses and interventions in order to provide safe nursing care. The test plan is based on the nursing process and areas of client needs.

NURSING PROCESS   Each of the five phases of the nursing process have equal importance. Each of the five phases—*assessing, analyzing, planning, implementing,* and *evaluating*—is weighted equally and constitutes approximately 15 to 25 percent of the questions.

CLIENT NEEDS   There are four categories of health needs as identified by the Job Analysis Study (Yocom, 1990). These are broken down into percentages which reflect the weight of that category on the NCLEX-RN.

- ◆ Safe, effective care environment: 25% to 31%
- ◆ Physiological integrity: 42% to 48%
- ◆ Psychosocial integrity: 9% to 15%
- ◆ Health promotion and maintenance: 12% to 18%

COMPUTER ADAPTIVE TESTING (CAT)

In August 1991, the Assembly of the National Council voted to implement computer adaptive testing for the national licensure examinations. This was decided after extensive research and field testing to determine the validity and reliability of computer testing. A licensure examination, either by paper and pencil or by computer, must be able to measure the competencies required for safe practice and distinguish consistently between candidates who demonstrate those competencies and those who do not (Issues, 1991).

As of April 1994, the National Council of State Boards of Nursing, Inc. is implementing CAT for the NCLEX, for both practical/vocational nurses (NCLEX-PN/VN) and registered nurses (NCLEX-RN). This represents a major advancement in the implementation and administration of the examination. NCLEX CAT is based on the same test plan as the paper and pencil NCLEX, multiple choice questions will be continued to be utilized. The same type of client care/nursing knowledge will be tested. The National Council has conducted extensive research in preparation for the transition from a paper and pencil test to a computer based examination. Sylvan/KEE Systems has contracted with the National Council to administer the NCLEX in the Sylvan Learning Systems centers. The information presented here is to introduce you to NCLEX-RN CAT. It is important that you carefully follow the information and instructions you receive from your state board of nurse examiners, as each state still has the responsibility for the administration of the examination.

What Does CAT Mean?

With CAT, each candidate receives a different set of questions via the computer. The computer develops an examination that is unique to that candidate. The questions to be presented to the candidate are determined by the response of the candidate to the previous questions. The number of questions each candidate receives and the testing time for each candidate will vary. The questions presented will continue to reflect the NCLEX plan based on the nursing process, client needs, and the job analysis survey. CAT is not to be confused with Computerized Clinical Simulation Testing (CST). CST presents a clinical situation in which the candidate may demonstrate problem solving and decision making ability; it is not multiple choice testing. CAT is all multiple choice questions. However, the examination is "adapted" to the individual candidate who is taking the examination (NCSBN, 1991).

"Tryout" questions will continue to be integrated into the examination. These are questions that allow the council to gather statistical information to determine whether a question is valid and can be added to the test bank of questions for future selection (NCSBN, 1993). Don't get alarmed—these questions are not counted in the grading of the examination and time has been allocated for the candidate to answer these questions. These questions were used in the paper and pencil test, and will continue to be used in CAT.

What Is the Application Process for CAT?

As in the past the school of nursing will have the candidates complete the application forms and submit them to the state board of nurse examiners. Each candidate will receive instructions as well as telephone numbers and addresses of the Sylvan Learning Systems centers that will be administering the examination. Read your instruction packet carefully. Candidates will also receive an "Authorization to Test," which will be required for admission into the testing centers. Application forms for the examination may be obtained by contacting the respective board of nurse examiners. All candidates will be thumbprinted and photographed at the testing location.

Where Do I Take the Test?

There will be approximately 200 testing sites, with at least one in each state. The candidate will receive information regarding the locations of the centers and may select the center that is most convenient. There will be approximately 10 testing stations at each center. A candidate may take the test at any of the testing sites in the United States; however, license to practice will be given only in the state in which the application was submitted.

When Do I Take the Test?

After receiving approval from the respective State Board of Nursing, a candidate may contact the Sylvan Learning Systems center to schedule the examination. The staff will schedule an appointment for the candidate. Testing center hours will be extended as necessary to accommodate the candidates.

How Much Time Do I Have and How Many Questions Are There?

Each candidate is scheduled for a 5-hour time slot. The candidate must answer at least 75 questions. The candidate may take up to 265 items, or test over a 5-hour time frame. CAT will end when the student:

- ◆ measures at a level of competence above or below the standard and at least 75 questions have been answered.
- ◆ completes a maximum of 265 questions.
- ◆ has been testing for the maximum time frame of 5 hours (NCSBN, 1993).

Do I Have to Be "Computer Literate"?

It is not necessary to study from a computer or that you be "computer literate." Research has demonstrated that candidates who were not accustomed to working on a computer did as well as those who were very comfortable with the computer. So prior computer experience is not a prerequisite to passing the NCLEX!

How Will I Keep the Computer Keys Straight?

There are only two keys to be concerned with, the ENTER key and the "space bar" key. All other keys will be turned off and will not affect the test. The space bar key will be used to move through the answer options. The ENTER key will allow the candidate to record the answer and the computer screen will automatically progress to the next question. At the testing site each candidate will be oriented to the computer and will go through a keyboard practice/orientation process. Every effort will be made to make sure that the candidate understands and is comfortable with the testing procedure.

What Is the Passing Score?

Every state requires the same passing criteria. Specific individual scores will not be available to you, your school, or your place of employment. Your score will be reported directly to you as pass or fail. A composite of student results will be mailed to the respective schools of nursing. There is no specific published "score" or number that represents passing.

How Will I Know I Have Passed?

The implementation of CAT makes results available on a more timely basis. The results from the testing centers will be wired directly to the state board of nurse examiners. It is anticipated that the candidates will be advised in writing by their board of nursing within 1 to 3 weeks of taking the examination. This is a projected time frame and may fluctuate somewhat as the new process is implemented and each state begins to change its system of reporting results to graduates.

What Difference Does a CAT Examination Make in How I Need to Study?

You should study in the same manner as you would for a paper and pencil test. Review courses and review books that reflect the NCLEX-CAT plan and focus on nursing care will continue to be very appropriate tools to assist you in preparation for the examination (McKay, 1990).

Will the Questions be Different From Those of the Paper and Pencil Test?

Since 1988, the new questions placed in the test bank have consisted of individual questions. This means there will not be a series of questions based on a situation. The questions on the paper and pencil test reflect the type of question to be found on CAT. The way the question is presented on the computer screen will be a little different from the way questions are traditionally presented on the paper and pencil test. (Fig. 18–1) (Bersky, 1992).

What Are the Technical Aspects of the NCLEX?

◆ All questions are multiple choice with four options. Some questions are "stand alone," and some relate to a situation and background information.

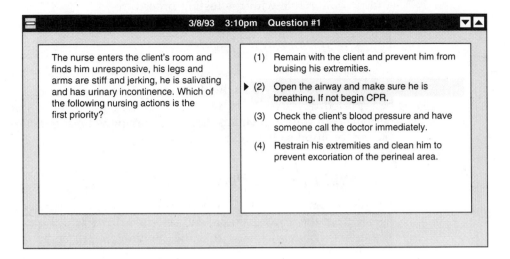

FIGURE 18–1   *Example of an NCLEX-RN CAT Question.*

In either type of question, all of the information for the question will be available on the computer screen.

◆ If you need scratch paper, it will be provided and you will be required to turn it in.

◆ You may not take calculators into the examination.

◆ Everyone will be tested on the same bank of questions and the same test plan.

◆ There is only one answer to each question; you do not get any "partial credit" for an answer—it is either right or wrong.

◆ All questions must be answered, even if you have to make a wild guess. The computer selects the next question based on the response to the previous question. (In other words, it would confuse the computer if you tried to skip questions.)

◆ You will not be able to go back to a previous question once that question has been removed from the screen. (You can't go back and change your answer to the wrong one!)

◆ There will be a mandatory 10-minute rest period after 2 hours of testing.

◆ If you need to take a break prior to the 2 hours, notify one of the testing administrators.

◆ There will be lockers at the testing site for your personal items (Issues, 1993).

What if I Need to Change the Time or Date I Have Already Scheduled?

You can change your testing date and time if you advise the testing center at least 3 business days in advance. You can then reschedule the test at no additional cost. If a candidate does not show at the scheduled testing time, then all testing fees will be forfeited and an additional registration form and fee will be required.

What Are the Advantages of CAT for the Candidate?

- ◆ An environment that is quiet and conducive to testing.
- ◆ The work surface will be large enough to accommodate both right- and left-handed people with adequate room for the computer and scratch paper.
- ◆ The time frame is much more relaxed—there is a total of 5 hours. Candidates can work at their own pace.
- ◆ Each person will have his or her own testing station or cubicle. You will not be distracted by the other candidates who are testing at the same time.
- ◆ Personal items will be safe at the testing site.
- ◆ Security will be easier to maintain, eliminating the distraction of proctors moving through the testing area.

The bottom line here on CAT: it is not something to be afraid of.

It is simply a different way of testing than you may be familiar with. The same type of nursing knowledge will be required to pass the NCLEX whether it is a computer test or on a paper and pencil test (Bersky, 1992).

PREPARING FOR THE NCLEX-RN

Where and When Should I Start?

Six Months Prior to the NCLEX

Make Sure You Know the Deadlines and Application Process for Your State. Your school will advise you as to the specific dates the forms are due to the state office. Make sure you follow the directions exactly. State boards of nursing do not respond favorably to applications that are not submitted on time or are submitted in an incorrect format. A listing of the state boards of nursing can be found in Appendix A. If you plan on applying for licensure in another state, it is your responsibility to contact the board of nursing in that state to obtain your papers for application. Plan early to investigate the feasibility of taking the examination in another state.

Investigate Formal Review Courses.   Review courses can assist you in organizing your study materials and identifying areas in which you need to focus your study time. The percentage of graduates passing the examination is higher for those who participated in a formal review course (Zerwekh, 1986).

Evaluate Your Goals and Preferences for Employment.   Working on a general medical-surgical unit will provide experience you may not have been able to obtain during school. The NCLEX-RN has a lot of questions based on common nursing care activities found on medical-surgical units. Some hospitals pay for a formal review, some only give time off to attend, and others do not offer any assistance.

Evaluate Hospital Orientation Programs Carefully.   An extensive orientation program with a preceptor will assist you in obtaining a different perspective on patient care. Remember, your nursing instructors do not write the NCLEX. An experienced nurse will help you to apply theory to patient care from a practicing perspective. A preceptor is an excellent resource for on-the-spot explanations and assistance. It is to your benefit to work with a preceptor or an experienced nurse to understand different perspectives, which leads ultimately to a better understanding of nursing care concepts and interventions. Once you have passed the NCLEX, then evaluate if you want to stay in the same environment or transfer to a specialty area.

Plan an Expense Account for the End of School and NCLEX.   Frequently students are caught at the end of school with unexpected expenses, one of which may be the fees for the NCLEX and another the travel/hotel expenses for staying at the testing site. Start a small "stash"—maybe $5 a week—to help defer these expenses. For inquiring friends who want to "give you something for graduation," you might start a "wish list" for those expenses incurred at graduation.

Two Months Prior to the NCLEX: What Do I Need to Do Now?

If You Have a Job, Discuss with Your Supervisor Your Anticipated NCLEX-RN Test Date and Submit Your Request for Days Off in Writing as Soon as Your Test Date Is Confirmed.   Hospitals may not be aware of the new scheduling procedure for the examination. In the past all new candidates took the examination on the same day; now each candidate schedules her or his own testing date. Plan on taking off the day before the examination and if possible the day after also. This will allow you time to relax and, if necessary, travel to and from the testing site.

BOX 18–1

Budget for End of School and NCLEX

How Much Is It Going to Cost Me to Get Out of School?

◆ *Required Expenses*

Graduating fees from college or university   _____

Application fees for NCLEX-RN   _____

Passport-type picture (may be required for state application)   _____

◆ *Expenses to Take NCLEX-RN*

Travel—car, bus, airfare   _____

Hotel accommodations at NCLEX testing site   _____

Miscellaneous (food, transportation to site, etc.)   _____

◆ *Optional Expenses*

Assess test (e.g., Mosby or NLN)   _____

School pin   _____

Uniform or cap and gown for graduation   _____

Graduation expenses passed on to graduate   _____

Graduation pictures (class or individual)   _____

Graduation invitations   _____

NCLEX-RN review course (need to plan this before school is out)   _____
NCLEX-RN review book(s) (get these early— really helps with the last year of nursing school!)   _____

◆ *Expenses After Graduation (It's Not Over Yet!)*

Professional organizations (most organizations will give a discount on new membership to the graduate nurse)   _____

Professional journals   _____

Uniform, scrub suits, shoes to begin new job   _____
Professional liability insurance (check with the school regarding transfer from school policy to individual policy)   _____

Decide How You Are Going to Get to the Test Site and Where You Will Stay.   If the closest testing site is not easily accessible, is more than a 1-hour drive away, or involves driving through a heavily congested traffic area, you may need to consider staying overnight in a hotel room close to the site. For some graduates this will prevent unnecessary hassle and increased anxiety on the day of the examination. If you are going to fly, you need to make your reservations early to get the best deal on the ticket. Be aware, though, that bargain fares frequently have restrictions. How will you get from the airport to the hotel, and to the testing site?

Be sure to guarantee your room with a credit card so the hotel will not give it up to someone else if you are late coming in. If a group of graduates are traveling together and have been able to schedule the examination on the same day, consideration should be given to planning the hotel accommodations. Don't have a crowd in your room. Plan on having a bed to sleep in. Five people in a room designed for two or four will not be conducive to sleep the night before the examination! If you are rooming with another person, select someone you like and can tolerate in close quarters for a short period of time. Surround yourself with people who have a positive attitude; you don't need complainers and negative thinkers.

Develop a Plan for Studying.   Do you need to study alone, or do you benefit from group study time? Set yourself a study schedule that you can realistically stick to. Two to three hours a day for 2 or 3 days a week is realistic; 8 hours a day on your days off doesn't work. If you take a formal review course, plan your study time to gain the most from the review course. A review course is not meant to be your only study time. There will be areas you need to focus on for your individual learning needs. Priority areas to study are those you are the weakest in; focus on these first.

One Week to the NCLEX

Make Sure You Have All of Your Papers Required for Admission.   Read your information packet again. The "authorization to test" that you receive from the Educational Testing Service (ETS) will be required at the testing site. The information packet that you receive from the ETS should have all of the necessary information and directions needed for the test site. Check to see if there is anything else you will need to take with you to the site.

The Day Before the BIG DAY

Don't Take All of Your Class Notes From the Past 3 Years and All of Your Nursing Textbooks to the Hotel or to the Test Site.   Last-minute cramming will increase your anxiety, and you cannot take any type of study materials into the testing area.

Make a "Test Run" to the Site the Evening Before the Test.   Find the parking areas. If your hotel is within four to six blocks of the test site, the walk will be a terrific way to help reduce anxiety and get the blood circulating to your brain! Whether you drive or walk to the site, go the day before to make sure you know where you are going.

Go to Bed Early, Don't Study or Party.   Plan on eating a light dinner, something that will not disagree with your stomach—you don't need to be up half of the night with heartburn and/or diarrhea!

The BIG DAY Is Here

Eat a Good Breakfast, Not Sweet Rolls and Coffee.   Protein and complex carbohydrates will help sustain you during the examination. Don't drink a lot of coffee—you don't need to be distracted by frequent bathroom trips. Security is strict, if you need to go to the bathroom, a security person may go with you.

Dress Comfortably.   Anticipate that the temperature at the testing sites will be a little cool rather than too warm. Don't wear tight clothes that restrict your breathing when you sit down! Dress casually and comfortably, and be prepared with a sweater or light jacket just in case you need it.

Arrive At the Test Site a Little Early.   This will allow you time to get checked in and prevent anxiety about being late.

HOW DO I SELECT AN NCLEX REVIEW COURSE?

There are many review courses available to assist the graduate nurse in preparing for the NCLEX. Before you sign up, evaluate which course will be most beneficial to you. In considering a review course, remember the objective is to review, not primary learning.

What Type of Review Courses Are Available?

Evaluate your geographic location. Which review courses are easily accessible? Are you considering traveling to another city to attend a review course? Collect data on all of the courses, then compare to see which best meets your needs and budget. Check with your prospective employer regarding time off and scheduling. Plan ahead and make an intelligent decision regarding review courses. Do not feel that you must sign up with the first review company that contacts you!

Carefully evaluate your need for a review course. Are you the type of student who can plan study time, establish a study review schedule, and stick to it? Were you in the top 25% of your graduating class? Have you had experience working in a hospital with adult medical-surgical clients, other than while you were in school? As a new graduate do you feel comfortable and ready for the examination? If you can answer "yes" to all of these questions, you may not want to consider a review course in your preparation for the NCLEX-RN. The majority of nursing students and/or graduates are able to say "yes" to one or two of these questions, but not all of them.

What Are the Qualifications of the Review Course Instructors?

In order to teach a review course effectively, the instructor needs to be familiar with the NCLEX. That ability is most often found in instructors who have recent teaching experience in a school of nursing. Some hospitals provide "in-house" review courses taught by excellent clinical specialists. Determine if these instructors are familiar with the NCLEX plan. If the information is not a focus of the NCLEX plan, it does not need to be included in a review course. It is also important to find out if the review faculty is from a school of nursing in your immediate area. It is possible you will be paying for a review course to be taught by your same nursing school faculty. A review course should be taught from a different perspective. This different perspective helps to anchor information and promote reinforcement of previous learning. Look for a course that brings faculty in from areas outside your school.

How Many Instructors Teach the Course?

There may be a new instructor every day, there may be two instructors for the course, or there may be only one instructor for the entire course. If you like variety, you may prefer a new instructor every day. If you like time to adjust to how a person teaches, then two instructors for the course may be better suited to your learning style. Having one person to teach the entire course is a questionable practice, they have to have excellent teaching skills, a very wide knowledge base, a strong voice, and exceptional endurance to teach the entire course. There are, however, some review course faculty who can do this exceptionally well.

What Type of Instructional Materials Are Used in the Course?

Are the materials an additional course expense? Do you get to keep the materials after the course is over? Are handouts, workbooks, audio tapes, books, and other materials used to enhance learning? Be concerned if there are no course outlines, workbooks, handouts, or books; you might spend all of your time writing and miss listening to the necessary information. Do the course materials include practice test questions that are similar in format to the NCLEX? Ask how the material is organized, what is the format (integrated, blocked, systems, etc)? How does the format compare to the NCLEX plan of client needs and nursing process? These are all important questions to ask. Each graduate needs to determine which of these areas are the most important to their learning style.

How Is the Course Taught?

Are overhead transparencies or slides used to enhance learning? Is the presentation given by a "live person"? Some courses may have video and audio tapes rather than a person you can actually speak to and ask questions.

Does the Course Include Instruction in Test-Taking Skills and Practice?

Test taking skills and practice are a very important aspect of a review course. The graduate needs to begin to practice taking a test written by someone other than their nursing school faculty.

How Much Does the Course Cost?

Most review courses cost about $200 to $250. Frequently there is a discount for early registration, and there may also be a discount for group registration. Make sure you understand the review company policy regarding "deposit" and/or "registration fee." Sometimes there are hidden charges that may be tacked on to the end. Make sure you understand the cancellation policy. Some companies will let you pay a deposit, with the total amount due by a certain date. Check out the possibility of organizing a group; some courses give a free review or a discount to the group organizer.

How Long Does It Last?

Is the course 3, 4, or 5 consecutive days? Is it given only in the evenings? Is it taught only on the weekend for 6 weeks? This is very important to determine early in your evaluation of review courses. Compare the price with the length of the course; are you getting your money's worth? Notify your employer as soon as possible if you need to fit the review into your work schedule. Most hospitals will arrange the new graduate's schedule to allow attendance at a review course. Some hospitals even provide a review course as a benefit to the new graduate nurse employee! Once you have determined which review course you wish to take, discuss it with your prospective employers, or notify your current employer as soon as possible. It is important to provide adequate advance notice to your employer in order that staffing schedules may be planned.

Where Is the Course Held?

Are you going to have to drive for an hour every day? Will you need to obtain a hotel room? Ask about parking. Is there going to be a charge for parking? What is the availability of inexpensive restaurants in the area? Is food going to be a major expense?

What Are the Statistics Regarding the Pass Rate for the Company?

The national average for first time test-takers is approximately 87%. It is very appropriate to inquire about how the pass rate statistics are determined by the company. The review company must obtain the results directly from course participants or from schools of nursing. The National Council does not make this information available to the review companies. Find out if the advertised pass rate is based on actual responses from participants or from projected figures from the company.

Does the Review Company Offer Any Type of Guarantee?

Some review companies will offer you a free review course and/or a home study guide if you are not successful on the examination. Find out what the guarantee means and who is eligible for it. Make sure you get in writing what you must do in order to be eligible and to file for the benefit, if necessary.

What Is the Size of the Class?

Some review course classes will have several hundred participants. One problem resulting from a large class is that if you don't get there an hour early, you don't get a seat where you can see or hear. There are some review companies that limit the enrollment depending on the classroom environment. Ask about the size of the class and the classroom environment.

When Is the Course Offered?

Some graduates prefer to take a review course just before the examination so the information is still fresh in their minds. The majority of graduates prefer to take the review within 2 to 3 weeks prior to the examination. This allows time to organize and study those areas that are the weakest. With CAT it is important to determine when you want to schedule your NCLEX-RN date and plan your review course accordingly. If you have only one review course available, how does it fit with your plans for scheduling the examination? Another aspect to consider is your employment schedule. Can you get time off from work? If your employer will not give you the time off, you may need to take a review course as early in the day as possible so you can go to work. Try to arrange your review course time so you can focus on reviewing the information. If you have to work nights or evenings during the course, you will not benefit as much from the review. Frequently review programs will have home study assignments during the course.

Call the review company to get your questions answered. Do they spend time on the phone with you, or are they in a rush to get you off the phone? Ask what makes their course better than another course. Is the company representative friendly and knowledgeable, and does that person demonstrate concern for answering all of your questions?

Ultimately, each graduate must decide whether or not to take a review course and which review course is right. The more informed you are regarding a review course, the more intelligent a decision you can make.

NCLEX-RN REVIEW BOOKS

Which One Is Right for You?

It is important to select a review book that meets your study needs. The first step is to check out your choices. Nursing faculty, friends with review books,

---

BOX 18–2

Selecting an NCLEX Review Course: Questions I Need to Answer

Courses Available in Area	Dates	Location	Telephone Number
1.			
2.			
3.			

Courses Outside Immediate Area	Dates	Location	Telephone Number
1.			
2.			
3.			

Continued

BOX 18–2

Selecting an NCLEX Review Course: Questions I Need to Answer Continued

Where am I going to work? _____

Will the institution pay for the review? _____

Will the institution pay the initial fee or do I need to plan for reimburse-ment? _____

Does the Institution Provide an On-Site Review?

Who teaches it? _____

Is it an independent company or hospital employees? _____

Review Course Instructors

What type of degrees do the instructors have?

Bachelors in Nursing _____

Masters Degree _____

Doctorate Degree _____

How much teaching experience? _____

Was experience in a school of nursing or in hospital inservice? _____

Where is the instructor currently employed or teaching? _____

How many instructors teach the review course? _____

What Type of Instructional Material Is Used?

Does it cost extra from the registration fee? _____

If it is additional to registration fee, where do I get it? _____

Can I keep all of the instructional materials? (books, testing booklets, audio tapes, etc.) _____

Does the instructional material include practice test questions in the NCLEX format? _____

Can I get any of the course materials ahead of time to begin study-ing? _____

BOX 18–2

Selecting an NCLEX Review Course: Questions I Need to Answer
Continued

How Are the Classes Conducted?

How many days? _____

Are days consecutive or spread over several weeks? _____

What are the hours each day? _____

What type of audio visual aids are used? _____

What is the teaching style: (group work, lecture, home study, group participation, testing practice, etc.) _____

_____

_____

What is the average size class for the area? _____

How Much Does It Cost?

What is the total price? _____

Does this include all of the class materials? _____

What is the per hour or per day cost? (this will help to evaluate cost effectiveness of various types of programs) _____

Are there group rates and what are they? _____

Are there early registration discounts? _____

When does the money have to be in? _____

Are there any "extra incentives"? _____

How Do I Pay for It?

Credit card _____

Personal check _____

Money order/cashiers check _____

Is there a payment plan? _____

Continued

BOX 18–2

Selecting an NCLEX Review Course: Questions I Need to Answer
Continued

Can I make an early deposit to hold my space? _____

When is the deposit due? When is the final amount due? _____

If I change my mind after I make the deposit, can I get the deposit

back? _____

Is There a Guarantee?

What is the guarantee? _____

Can I take the review over again? _____

Does it have to be in the same location as first time? _____

What do I have to do to qualify for the guarantee? _____

Do I get further assistance in identifying areas of need and studying for

next time? _____

What Is the Pass Rate and How Is It Determined?

Is it based on all new graduates who took review? _____

Is it a company survey of participants after NCLEX? _____

Is it based on all participants, or only the first time takers? _____

Is it based on direct response from students, and if so how many were

surveyed? _____

Is it based on the company projected success rate of course? _____

Did the review company answer all of my questions in a courteous manner

and seem interested in my business? _____

Do you know anyone who has taken a review? _____

What are their recommendations? _____

_____

_____

_____

_____

the school library, and the local nursing textbook stores are all sources of information regarding review books. There are two primary kinds of nursing review books, those with content review, and those that consist totally of review questions. Evaluate how the book should be used: is it for study during school, or is it specifically for review for the NCLEX? For example, if you bought the review book to study pediatric nursing, you may be disappointed. The focus of the NCLEX is not on pediatrics, therefore it is not often a strong component in review books. If you wish to use a review book to identify priority aspects of care in the medical-surgical client, however, a review book can be of great benefit. The following discussion of review book selection is directed primarily toward review books that contain content review. Take notes as you review the different selections; it is hard to remember all the positive and negative points of each book (Box 18–3). Plan on purchasing a review book while you are still in nursing school. Review books are revised about every 3 years.

Do an Overview

Is the type style and size comfortable to read? Does the page layout enhance reading and finding information? Are there graphics, charts, and/or diagrams? Is the information outlined or is it narrative style? Is it difficult to read a constant narrative text?

Scan the Table of Contents

Is the information presented in a logical sequence? How is the information organized? Review books generally follow two basic formats. The *block format* presents information according to medical-surgical, psychosocial, pediatric, and obstetric nursing content. You may find that information is repeated with the block format, for example, respiratory concepts and care are discussed in three different areas: adult medical-surgical client, obstetric client, and pediatric client.

The second format for organization of information is the *integrated format*. There are many different ways of presenting information in an integrated format. It is important that the information be organized in a manner that is logical to you. The NCLEX is based on an integrated format using the nursing process and client needs. Read the introduction to see how these areas were considered in the organization of the text.

Quickly scan the table of contents and check the number of pages in various areas of subject material. Where is the focus of the material?

Check Out the Authors

Are the authors currently involved with preparing the graduate nurse to take the NCLEX? Professional backgrounds are important in evaluating whether or not the author is likely to be most knowledgeable about the current status of the NCLEX.

Evaluate Chapter Layout

How well is the material organized within the chapter? Are there major headings and subheadings to assist you in finding information quickly? Some texts use two-toned shading, boxes, or a second color to highlight divisions of content or priority information. These may not be points you have identified in previous textbooks, however, it helps to decrease the monotony of constant reading and to increase interest in the material presented.

Evaluate Content

Select a topic(s) you would like to read in each of the review books you are considering. Select the priority nursing concepts and interventions you want to identify (for example, nursing care of the diabetic client is a high-priority area). Evaluate the information regarding the adult, pediatric, obstetric client. How does the information compare in the review books you are considering? Is the material logically organized, does it contain the major concepts of care for that particular concept? The focus of the book should be toward nursing care, not medical diagnosis, pharmacology, or pathophysiology. In evaluating the currency of content, keep in mind that you can't expect information that came out last month to be reflected in any textbook. Remember, the NCLEX is more heavily weighted toward the medical-surgical client.

Evaluate the Index

Take several common topics and look them up in the index. A good index is critical to finding information in a timely manner.

Test Questions

Are test questions included in the text? Questions may be found after each of the main chapters, or grouped together at the end of the book. Check to see if a rationale for the correct answer is included for each question.

Test-Taking Strategies

Does the book include information on test-taking strategies for multiple choice questions? Test-taking strategies help you to be more "test wise." These strategies can be of great benefit while you are still in school, as well as while you prepare for the NCLEX.

BOX 18–3

Selecting a Review Book—Where Do I Start?

What is available?   Content review   Questions Only   Cost

    1. _____

    _____

    2. _____

    _____

    3. _____

    _____

    4. _____

    _____

References from other students and faculty: _____

_____

_____

_____

For use during school or only for NCLEX Review? _____

Does the review course I am considering provide a review book? _____

What does the review book look like?

    Type style, is it easy to read? _____

    Outline or narrative format? _____

    Quality of the paper—does it bleed through when highlighted? ____

    Is the Table of Contents helpful? _____

What is the organization pattern of the book? _____

Is the information blocked or integrated? _____

What is in the content? _____

Is the primary focus on nursing care? _____

Are the high priority areas easily identified and adequately covered? ____

Is there a comprehensive index? _____

Continued

BOX 18–3

Selecting a Review Book—Where Do I Start? Continued

Evaluate each book being considered for these areas:

     Care of diabetic client (OB, pedi, and adult) _____

     Care of client with myocardial infarction _____

     Care of pediatric respiratory problems _____

     Nursing care in the labor client _____

How easy is the information to find and to understand? _____

Does it cover the priorities of nursing care? _____

Where are the medications, treatments, and diagnostics for each of these topics? _____

Are there test questions included in the content review book? _____

Are the questions at the end of each chapter? _____

Are the questions in a study guide format? _____

Are there sample test(s) to practice test taking skills? _____

Are the sample tests integrated, blocked (pedi, OB, medical), or reflective of previous chapter material? _____

Does the book include the correct answers and rationale for all of the test questions? _____

Is information repeated in different areas? _____

Where is the focus of the content? _____

Test taking strategies—are they included in the book? _____

Are the testing strategies easy to understand and to apply? _____

Can you identify immediate application of testing strategies? _____

_____

_____

WHAT DIFFERENCE DOES TEST-TAKING STRATEGIES MAKE?

This information can be of benefit to you now, and later. Start putting into practice some of these tips, and they will be second nature when you take the NCLEX.

Knowing how to take an examination is a skill that is developed through practice. Look back at the beginning of nursing school and your first nursing examination—have you come a long way from there! How many times during school have you reviewed a test and discovered you knew the right answer, but marked the wrong one? Nursing faculty and those responsible for the NCLEX are not sympathetic to your claim that you "really meant this answer and not the one you marked." How many times did you go back and change an answer from the correct response to the wrong one? Perhaps the reason you have missed questions you know the answer to is because your testing practices are faulty. Some of the testing practices you have developed over the years may be positive, some may be negative. Analyze where you are with testing skills, get rid of the negative, and retain the positive.

Test Anxiety—What Is the Disease? How Do You Get Rid of It?

Frequently students and graduates focus on their "test anxiety" as the reason for not doing well on examinations. Test anxiety is something that you can change. You are the one allowing the anxiety to affect you in a negative way. The only person responsible for your test anxiety is yourself and the only one who can do anything about it is you. Look at some simple steps to decrease your anxiety regarding testing.

Plan Ahead.   Don't wait till the last minute to read the 150 pages in your textbook, review all your classroom notes, and read the 10 articles assigned for the test. Plan study time and stick to it!

Set Aside Study Time When You Are At Your Best.   Frequently study time is scheduled at a time when everything else (laundry, meals, housecleaning, yard work, etc.) is taken care of. You are defeating your purpose and increasing anxiety when you try to study at a time when you are not receptive to learning.

Give Yourself a Break!   Plan your study time to include a break about every hour. Your retention of information begins to decrease after about 30 minutes and is significantly decreased after an hour.

Think Positive!   If your friends are "negative thinkers," don't plan on studying with them. Go to the movies or play sports with them, but don't study with them. Anxiety and negative thinking are contagious—don't expose yourself to the disease!

Don't Cram.   Exams during nursing school and the NCLEX are not written to evaluate memory-based information. Frequently, tests focus on the application of principles and the analysis of information in order to determine an appropriate nursing response or action. Don't jeopardize your critical thinking skills by staying up late and cramming.

Just thinking about an examination can cause some students an increase in anxiety. It seems as though during the last year of school, particularly the last semester, tests become a major source of anxiety. Everyone knows fellow students who become obsessed with the idea they are going to fail an important examination. It is essential that examinations be viewed in a positive manner—get rid of those negative thought tapes! Put yourself in charge of your feelings. Replace those negative thoughts and ideas with positive ones: "I will pass this test." Write down positive affirmations and put them on your bathroom mirror, on your refrigerator, anywhere you will see them often. Potential employers, state boards of nursing, your preacher, and your neighbors are not going to think less of you if you are not at the top of the class. Keep in mind that your employers and the state board do not care what your grades were in school or on the NCLEX, they just want to know that you can practice nursing safely. So back off, give yourself permission to be in the middle, an average student on grades, but one who is concerned about professional safe nursing practice.

What Are Strategies for Answering Multiple Choice Questions?

On the NCLEX, multiple choice test questions have a stem where the question is presented and four options from which to choose an answer. Of these four options, three are meant to distract you from the correct answer. There is only one correct answer. (Unlike during school, you cannot bargain for any extra points!) The NCLEX will contain multiple choice questions where the options give you the choice of four answers (for example, 1. A; 2. B), not a combination of the four options (for example 1.A, B, C).

Read the Question (Stem) Carefully.   DO NOT read extra meaning into the question. Make sure you read the stem correctly and understand exactly what information is being requested (do you tend to make the client sicker than he really is by the time you finish the question?).

Create a Pool of Answers.   What do you anticipate the answer to include? Get a general idea before you read the options.

Evaluate All the Options in a Systematic Manner.   Focus on what information is being requested, then carefully go through each option. Do not stop with the first correct answer; the last option may be more correct or more inclusive of information.

Eliminate Options You Know Are Not Correct.   *And leave them alone!* Once you have eliminated an option, don't go back to it unless you have gained more insight into the question. Frequently your initial response to a question is correct.

Identify Similarities in the Options.   Find the one that is different. The option that is different may be the correct answer. For example, in a question dealing with a low-residue diet, three of the options might contain a vegetable with a peeling, but one option does not, that one is probably the correct answer. Evaluate options that contain several suggested client activities; are the activities similar, but one different?

Evaluate Priority Questions Very Carefully.   Keep in mind the nursing process and Maslow's Hierarchy of Needs. You must obtain adequate assessment information before proceeding with the nursing process. According to Maslow, physical needs must be met before psychosocial needs—your mental health client needs his basic physical needs met before you can focus on mental health. Of the physical needs, respiratory needs are a priority. (You've got to breathe first!)

Select Answers That Focus On the Client.   Choices that focus on hospital rules and polices are most often not correct (Zerwekh, 1991).

Analyze your testing skills so that you will know where to start to improve them. Once you have identified your testing weaknesses, then organize a plan to correct the problem areas. One of the most difficult things to do is to change the way you are used to doing something, even when it makes life easier. Get an early start on evaluating testing skills; it can make a significant difference in the remaining examinations in nursing school.

Wow! NCLEX deadlines, review courses, testing skills, review books, money, license . . . and all you thought you needed to do was graduate from nursing school! There are a lot of steps in between graduating from nursing school and being successful on the NCLEX. The key to surviving it all with a smile is careful planning and implementing those plans during your role transition. (That sounds a lot like the nursing process doesn't it?) The NCLEX-RN is one of the most incredible opportunities of your life. This examination will open the doors for you as you begin one of the most fantastic experiences of a lifetime: a career in nursing.

REFERENCES

Bersky, A: *Computerized Adaptive Testing*. National Council of State Boards of Nursing, Inc. NCLEX Third Regional Invitational, New Orleans, April 22–23, 1992.

Bouchard, J: Future directions for the National Council: The Computerized Adaptive Testing Project. *Issues* 11, No. 4 (1990): 1–3.

Burckhardt, JA: NCLEX—fact or fiction? *Graduating Nurse*. Fall (1991): 15.

Colombraro, GC: Preparing for state boards—which review course is right for you? *Nursing 91* October (1991): 12–14.

Lagerquist, S: The NCLEX Game Plan. *Graduating Nurse* Spring (1992): 9.

McKay, M: The experience of a CAT field test State. *Issues* 11, #4 (1990).

National Council of State Boards of Nursing, Inc: *The NCLEX Process*. Chicago, 1991a.

National Council of State Boards of Nursing, Inc: Work plan for CAT transition. *Issues* 12; No. 4 (1991b): 3.

National Council of State Boards of Nursing, Inc: NCLEX Third Regional Invitational, New Orleans, April 22–23, 1992.

National Council of State Boards of Nursing, Inc: *Introduction to Computerized Adaptive Testing (CAT) for NCLEX*. National Council of State Boards of Nursing, Inc., Chicago: 1992, video.

National Council of State Boards of Nursing, Inc: Field tests of NCLEX using computerized adaptive testing. *Issues* Special Edition (1993).

Rayfield, S: Countdown to the NCLEX-RN exam. *Nursing 91*, October (1991a): 6–10.

Rayfield, S: What you should know about the NCLEX-RN exam. *Nursing 91* October (1991b): 10–11.

Stockert, P: Konaradi, D: NCLEX-RN preparation: Three steps for success. *Imprint* January (1992): 6–9.

Wendt, A., et al: Computer simulation: The time is now. *Issues* 12, No. 1 (1991): 5.

Yocom, C: et al: *Job Analysis for Newly Licenses Registered Nurses—1989*. National Council of State Boards of Nursing, Inc., Chicago, 1990.

Yocom, C: Progress report—job analysis study of entry level registered nurses. National Council of State Boards of Nursing, Inc. *Issues* 14, No. 1 (1993).

Zerwekh, J: *A Delphi Study of Factors Influencing Nursing Students to Enroll in Review Courses*. Dissertation, East Texas State University, 1986.

Zerwekh, J., Claborn, JC: *NCLEX-RN: A Comprehensive Study Guide*. Nursing Education Consultants, Dallas, 1991.

APPENDICES

Appendix A

Boards of Nursing

Alabama Board of Nursing
Ste. 203, 500 Eastern Blvd.
Montgomery, AL 36117
(205)261-4060

Alaska Board of Nursing
Dept. of Comm. & Econ.
Develop.
Div. of Occupational
Licensing
3601 C St., Ste. 722
Anchorage, AK 99503
(907)561-2878

American Samoa Health
Services Regulatory Board
LBJ Tropical Medical
Center
Pago Pago, American
Samoa 96799
(684)633-1222 Ext. 206

Arizona Board of Nursing
1651 E. Morten Ave.,
Suite 150
Phoenix, AZ 85020
(602)255-5092

Arkansas Board of Nursing
1123 South University
Little Rock, AR 72204
(501)371-2751

California Board of
Registered Nursing
P.O. Box 944210
Sacramento, CA 94244-
2100
(916)322-3350

Colorado Board of Nursing
1560 Broadway, Suite 670
Denver, CO 80202
(303)894-2430

Connecticut Board of
Nursing
150 Washington St.
Hartford, CT 06106
(203)566-1041

Delaware Board of Nursing
Margaret O'Neill Bldg.
P.O. Box 1401
Dover, DE 19901
(302)736-4522

District of Columbia Board
of Nursing
614 H St. NW
Washington, DC 20001
(202)727-7468

Florida Board of Nursing
111 Coastline Dr., East
Jacksonville, FL 32202
(904)359-6331

Georgia Board of Nursing
166 Pryor St. SW
Atlanta, GA 30303
(404)656-3943

Guam Board of Nursing
P.O. Box 2816
Agana, Guam 96910
(671)734-2950

Hawaii Board of Nursing
P.O. Box 3469
Honolulu, HI 96801
(808)548-5086

Idaho Board of Nursing
500 South 10th St., Suite 102
Boise, ID 83720
(208)334-3110

Illinois Board of Nursing
320 W. Washington St., 3rd Fl.
Springfield, IL 62786
(217)782-4386

Indiana Board of Nursing
One American Square
Suite 1020, Box 82067
Indianapolis, IN 46282-0004
(317)232-2960

Iowa Board of Nursing
Executive Hills East
1223 East Court
Des Moines, IA 50319
(515)281-3256

Kansas Board of Nursing
Landon State Office Bldg.
900 SW Jackson, Ste. 551S
Topeka, KS 66612-4929
(913)296-4929

Kentucky Board of Nursing
4010 Dupont Circle
Suite 430
Louisville, KY 40207
(502)897-5143

Louisiana Board of Nursing
907 Pere Marquette Bldg.
150 Baronne St.
New Orleans, LA 70112
(504)568-5464

Maine Board of Nursing
295 Water St.
Augusta, ME 04330
(207)289-5324

Maryland Board of Nursing
201 W. Preston St.
Baltimore, MD 21201
(301)225-5880

Massachusetts Board of Nursing
Leverett Saltonstall Bldg.
100 Cambridge St., Rm. 1519
Boston, MA 02202
(617)727-7393

Michigan Board of Nursing
P.O. Box 30018
Lansing, MI 48909
(517)373-1600

Minnesota Board of Nursing
2700 University Ave., West #108
St. Paul, MN 55114
(612)642-0567

Mississippi Board of Nursing
239 N. Lamar St., #401
Jackson, MS 39206-1311
(601)359-6170

Missouri Board of Nursing
P.O. Box 656,
3523 N. Ten Mile
Jefferson City, MO 65102
(314)751-2334, Ext. 141

Montana Board of Nursing
Dept. of Commerce, Prof. Lic.
1424 9th Ave.
Helena, MT 59620-0407
(406)444-4279

Nebraska Board of Nursing
Bureau of Examining Boards
P.O. Box 95007
Lincoln, NE 68509
(402)471-2115

Nevada Board of Nursing
1281 Terminal Way, Ste. 116
Reno, NV 89502
(702)786-2778

New Hampshire Board of Nursing
Health and Welfare Building
6 Hazen Dr.
Concord, NH 03301
(603)271-2323

New Jersey Board of Nursing
1100 Raymond Blvd., Room 508
Newark, NJ 07102
(201)648-2570

New Mexico Board of Nursing
4253 Montgomery Blvd., Ste. 130
Albuquerque, NM 87109
(505)841-8340

New York Board of Nursing
Cultural Education Center
Room 3013
Albany, NY 12230
(518)474-3843

North Carolina Board of
Nursing
P.O. Box 2129
Raleigh, NC 27602
(919)782-3211

North Dakota Board of
Nursing
919 South 7th Street
Suite 504
Bismarck, ND 58504
(701)224-2974

Northern Mariana Islands
Board of Nurse Examiners
Public Health Center
P.O. Box 1458
Saipan, MP 96950
0-11-670-234-8950

Ohio Board of Nursing
65 S. Front St., Ste. 509
Columbus, OH 43266-0316
(614)466-3947

Oklahoma Board of Nursing
2915 N. Classen Blvd.,
Ste. 524
Oklahoma City, OK 73106
(405)525-2076

Oregon Board of Nursing
1400 SW 5th Ave., Room
904
Portland, OR 97201
(503)229-5653

Pennsylvania Board of
Nursing
Department of State
P.O. Box 2649
Harrisburg, PA 17105
(717)787-8503

Rhode Island Board of
Nursing
75 Davis St., Room 104
Providence, RI 02908-2488
(401)277-2827

South Carolina Board of
Nursing
1777 St. Julian Pl., Ste.
102
Columbia, SC 29204-2488
(803)737-6594

South Dakota Board of
Nursing
304 S. Phillips Ave., Ste.
205
Sioux Falls, SD 57102
(605)335-4973

Tennessee Board of Nursing
283 Plus Park Blvd.
Nashville, TN 37217
(615)367-6232

Texas Board of Nurse
Examiners
P.O. Box 140466
Austin, TX 78714
(512)835-4880

Utah Board of Nursing
Heber M. Wells Bldg., 4th
Fl.
160 E 300 South, P.O. Box
45802
Salt Lake City, UT 84145
(801)530-6628

Vermont Board of Nursing
Redstone Building
26 Terrace St.
Montpelier, VT 05602
(802)828-2396

Virgin Islands Board of
Nursing
Knud Hansen Complex
Charlotte Amalie
St. Thomas, Virgin
Islands 00801
(809)776-7397

Virginia Board of Nursing
1601 Rolling Hills Dr.
Richmond, VA 23229-5005
(804)662-9909

Washington Board of
Nursing
P.O. Box 9012
Olympia, WA 98504
(206)586-1923

West Virginia Board of
Nursing
922 Quarrier St., Ste. 309
Charleston, WV 25301
(304)348-3596

Wisconsin Board of Nursing
1400 East Washington
Ave.
P.O. Box 8935
Madison, WI 53708 8935
(608)266-3735

Wyoming Board of Nursing
Barrett Bldg., 4th Floor
2301 Central Ave.
Cheyenne, WY 82002
(307)777-7601

Appendix B

Specialty Nursing Organizations

The NFSNO member organizations are excellent resources for nurses interested in receiving information on nursing specialties. For more information, call NFSNO at (609)848-5932.

American Urological
Association Allied
11512 Allecingie Parkway
Richmond, VA 23235
(894)379-1306

American Academy of
Ambulatory Nursing
Administration
N. Woodbury Road,
Box 56
Pitman, NJ 08071
(609)582-9617

American Association of
Critical-Care Nurses
101 Columbia
Aliso Viejo, CA 92656
(714)362-2000

American Association of
Diabetes Educators
600 N. Michigan Ave.,
Suite 1400
Chicago, IL 60661
(312)661-1700

American Association of
Neuroscience Nurses
218 N. Jefferson, #204
Chicago, IL 60661
(312)993-0043

American Association of
Nurse Anesthetists
216 Higgins Road
Park Ridge, IL 60068
(708)692-7050

American Association of
Occupational Health
Nurses
50 Lenox Pointe
Atlanta, GA 30324
(404)262-1162

American Association of
Spinal Cord Injury Nurses
75-20 Astoria Boulevard
Jackson Heights, NY
11370-1178
(718)803-3782

American College of Nurse-
Midwives
1522 K. St. N.W.,
Suite 1000
Washington, D.C. 20005
(202)289-0171

American Nephrology
Nurses' Association
N. Woodbury Rd. Box 56
Pitman, NJ 08071
(609)589-2187

American Psychiatric
Nurses' Association
6900 Grove Road
Thorofare, NJ 08086
(609)848-7990

American Public Health
Association/Public Health
Nursing Section
1015 Fifteenth St. N.W.
Washington, D.C. 20005
(202)789-5600

American Society of
Opthalamic Registered
Nurses
P.O. Box 193030
San Francisco, CA 94119
(415)561-8513

American Society of Plastic
and Reconstructive
Surgical Nurses
North Woodbury Road,
Box 56
Pitman, NJ 08071
(609)589-5516

American Society of Post
Anesthesia Nurses
11512 Allecingie Parkway
Richmond, VA 23235
(804)379-5516

Association for Practitioners
in Infection Control
505 E. Hawley St.
Mundelein, IL 60060
(789)949-6052

Association of Operating
Room Nurses
11512 Alecingie Parkway
Richmond, VA 23235
(804)379-9150

Association of Rehabilitation
Nurses
5700 Old Orchard Rd.,
1st Floor
Skokie, IL 60077
(708)966-3433

Dermatology Nurses'
Association
North Woodbury Road,
Box 56
Pitman, NJ 08071
(609)582-1915

Emergency Nurses
Association
230 East Ohio, Suite 600
Chicago, IL 60611-3297
(312)649-0297

Intravenous Nurses Society
Two Brighton St.
Belmont, MA 02178
(617)489-5205

National Association for
Health Center
Recruitment
P.O. Box 5769
Akron, OH 44372
(216)869-3088

National Association of
Neonatal Nurses
191 Lynch Creek Way,
Suite 101
Petaluma, CA 94954
(707)762-5588

National Association of
Nurse Practitioners in
Reproductive Health
325 Pennsylvania Ave.
S.E.
Washington, D.C. 20003
(202)544-3208

National Association of
Orthopaedic Nurses
North Woodbury Road,
Box 56
Pitman, NJ 08071
(609)582-0111

National Association of
Pediatric Nurse Associates
& Practitioners
1101 Kings Highway N.,
Suite 206
Cherry Hill, NJ 08034
(609)667-1773

National Association of
School Nurses
P.O. Box 1300
Scarborough, ME
04070-1300
(207)883-2117

National Flight Nurses
Association
6900 Grove Road
Thorofare, NJ 08086
(609)384-6725

National Nurses Society on
Addictions
5700 Old Orchard Road,
1st Floor
Skokie, IL 60077
(708)966-5010

National Student Nurses
Association
555 West 57th St.,
Suite 1325
New York, NY 10019
(212)581-2211

Oncology Nursing Society
1016 Greentree Road
Pittsburg, PA 1520-3125
(412)921-7373

Society of Gastroenterology
Nurses and Associates
1070 Sibley Tower
Rochester, NY 14604
(716)546-7241

Society of
Otorhinolaryngology and
Head-Neck Nurses
439 N. Causeway
New Smyrna Beach, FL
32169
(904)428-1295

The Organization for
Obstetric, Gynecologic,
Neonatal Nurses
409 12th Street, SW
Washington, DC
20024-2191
(202)863-2442

From *Graduating Nurse* (Spring, 1992), p. 13.

Appendix C

State Nurses Associations

Alabama State Nurses
Association
360 North Hull Street
Montgomery, Alabama
36197
(205)262-8321

Alaska Nurses Association
237 East Third Avenue
Anchorage, Alaska 99501
(907)274-0827

Arizona Nurses Association
Suite #1
1850 E. Southern Avenue
Tempe, Arizona 85282
(602)831-0404
FAX (602)831-0537

Arkansas State Nurses
Association
117 South Cedar Street
Little Rock, Arkansas
72205
(501)664-5853

California Nurses
Association
1855 Folsom Street, Room
670
San Francisco, California
94103
(415)864-4141
FAX (415)431-1011-San
Francisco
FAX (916)446-6319-
Sacramento

Colorado Nurses
Association
5453 East Evans Place
Denver, Colorado 80222
(303)757-7484

Connecticut Nurses
Association
Meritech Business Park
377 Research Parkway,
Suite 2D
Meriden, Connecticut
06450
(203)238-1207

Delaware Nurses
Association
2634 Capitol Trail, Suite C
Newark, Delaware 19711
(302)368-2333

District of Columbia Nurses
Association, Inc.
5100 Wisconsin Avenue,
N.W., Suite 306
Washington, D.C. 20016
(202)244-2705
FAX (202)362-8285

Florida Nurses Association
P.O. Box 536985
Orlando, Florida 32853-
6985
(407)896-3261
FAX (407)896-9042

Georgia Nurses Association,
Inc.
1362 West Peachtree
Street, N.W.
Atlanta, Georgia 30309
(404)876-4624

Guam Nurses Association
Post Office Box 3134
Agana, Guam 96910
(671)646-5801

Hawaii Nurses Association
677 Ala Moana Boulevard,
Suite 301
Honolulu, Hawaii 96813
(808)531-1628

Idaho Nurses Association
200 North 4th Street,
Suite 20
Boise, Idaho 83702-6001
(208)345-0500

Illinois Nurses Association
Suite 2520
20 North Wacker Drive
Chicago, Illinois 60606
(312)236-9708

Indiana State Nurses
Association
2915 North High School
Road
Indianapolis, Indiana
46224
(317)299-4575/4576

Iowa Nurses Association
100 Court Avenue, 9LL
Des Moines, Iowa 50309
(515)282-9169

Kansas State Nurses
Association
700 Jackson, Suite 601
Topeka, Kansas 66603
(913)233-8638

Kentucky Nurses
Association
1400 South First Street
P.O. Box 2616
Louisville, Kentucky
40201
(502)637-2546/2547
FAX (502)637-8236

Louisiana State Nurses
Association
712 Transcontinental
Drive
Metairie, Louisiana 70001
(504)889-1030

Maine State Nurses
Association
P.O. Box 2240
Augusta, Maine 04330
(207)622-1057

Maryland Nurses
Association, Inc.
5820 Southwestern
Boulevard
Baltimore, Maryland
21227
(301)242-7300
FAX (301)242-7307

Massachusetts Nurses
Association
340 Turnpike Street
Canton, Massachusetts
02021
(617)821-4625
FAX (617)821-4445

Michigan Nurses
Association
120 Spartan Avenue
East Lansing, Michigan
48823
(517)337-1653
FAX (517)337-1757

Minnesota Nurses
Association
1295 Bandana Boulevard
North
Suite 140
St. Paul, Minnesota 55108-
5115
(612)646-4807

Mississippi Nurses
Association
135 Bounds Street, Suite
100
Jackson, Mississippi 39206
(601)982-9182/9183

Missouri Nurses Association
206 East Dunklin Street,
Box 325
Jefferson City, Missouri
65101
(314)636-4623

Montana Nurses Association
104 Broadway, Suite G-2
P.O. Box 5718
Helena, Montana 59601
(406)442-6710

Nebraska Nurses
Association
941 O Street, Suite 707-
711
Lincoln, Nebraska 68508
(402)475-3859

Nevada Nurses Association
3660 Baker Lane, Suite #104
Reno, Nevada 89509
(702)825-3555

New Hampshire Nurses
Association
48 West Street
Concord, New Hampshire
03301
(603)225-3783

New Jersey State Nurses
Association
320 West State Street
Trenton, New Jersey
08618
(609)392-4884 or 392-2031
FAX (609)396-2330

New Mexico Nurses
Association
525 San Pedro, N.E.,
Suite 100
Albuquerque, New
Mexico 87108
(505)268-7744

New York State Nurses
Association
2113 Western Avenue
Guilderland, New York
12084
(518)456-5371, FAX
(518)456-0697

North Carolina Nurses
Association
103 Enterprise Street
Box 12025
Raleigh, North Carolina
27605
(919)821-4250

North Dakota Nurses
Association
Green Tree Square
212 North Fourth Street
Bismarck, North Dakota
58501
(701)223-1385

Ohio Nurses Association
4000 East Main Street
Columbus, Ohio 43213-
2950
(614)237-5414

Oklahoma Nurses
Association
6414 North Santa Fe,
Suite A
Oklahoma City,
Oklahoma 73116
(405)840-3476

Oregon Nurses Association,
Inc.
9600 S.W. Oak, Suite 550
Portland, Oregon 97223
(503)293-0011
FAX (503)293-0013

Pennsylvania Nurses
Association
2578 Interstate Drive
P.O. Box 8525
Harrisburg, Pennsylvania
17105-8525
(717)657-1222
FAX (717)657-3796

Rhode Island State Nurses
Association
Hall Building South
345 Blackstone Boulevard
Providence, Rhode Island
02906
(401)421-9703

South Carolina Nurses
Association
1821 Gadsden Street
Columbia, South Carolina
29201
(803)252-4781

South Dakota Nurses
Association, Inc.
1505 South Minnesota,
Suite 6
Sioux Falls, South Dakota
57105
(605)338-1401

Tennessee Nurses
Association
545 Mainstream Drive,
Suite 405
Nashville, Tennessee
37228-1207
(615)254-0350

Texas Nurses Association
Community Bank
Building
300 Highland Mall
Boulevard, Suite 300
Austin, Texas 78752-3718
(512)452-0645
FAX (512)452-0648

Utah Nurses Association
1058A East 900 South
Salt Lake City, Utah 84105
(801)322-3439/3430

Vermont State Nurses
Association, Inc.
500 Dorset Street
South Burlington,
Vermont 05403
(802)864-9390

Virgin Islands Nurses
Association
P.O. Box 583
Christiansted
St. Croix, U.S. Virgin
Islands 00820
(809)773-2323, Ext. 116/
118

Virginia Nurses Association
1311 High Point Avenue
Richmond, Virginia 23230
(804)353-7311

Washington State Nurses
Association
2505 Second Avenue,
Suite 500
Seattle, Washington 98121
(206)443-WSNA
FAX (206)728-2074

West Virginia Nurses
Association, Inc.
2 Players Club Drive, Bldg
#3
P.O. Box 1946
Charleston, West Virginia
25327
(304)342-1169

Wisconsin Nurses
Association, Inc.
6117 Monona Drive
Madison, Wisconsin 53716
(608)221-0383
FAX (608)221-2788

Wyoming Nurses
Association
Majestic Building, Room
305
1603 Capitol Avenue
Cheyenne, Wyoming
82001
(307)635-3955

Appendix D

Canadian Registration/ Licensure Authorities

To obtain information on writing the Nurse Registration/Licensure Examination, contact any of the provincial registering/licensing authorities.

Alberta Association of
  Registered Nurses
11620 - 168th Street
Edmonton, Alberta
T5M 4A6
| | (403)451-0043 |
| Fax: | (403)452-3276 |

Association of Nurses of
  Prince Edward Island
17 Pownal Street, Box
1838
Charlottestown
Prince Edward Island
C1A 7N5
| | (902)368-3764 |
| Fax: | (902)628-1430 |

Association of Registered
  Nurses of Newfoundland
55 Military Road
P.O. Box 6116
St. John's, Newfoundland
A1C 5X8
| | (709)753-6040 |
| Fax: | (709)753-4940 |

College of Nurses of
  Ontario
101 Davenport Road
Toronto, Ontario
M5R 3P1
	(416)928-0900
Fax:	(416)928-6507
Toll Free:	1-800-387-5526

Manitoba Association of
  Registered Nurses
647 Broadway Avenue
Winnipeg, Manitoba
R3C 0X2
| | (204)774-3477 |
| Fax: | (204)775-6052 |

Northwest Territories
  Registered Nurses
  Association
P.O. Box 2757
Yellowknife, Northwest
  Territories
X1A 2R1
| | (403)873-2745 |
| Fax: | (403)873-2336 |

Nurses Association of New
Brunswick
165 Regent Street
Fredericton, New
Brunswick
E3B 3W5
          (506)458-8731
Fax: (506)459-2857

Order of Nurses of Québec
4200 Quest, Boulevard
Dorchester
Montréal (Québec)
H3Z 1V4
          (514)935-2501
Fax: (514)935-1799
Toll Free: 1-800-363-6048

Registered Nurses
Association of British
Columbia
2855 Arbutus Street
Vancouver, British
Columbia
V6J 3Y8
          (604)736-7331
Fax: (604)738-2272

Registered Nurses
Association of Nova
Scotia
Suite 104, 120 Eileen
Stubbs Ave.
Dartmouth, Nova Scotia
B3B 1Y1
          (902)468-9744
Fax: (902)468-9510

Saskatchewan Registered
Nurses Association
2066 Retallack Street
Regina, Saskatchewan
S4T 2K2
          (306)757-4643
Fax: (306)525-0849

Yukon Nurses Society
P.O. Box 5371
Whitehorse, Yukon
Y1A 4Z2
          (403)667-4062

Index

Note: Page numbers in italics refer to illustrations, page numbers followed by b refer to boxed material, those followed by t refer to tables.